BLOOD DISORDERS IN PREGNANCY

BLOOD DISORDERS IN PREGNANCY

RUSSELL K. LAROS, JR., M.D.

Editor

Department of Obstetrics, Gynecology and Reproductive Sciences
University of California, San Francisco
San Francisco, California

LEA & FEBIGER PHILADELPHIA

1986

Lea & Febiger
600 Washington Square
Philadelphia, PA 19106-4198
U.S.A.
(215) 922-1330

Library of Congress Cataloging-in-Publication Data
Main entry under title:

Blood disorders in pregnancy.

Includes bibliographies and index.
1. Blood—Diseases. 2. Pregnancy, Complications of.
I. Laros, Russell K., 1936- . [DNLM: 11. Hematologic
Diseases—in pregnancy. 2. Pregnancy Complications,
Hematologic—diagnosis. 3. Pregnancy Complications,
Hematologic—therapy. WQ 252 B655]
RG580.H47B55 1986 618.3 85-24012
ISBN 0-8121-1009-9

PRINTED IN THE UNITED STATES OF AMERICA

Print No. 4 3 2 1

DEDICATION

This text is dedicated to my family and to the scores of students, residents, and fellows who have asked provocative questions over the years. Without the stimulation and support of these two groups my life would indeed be far less fulfilling.

PREFACE

The purpose of this text is to provide the obstetrician with a reference volume dealing with those hematologic problems most commonly associated with pregnancy. We have not tried to be all-inclusive but have emphasized a practical and systematic approach to diagnosis and treatment. For each disease entity, we have tried to provide enough basic pathophysiology to enhance the reader's understanding of the diagnostic and therapeutic steps recommended. This text differs from the standard obstetric references by providing far greater detail about hematologic problems and from the standard hematologic text by focusing on those considerations specific to the parturient.

Chapter 1 stresses a systematic approach to the evaluation of the anemic patient and reviews the various laboratory studies useful in reaching a specific diagnosis. Similarly, chapter 8 reviews the physiology of clotting and highlights those laboratory studies commonly used in clinical practice. These two chapters serve as an essential framework for logical diagnosis and treatment of specific hematologic disorders.

Each of my coauthors is both an understanding teacher and a recognized authority in the field of hematology or transfusion therapy. Each has shared generously of his or her knowledge and skill in preparing the text.

Finally, I wish to acknowledge the excellent editorial assistance of my secretarial staff, including Claudia Schumann, Bonnie Davidson, and John Waldman.

Russell K. Laros, Jr.

CONTRIBUTORS

Laurence Corash, M.D.
Department of Laboratory Medicine
University of California, San Francisco
San Francisco, CA

Kathy S. Gookin, M.S.N.
Division of Maternal-Fetal Medicine
University of Mississippi Medical Center
Jackson, MS

Roland G. Hiss, M.D.
Department of Postgraduate Medicine
The University of Michigan Medical Center
The Towsley Center for Continuing Medical Education
Ann Arbor, MI

Russell K. Laros, Jr., M.D.
Department of Obstetrics, Gynecology and Reproductive Sciences
University of California, San Francisco
San Francisco, CA

Brian J. Lewis, M.D.
Department of Medicine
University of California, San Francisco
San Francisco, CA

Charles A. Linker, M.D.
Department of Medicine
University of California, San Francisco
San Francisco, CA

John C. Morrison, M.D.
Division of Maternal-Fetal Medicine
University of Mississippi Medical Center
Jackson, MS

Harold A. Oberman, M.D.
Department of Pathology
The University of Michigan Medical Center
Pathology Building
Ann Arbor, MI

CONTENTS

Chapter 1

EVALUATION OF THE ANEMIC PATIENT

Roland G. Hiss

There is general agreement that anemia is the most frequent medical complication occurring as a consequence of, or in association with, pregnancy.[1–3] The evaluation of the hematologic system and some attention to its variations during pregnancy are a routine part of the care provided to the pregnant patient, and the hematologic system receives more attention than any other nonreproductive system.

This chapter describes the normal and physiologic events associated with pregnancy that affect the hematologic system and differentiates these normal events from similar-appearing manifestations that are not normal and require therapeutic intervention. This entails description of a scheme to differentiate the physiologic from the pathologic condition and to determine both the severity and the nature of the abnormality. This chapter is intended to provide a framework for understanding the hematologic events associated with pregnancy so that the common, mild hematologic abnormalities can be dealt with in a routine way and the rare, more severe hematologic abnormalities (described in later chapters) can be selected out and dealt with energetically.

NORMAL HEMATOLOGIC EVENTS ASSOCIATED WITH PREGNANCY

PLASMA AND RED BLOOD CELL VOLUME CHANGES

The "plethora of pregnancy" has been recognized clinically for many centuries and was commented upon in the scientific literature of the early part of this century by Williams.[4] The "plethora" results from an expanded blood volume in pregnancy and produces a tolerance for hemorrhage and for the sequestration of blood in the lower extremities, which are common features of pregnancy. This hypervolemia has several other benefits, as summarized by Peck and Arias.[5]

The increase in blood volume associated with pregnancy totals between 1 and 2 L, depending on the size of the patient and several other variables that may enhance or cancel one another. The variation of the range of "normal" is quite broad as a result of the interaction of these several factors. The two variables that have the greatest effect on blood volume changes are the independent variation of the plasma volume and the red blood cell volume. These are not at all synchronous, and their discordance accounts for most of the apparent "anemia" associated with pregnancy.

Figure 1–1 shows the general relationship between plasma volume, red cell volume, and total blood volume associated with the progressive stages of pregnancy. Plasma volume increases first, beginning part way through the first trimester, and reaches a

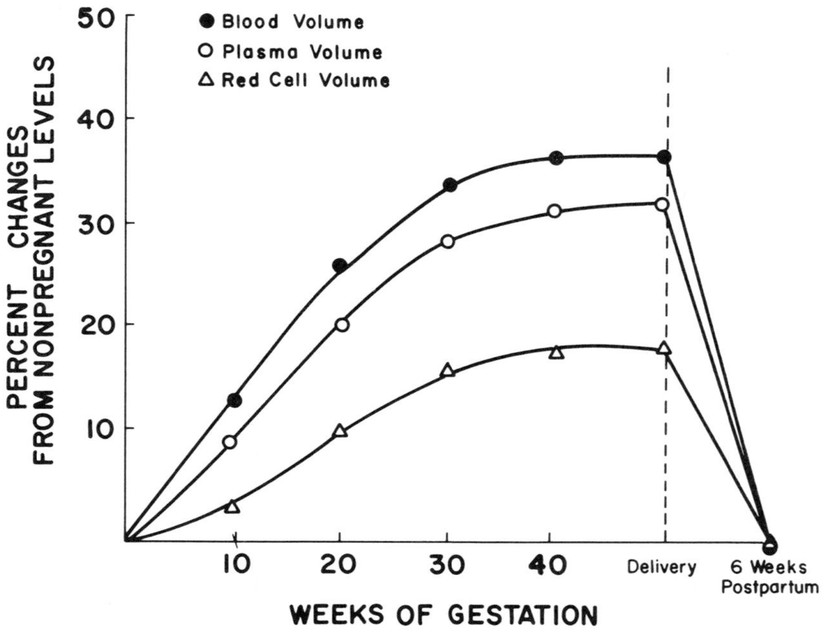

Figure 1–1. Changes in blood volume and its components (plasma and red cell volumes) during pregnancy and post partum. Graph constructed from several reports in the literature. (Redrawn from Peck, T.M., and Arias, F.: Hematologic changes associated with pregnancy. Clin Obstet Gynecol *22*:785, 1979. By permission of Harper & Row, Publishers.)

peak about the 28th to 30th week. From then on it slowly rises until term, but the rate of rise is so slow that it simulates a plateau effect. The total plasma volume expansion ranges from 25 to 50%, the wide range resulting from individual variation among normal pregnancies, and not from scientific contradictions among the methods of measurement used by various investigators. (One source of variation in plasma volume dynamics that did result from methodologic considerations was the difference in plasma volumes measured with pregnant subjects in the decubitus as opposed to the supine position. The supine position created erroneous results because of the effect of compression of venous return from the lower extremities by the gravid uterus. This was corrected when the studies were done with the patients on their sides.)[6]

The red cell volume begins to rise in pregnancy late in the first trimester and continues to rise throughout pregnancy, following a different curve from that of the plasma volume. The total increase in red cell mass during pregnancy approximates 20 to 40%.[7] For the individual woman, the expansion of red cell mass is less than the proportional expansion of plasma volume. Because the increase in red cell mass in pregnancy lags behind and is of smaller magnitude than the expansion of plasma volume, pregnancy demonstrates "an anemia of dilution." The hemoglobin concentration in blood, measured with the standard laboratory assessment (g/dl), records what appears to be an anemia if judged by standards applicable to the nonpregnant female. There is in fact an *expanded* total body hemoglobin during pregnancy, so that the term "anemia" is only relative and does not have the same significance in the pregnant female as in the nonpregnant female or adult male.

At approximately the 30th week of pregnancy, plasma volume expansion plateaus and the progressive decline of hemoglobin concentration stops. During the last trimester a slight rise in the hemoglobin concentration toward (but usually not reaching) the prepregnant level may occur. The effects of these red cell and plasma volume changes upon laboratory assessments of the hematologic system and on the iron kinetics of the pregnant patient are noted in sections following. A review of the subject of plasma and red cell volumes during pregnancy is provided by Chesley,[7] who cites numerous studies on the subject of red cell and plasma volumes done by various investigators. The field has been thoroughly studied by many authors.[8, 9]

With delivery, there is loss of some of the expanded blood volume associated with pregnancy, averaging 500 ml for a normal vaginal delivery[8] and larger amounts if delivery is by cesarean section. This expected and normal loss associated with delivery leaves the newly delivered woman still relatively hypervolemic, which accounts for the tolerance for hemorrhage characteristic of pregnant patients. During the puerperium, there is rapid restoration to prepregnant blood, plasma, and red cell volume levels, which takes place as rapidly as within one week.[5] The most interesting of these events of volume contraction is the fate of the expanded red cell mass, with its precious iron content. This subject will be addressed in a later section.

IRON STORES AND KINETICS IN PREGNANT AND NONPREGNANT WOMEN

The classic studies of Scott and Pritchard[10] have shown that iron stores in young, healthy women are marginal, and this fragile state has implications for the hematologic response to pregnancy, which requires an increased utilization of iron for both mother and fetus. Approximately two thirds of young, white college students who had never hemorrhaged, donated blood, been pregnant, or taken medicinal iron showed bone marrow iron stores in either trace or absent amounts (Fig. 1–2). Scott and Pritchard also demonstrated that nearly one half of 133 primigravida women tested during the first half of pregnancy had no storage iron on bone marrow examination.[11] Monsen and coworkers[12] have similarly shown a negative iron balance state in young, healthy women.

The reason for marginal iron stores in young women is largely attributed to menstruation and the continual related loss of iron from puberty to menopause. With the growth spurt of the teenage years, the blood volume expands to reach its adult level, and the iron required for this hemoglobin expansion appears to consume the storage iron accumulated in childhood. The onset of menses interferes with restoration of storage iron via the normal dietary route. A normal menstrual period results in approximately 25 to 30 ml of whole blood loss, which is 12 to 15 mg of elemental iron, since each milliliter of whole normal blood contains 0.5 mg of this metal. This additional 15 mg requirement must be prorated over a month and represents an increased dietary iron requirement above the 1 to 1.5 mg per day that is needed to replace non–red cell losses. Depending on the size of the woman and whether or not her menstrual loss actually is a normal 25 to 30 ml per month (menstrual irregularities often lead to greater losses), the daily iron requirement for the nonpregnant female will be between 1.5 and 2.0 mg of iron. Although the average American diet contains 6 mg of iron per 1000 kilocalories, only 10% of dietary iron is absorbed under normal circumstances,[13] and the combination of these factors results in a negative iron balance, or at least a precarious one, for most menstruating females.

With pregnancy, there is expansion of the red cell volume in maternal circulation, and the iron required for this expansion of hemoglobin mass comes from iron stores present at the onset of pregnancy, to the extent that they exist. Pregnancy is similar to the polycythemic conditions in which red cell mass is expanded at the expense of iron stores. Increase in absorption of dietary iron is another potential source of additional iron, but this doesn't occur to any appreciable extent in the first half of pregnancy.[14] It does occur, however, during the last half of pregnancy, when fetal demands for iron occur. Increased iron absorption in late pregnancy parallels that seen in any condition of increased iron demand, such as in iron deficiency when the efficiency of gastrointestinal absorption of dietary iron is increased (apparently as a compensatory response).

If there is insufficient iron available to supply the demands of an increasing hemoglobin mass, the result is iron-deficient erythropoiesis. The situation *simulates* hemorrhagic loss in an iron-depleted person, namely, new red blood cells are produced whose hemoglobin content is below normal, the hallmark of iron deficiency anemia. Whether or not this occurs in a particular pregnancy and the degree to which it occurs depend upon the available iron stores at the beginning of pregnancy and the adequacy of the increased dietary absorption during pregnancy. The entire system appears to be remarkably efficient in view of the high incidence of marginal iron stores in women in the reproductive age range and the mildness of the anemia that attends pregnancy, if a real anemia occurs at all.

The increased iron assigned to the expanded red cell volume of the pregnant circulation is retrieved, in part at least, during the postpartum period when the expanded red cell mass decreases and the surfeit of iron is returned to stores. There are, however, definite permanent iron losses from the maternal economy associated

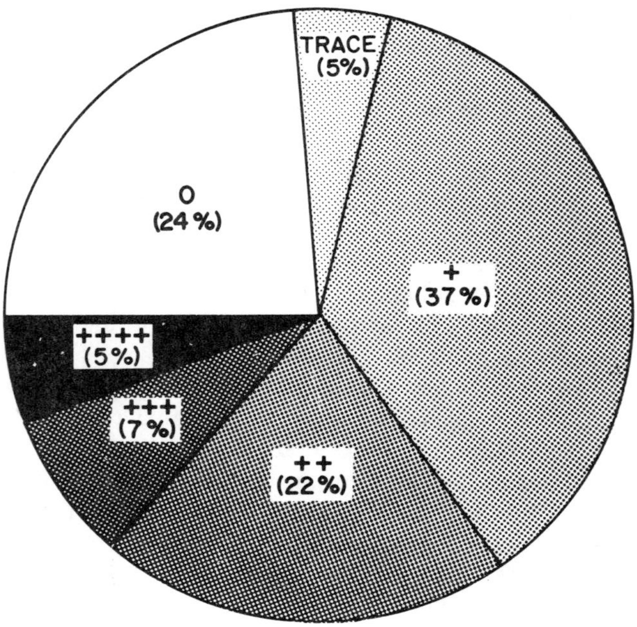

Figure 1–2. Distribution of marrow storage in iron in 114 healthy young college students who had never hemorrhaged, donated blood, or been pregnant. (Redrawn from Scott, D.E., and Pritchard, J.A.: Iron deficiency in healthy young college women. JAMA *199*:147, 1967. By permission of the American Medical Association.)

with the full events of pregnancy. Scott and Pritchard[1] list categories of iron loss associated with pregnancy that are in general agreement with several other authors who have studied the subject.[15–17] There is approximately a 300 mg transfer of iron to the average-sized single fetus and placenta, a 200 mg loss through various secretions during pregnancy (the continuing normal human loss of approximately 1 mg per day), and about 250 mg of iron lost as whole blood with normal vaginal delivery. There are, thus, about 750 to 800 mg of iron permanently lost during pregnancy that is over and above that iron used to expand the maternal red cell volume.

FOLIC ACID

Folic acid is another nutrient utilized by proliferating cells (in the case of pregnancy, those in both maternal and fetal tissues). The daily requirement for normal nonpregnant women has been determined to be between 50 to 100 μg of folate per day,[18] and this increases approximately threefold during pregnancy.[19] The vigorous growth of fetal tissues is responsible for most of this increased demand, but the expansion of some maternal tissues, particularly blood tissues, accounts for a bit of it. Whatever the reasons for the increased demand, it is maternal needs that are compromised if a deficiency state occurs, not those of the fetus. The normal stores of folate in the adult human are found largely in the liver, approximately a four-month supply if dietary sources have been adequate. Dietary supply of folate may be compromised by socioeconomic factors, personal eating habits, and food preferences. The number of folate-containing foods is not extensive. Furthermore, vigorous cooking of foods destroys whatever folate content they may have. As a result of all these factors, there are many women who enter pregnancy with a marginal folate reserve and are ill-prepared to face the increased requirement for this vitamin.

Available folate supply is usually sufficient to meet the modest increases in red cell production early in pregnancy, and fetal requirements do not become large until later in pregnancy. Accordingly, folate deficiency leading to an overt anemia (and neutropenia and thrombocytopenia) is rare prior to the third trimester. Whether it occurs at all is largely dependent upon the folate reserve at the beginning of pregnancy and the dietary habits of the pregnant woman.

VITAMIN B_{12}

Vitamin B_{12} is a folate associate in several steps of DNA synthesis. However, vitamin B_{12} supply in the adult human is very extensive in all except those who are strict vegetarians, in which case the somewhat increased demands for vitamin B_{12} associated with pregnancy can result in a deficiency of this vitamin as well. Pregnancy-precipitated vitamin B_{12} deficiency implies very long-standing severe dietary restriction of vitamin B_{12}—an extremely unusual circumstance in the United States. Vitamin B_{12} deficiency associated with failure of dietary absorption secondary to inadequate gastric production of the intrinsic factor (pernicious anemia) is extremely rare in the young age group of pregnancy. It has occurred, however, at case report frequency.[20, 21]

VARIATIONS IN LABORATORY TESTS ASSOCIATED WITH PREGNANCY

ERYTHROID VALUES

The components of the complete blood count are a standard part of the evaluation of virtually any patient, including the pregnant patient. They are available in all clinical laboratories and are performed with automated methods that are reliable and inexpensive. These components include the hemoglobin (g per dl), hematocrit, red blood cell count (of value primarily as an intermediate for calculation of red blood cell indices), the mean corpuscular volume (average volume of red cells), and the mean corpuscular hemoglobin concentration.

The hemoglobin value in the nonpregnant healthy adult female is 14 ± 2 g/dl in most laboratories.[22] Although this is the generally stated "normal" range, a large majority of women in the reproductive age range have hemoglobins in the lower end of this range—e.g., 12 to 13 g/dl—and many fall a few tenths of a gram below the level of 12 without clear-cut evidence of hematologic pathology. With pregnancy, the hemoglobin concentration begins to fall during the first trimester because of the greater expansion of plasma volume compared with red cell mass that characterizes the first two thirds of pregnancy. Virtually all pregnant women experience a lowering of hemoglobin (and the other erythroid values) from this phenomenon, and this "anemia of pregnancy" must be considered a physiologic, not a pathologic event. How far this fall in hemoglobin value can go and still be considered physiologic, however, is difficult to precisely define because of the multiple variables at play; the value of 10 g/dl has been suggested as approximating the demarcation between the physiologic fall of hemoglobin concentration and the presence of true anemia.[1] Therefore, pregnant women with hemoglobin values higher than 10 can be operationally considered free of anemia requiring investigation, and those with values below 10 should be evaluated for anemia.

The other erythroid values—hematocrit and red blood cell count—decrease in approximate parallel to the hemoglobin. The classic ratios between erythroid values, the mean corpuscular volume, and the mean corpuscular hemoglobin concentration show minor variations in pregnancy that are important only for recognition that they do not represent an abnormal process. The mean corpuscular volume (MCV) rises slightly during pregnancy, an average of 4 fl.[23,24] However, the increase does not put the MCV values outside the normal range—that is, it does not produce a macrocytosis by usual standards. Nonpregnant women whose red cell erythroid values show microcytosis, such as those with β-thalassemia, also show a slight rise in the MCV with pregnancy, but this is of lesser magnitude than for the hematologically normal woman and does not eradicate the microcytosis present in the prepregnant state.[25] The "normal" macrocytic change of pregnancy is best seen in pregnant women who are taking iron supplements[26] and may be so trifling as to be undetected in those who are not.

There is a minor reduction in the mean corpuscular hemoglobin concentration (MCHC), in part explained by the concurrent macrocytic tendency, but it is extremely small and without clinical significance. A fall in the MCHC associated with the onset of iron deficiency anemia is of greater importance and of greater magnitude than the physiologic decrease of the MCHC. For clinical purposes, appreciable lowering of the MCHC should be considered evidence suggestive of iron deficiency rather than a physiologic event.

ASSESSMENT OF IRON KINETICS

The effects of pregnancy on laboratory studies used in the evaluation of anemia are important to note, so that differences in interpretation of results between the pregnant and nonpregnant state can be appreciated. The serum iron level and iron-binding capacity, for instance, are frequent assessments in the pursuit of an anemia, and they usually provide convincing evidence for the presence of iron deficiency anemia in a nonpregnant subject. In pregnancy, physiologic changes in both the serum iron concentration and iron-binding capacity that simulate iron deficiency, occur, however, and it is difficult to reliably distinguish between the physiologic effects and those of the pathologic condition. The serum iron tends to be decreased in the early part of pregnancy as a result of the mobilization of iron from stores to feed the expanding red cell mass. Later in pregnancy, the fetal demands for iron keep the increased rate of iron utilization going and the serum iron level down. (A decreased serum iron level is an expected finding in any condition in which iron is being utilized at a greater than usual rate.) Most binding proteins are increased in pregnancy, and the iron-binding protein transferrin is included among those producing conditions that mimic iron deficiency. The combination of a decreasing serum iron and a rising transferrin level produces a lowering of the saturation (ratio of serum iron to transferrin), which *also* mimics the conditions seen in iron deficiency. As in the case of hemoglobin, where an arbitrary lower limit has been set to distinguish the physiologic from the pathologic state (10 g/dl), the value of 15% transferrin saturation has been arbitrarily set as distinguishing normal from abnormal.[1, 17] The clinician should appreciate that arbitrarily set demarcation levels are only approximations and can show error in either direction. A transferrin saturation of less than 15% is *probably* indicative of iron deficiency, and values above this level are *probably* not associated with that diagnosis; however, values near the 15% mark could be either in a given case.

The oral administration of iron during pregnancy modifies the serum iron kinetics considerably, and the expected fall in serum iron can be reduced or even eliminated.[26] The usual rise in transferrin levels with pregnancy does occur if iron supplementation is given, but to a somewhat lesser degree. The sum of these variations in serum iron and iron-binding capacity in pregnancy, and their physiologic simulation of iron deficiency which they otherwise would be used to confirm, reduce the utility of these two laboratory tests in evaluating anemias of pregnancy.

The evaluation of iron status in pregnancy (and indeed in all other conditions) has been materially improved by the availability of measurement of the serum ferritin level. Using a radioimmunoassay test, this determination is directly correlated with the reticuloendothelial stores of iron,[27] and the assessment of iron stores such as those in marrow is the ultimate standard upon which the diagnosis of iron deficiency, or overload, has always rested.

The correlation of serum ferritin with bone marrow iron stores in pregnancy has been confirmed by Puolakka and associates,[28] who showed that the serum ferritin value could accurately diagnose iron deficiency (as determined by bone marrow iron assessment) and differentiate it from anemia due to infection, which also lowers the serum iron level. The anemia of infection produces a low serum iron concentration, a decreased iron-binding capacity, and sometimes a mild hypochromia of the red cells; it can be confused with mild iron deficiency anemia. Since some of the characteristics of iron deficiency anemia are produced by pregnancy, the differentiation of the independent effects of chronic infection, true iron deficiency, and pregnancy was very problematic until the availability of serum ferritin determinations.

The normal range for serum ferritin is quite broad,[29] apparently because of the wide range of body iron stores in individuals of various circumstances. The lower limit is generally considered to be 12 ng per ml, and values below that are judged diagnostic of iron deficiency. This holds true in pregnancy as well. The serum ferritin level progressively falls in pregnancy from whatever prepregnant level existed to a low in about the 30th week. This fall correlates with the depletion of the maternal iron stores associated with the expanding red cell volume and, in the latter part of pregnancy, with transfer of iron to the fetus. Figure 1–3 demonstrates typical curves for the serum ferritin concentration through pregnancy in women who are receiving supplemental iron and in those who are not.[26] The supplemented women avoided iron deficiency (ferritin levels below 12 ng per ml) and actually showed a rise in serum ferritin levels toward term. Those without supplementation approached the iron-deficient level. The curves demonstrated in Figure 1–3 were previously determined (prior to the advent of serum ferritin reference values) by deLeeuw,[30] who used bone marrow iron assessments serially in pregnancy to show the progressive fall in stores, reaching the nadir at the 28th to 30th weeks. Ferritin levels are able to provide the same information as marrow iron assessments using much less expensive and less invasive testing procedures. The clinician can reliably diagnose iron deficiency at any point in pregnancy with the serum ferritin value.

Puolakka also demonstrated that the hematologic status of a woman early in pregnancy does not necessarily predict whether she will develop iron deficiency later on.[28] Those women who are iron-deficient at the outset, by whatever criteria, will, of course, only become more so as pregnancy proceeds if supplementation is not provided. However, it is quite possible for women who are hematologically normal at the beginning of pregnancy (including their serum ferritin levels) to develop iron deficiency later in the pregnancy (as measured by serum ferritin) without the intercession of any untoward event.

The serum ferritin value has permitted evaluation of fetal iron status, which previously usually appeared normal regardless of the mother's condition. The cord blood ferritin levels of newborns whose mothers' serum ferritin was in the iron-deficient range was reduced below that of infants whose mothers were not iron-deficient;

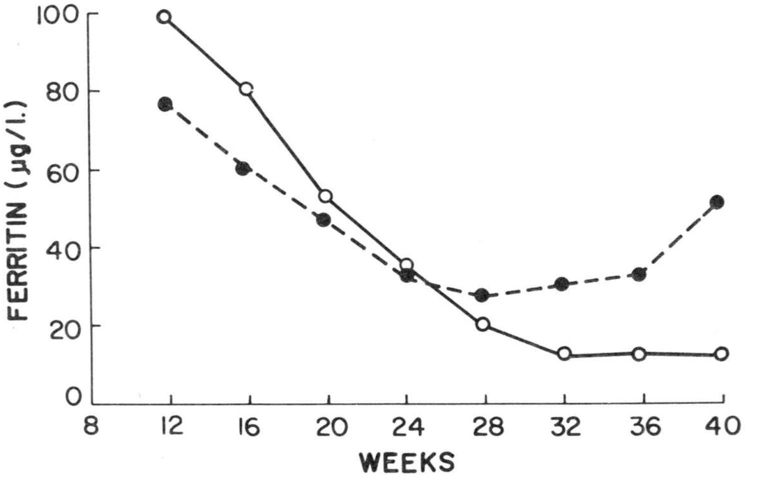

Figure 1–3. Serum ferritin levels during pregnancy in (a) women given oral iron supplements ●, and (b) untreated women ○. (Redrawn from Fenton, V., Cavill, J., and Fisher, J.: Iron stores in pregnancy. Br J Haematol *37*:145, 1977. By permission of Blackwell Scientific Publishers, Ltd.)

however, the infants low in ferritin were not anemic, had normal iron kinetics, and their serum ferritin values were not in the iron-deficiency range or even close to it.[26] They were in fact normal, just lower than the values of infants from non–iron-deficient mothers.

The serum ferritin level can be inaccurate in conditions of iron overload when the body iron stores are excessive. This is the result of a technical aberration known as the "high dose hook effect."[31] This laboratory peculiarity does not affect the utility of the serum ferritin in the diagnosis of iron deficiency, however, as it only applies to extremely high iron levels rarely seen in pregnancy. The serum ferritin reading will also be grossly influenced by recent parenteral administration of iron,[32] although it is believed that the distortion in serum ferritin levels created by intramuscularly or intravenously administered iron will stabilize in approximately one month. The determination of iron stores in someone who has recently been given iron parenterally, however, is most accurately assessed by totaling the dosage of elemental iron provided and not relying upon an indirect laboratory assessment.

FOLIC ACID ASSESSMENT

The serum folate activity in nonpregnant women is the same as for adult males, and the normal range varies somewhat from laboratory to laboratory. Most authorities consider values above 6 ng/ml to be normal, and most normal humans have double digit serum folate values. In pregnancy there is a progressive fall in the folate levels, reaching a mean value of 4.5 ng per ml,[33] probably representing mobilization and consumption of this coenzyme with kinetics that parallel those of iron during pregnancy. The lower limit for serum folate is usually 3 ng/ml, and values below this should be considered evidence of folate deficiency. Individual cases have been noted in which the serum folate level is in the diagnostic range but the patient is not anemic, or the anemia may not be megaloblastic. However, the reverse is not true; normal serum folate values are not found in a true folate-deficient megaloblastic anemia, and this finding suggests either laboratory error or another diagnosis. Serum vitamin B_{12} levels are not known to be affected by pregnancy.

OTHER CELLULAR ELEMENTS OF BLOOD

There is a moderate rise in the white blood cell count (WBC) during pregnancy, although the normal range (5000 to 10,000 per mm^3) may not be exceeded in all cases. This rise is caused by an increase in the percentage of neutrophils in the blood, some of which represent a relocation of cells from the endothelium into the circulation. There may be some change in the phagocytic and bacteriocidal capacity of polymorphonuclear neutrophils in pregnancy, and interestingly (although without apparent clinical importance), the leukocyte alkaline phosphatase is increased in the third trimester and falls sharply two days before delivery.[5]

The platelet count and life span are unaffected by pregnancy.

THE CASE FOR SUPPLEMENTATION DURING PREGNANCY

In previous sections, two hematologic factors associated with pregnancy were identified that are somewhat discordant. The first is the notion that a majority of women in the reproductive age range, regardless of socioeconomic status or other factors, have iron stores that are substantially decreased when compared with the male standard. (It might be argued philosophically that there is a flaw in evolutionary developments in that the adult female does not absorb a proportionally greater amount of dietary iron from the gastrointestinal tract to compensate for the regular menstrual loss.) The other feature is the expanded requirement for iron associated with increased red cell volume in pregnancy and iron losses to the fetus and at delivery. Purely from the point of view of her red cells, a woman enters pregnancy facing a challenge that she is poorly prepared to meet.

Because the iron reserves in many women are delicate, and because the iron demands of pregnancy are substantial, the event of pregnancy often precipitates iron deficiency anemia. The incidence of this occurrence depends upon the socioeconomic and ethnic population studied, because iron reserves are in part determined by diet and general health and these vary in different populations. However, it is clear that iron deficiency occurs in some pregnant women in all populations, and many women come very close to the iron-deficient state during normal pregnancy. Whether the advent of overt iron deficiency or its immediate precursor state (a total consumption of iron stores) has much significance in the overall health of the mother or in the obstetric aspects of the pregnancy has not been clearly demonstrated. In fact, the reverse has been repeatedly described, namely, we see normal pregnancies and healthy fetuses in women with definite and untreated iron deficiency anemia of various degrees.[34, 35] The importance of anemia caused by iron deficiency apparently is not great. However, several studies, such as those of deLeeuw,[30] have shown that iron supplementation in pregnancy can modify the otherwise progressive decline of hemoglobin during the first 30 weeks of pregnancy and during the last trimester and at delivery can produce erythroid values that are significantly higher than would have occurred without such supplementation. There is evidence that twice weekly administration of iron intramuscularly for 10 to 12 weeks was even more effective than iron taken orally in minimizing the reduction of hemoglobin associated with anemia.[36] It is apparent that supplemental iron given during pregnancy can have a positive effect, at least on laboratory values if not on the main event.

The question is whether supplementation should be given in view of what appear to be very modest consequences if it is not. Hemminki and Starfield[37] reviewed the world's literature for all controlled studies attempting to demonstrate whether routine administration of iron and vitamins during pregnancy had any beneficial effect on any aspect of pregnancy. This comprehensive review failed to demonstrate any benefit for routine iron supplementation. (Some studies reviewed showed slight modification of some nonhematologic outcomes, but these were of minor significance.) The issue of iron supplementation on a routine basis is a common editorial topic from time to time in the literature.[38] When the question "Do all pregnant women need iron?" is posed, the answer seems clearly to be "No, but it won't hurt." It may actually do some good, but this benefit will not be measurable in the usual terms selected to measure the outcome of pregnancy.

The requirement for iron supplementation during normal pregnancy is not a big issue in clinical medicine; it is a modest issue. Morbidity and mortality are not much affected one way or the other. However, the case for positively influencing some aspects of maternal health can be made. The pregnant woman is attempting to mobilize iron to meet increased demands, yet the storage bin is depleted. The fetal need for iron comes when the stores are at their lowest ebb at the beginning of the third trimester. If a greater supply of dietary iron is available (through oral ferrous compounds), it seems reasonable that the demands would be easier to meet, the permanent effect on iron stores would actually be improved, and the margin between depleted stores and frank iron deficiency would be widened. The only potential hazard would be iron overload, which is virtually impossible to produce with iron taken orally unless the individual has an independent iron absorption defect that forces her to absorb more iron than she needs. (Such individuals will develop iron overload anyway, and oral iron supplementation during pregnancy could not be blamed for causing this problem.) There is some symptomatic disadvantage to oral iron supplementation in the first trimester of pregnancy when gastrointestinal symptoms of the pregnancy are manifest and may be worsened by oral iron. For this reason, iron supplementation during pregnancy, when given, should not be commenced until the second trimester.

The dosage of iron supplementation is even less scientific than the recommendation. The World Health Organization recommends 60 mg/day of elemental iron,[39] but experienced clinicians have learned that this amount produces gastrointestinal side-effects in an appreciable percentage of patients. A lesser amount, such as 30 mg/day, probably has as much benefit, as shown by Scott and Pritchard[1] and by deLeeuw.[30]

The case for folic acid supplementation is similar in many respects but has certain unique features not shared by iron. In some populations folic reserves are even more tenuous than those of iron, and the precipitation of frank folic acid deficiency by pregnancy is a well-known event. The increased tissue growth inherent in pregnancy creates a very real increase in folate demands. Folate requirements are further increased in multiple pregnancies, with anticonvulsant therapy, with malabsorption, and in the presence of certain other hematologic disorders such as hemoglobinopathies. Women at greatest risk for pregnancy-induced folic acid deficiency are those with any of the risk factors just noted coupled with dietary and socioeconomic status factors resulting in marginal folate stores at the beginning of pregnancy.

It has been estimated that the folate requirement of the nonpregnant female is between 50 and 100 μg/day[18] and that this requirement increases to between 300 and 500 μg/day with pregnancy. Accordingly, a supplemental dose of folic acid approximating 350 μg/day is recommended,[19] with higher amounts if folic acid deficiency anemia is actually present. It is well known that megaloblastic anemia caused by vitamin B_{12} deficiency (such as pernicious anemia) may lead to acceleration of neurologic deficits if treated incorrectly with folic acid. There is no question that this is true, but the risk in the pregnant population is extremely small. Most cases of pernicious anemia (and that diagnosis encompasses most cases of vitamin B_{12} deficiency) occur in older populations who will not be pregnant. True vitamin B_{12} deficiency in pregnancy has been observed,[20] but so infrequently that it is virtually a nonissue, and the value of folic acid supplementation as a routine in pregnancy far outweighs the numerically tiny risk of harm to the very rare vitamin B_{12}-deficient patient. Awareness of the possibility of severely worsening a vitamin B_{12}-deficient patient by supplementation with folic acid is a sufficient caution for the clinician to observe.

The amounts of folic acid in prenatal formulations prepared by various pharmaceutical companies vary between 0.3 and 1 mg. As noted, somewhat less than half a milligram of folic acid per day is sufficient as a regular supplement during pregnancy. Supplementation with vitamin B_{12} is not needed and is a consideration only in a long-standing extremely strict vegetarian.

FETO-MATERNAL HEMATOLOGIC RELATIONSHIPS

There are certain interesting and unique characteristics of the supply of nutrients utilized by the fetus for its hematologic development. The fetal requirement for iron does not become significant until the last trimester, when most of fetal erythropoiesis occurs. (The increased pregnancy requirements for iron prior to the third trimester are those needed by the mother to expand her own red cell volume, not those of the fetus.) The fetal requirements for iron take great priority over any of those the maternal economy may have, and fetal requirements are supplied, against the gradient as it were, even when the mother is iron-deficient. In one study of African women, many of whom were iron-deficient prior to pregnancy, babies delivered by patients who were anemic actually had hematocrit levels in the upper limits of the normal range for newborns.[25]

From the maternal point of view, pregnancy represents a focus of bleeding. The mother loses iron as surely as if she had a steady hemorrhagic loss, and maternal blood assumes the characteristics brought on by chronic blood loss. There is a decrease in hemoglobin values, a fall in serum iron levels, and an increase in iron-binding capacity. These changes in iron kinetics simulate those seen in bleeding anemia. The serum ferritin level also falls progressively with pregnancy. In a sense, the mother is bleeding into the child. The fetus receives iron preferentially and usually is born with normal hemoglobin levels, although fetal iron stores as reflected by cord ferritin levels may be reduced if the mother is iron deficient.

The case for folic acid is similar. The fetus receives folate preferentially from the mother, and fetal folate deficiency is rare.[40] There are certain conditions, such as abruptio placentae, which are alleged to occur more frequently when there is folate deficiency in the mother, but these associations have not been firmly established.

Through passive transfer in the placental circulation, the fetus is the recipient of several maternal productions of potential hematologic importance. Immunoglobin G, involved in the common form of autoimmune hemolytic anemia, can cross the placental barrier and affect fetal red cells. This is also true for antiplatelet antibodies that the mother might have. Immune thrombocytopenia of the newborn is the consequence of this passive antibody transfer. Various plasma antibodies affecting blood group substances can be transferred, as discussed in Chapter 7.

THE DEFINITION OF ANEMIA DURING PREGNANCY

The diagnosis of anemia in clinical medicine is based on the hemoglobin concentration in blood, and only that. Hypervolemic states in which the plasma volume is expanded and hypovolemic states in which the plasma volume is restricted affect the hemoglobin value (by dilution and concentration, respectively) and reduce its accuracy as an index of total body hemoglobin. The hemoglobin concentration as provided by the usual laboratory assessment is an index of total body hemoglobin if the plasma volume is normal. The diagnosis of anemia can be made directly from the hemoglobin concentration value if it has not been altered by plasma volume changes or if the effect of these changes has been accounted for. For instance, a hemoglobin level of 11 g/dl in an edematous patient would probably be 13 or 14 g/dl if the plasma volume were normal. Similarly, a hemoglobin concentration of 14 g/dl in a dehydrated individual may actually represent anemia when the effects of the dehydration are considered.

The diagnosis of anemia during pregnancy is also based on an interpretation of the hemoglobin concentration. However, significant plasma volume changes occur during the course of pregnancy that affect the hemoglobin concentration in blood, and the standards for the diagnosis of anemia during pregnancy must be adjusted to reflect these continuing plasma volume changes. True anemia can be produced by the event of pregnancy, and the recognition of hemoglobin values that represent true anemia, in contradistinction to hemoglobin values that represent plasma expansion, is the important but somewhat difficult point.

Because plasma volume changes at various points in pregnancy, the definition of anemia (the hemoglobin value that can be used to define anemia) changes during pregnancy. The influence of this change during the first eight weeks of pregnancy is minimal, although there is evidence that it has already begun by this early date. The hematologic status of the pregnant woman prior to eight weeks should be judged by the same standards applied to the nonpregnant adult female. The normal hemoglobin range for adult women is 14 ± 2 g/dl. This produces a range of 12 to 16 g/dl. A normal nonpregnant woman, or a pregnant woman prior to eight weeks, can be considered anemic if her hemoglobin value is below 12 g/dl.

The red blood cell indices that accompany the hemoglobin on a routine complete blood count will show a normal mean corpuscular volume (MCV), which in most laboratories is between 85 and 95 fl, and a normal mean corpuscular hemoglobin concentration (MCHC), which ranges between 32 and 36%. Hematocrit and red blood cell counts are indirect measures of anemia and are not substitutes for the hemoglobin value in this regard. They are used in the evaluation of anemia to calculate red blood cell indices. The practice of using the hematocrit as a measure of anemia has arisen because of the convenience and availability of the microhematocrit centrifuge apparatus and the difficulty of doing hemoglobin determinations other than in established laboratories. The hematocrit value is a useful screening technique, but it only approximates the hemoglobin value. It should not be a substitute for the true hemoglobin value in the diagnosis of anemia.

There is one subtle aspect of red cell status that is not influenced by pregnancy and can be relied upon as an indicator of a bona fide erythroid problem whatever the status of the pregnancy. This measure is the red blood cell morphology, which should be reported on all blood counts and should not be abnormal unless a true anemia exists. The findings of anisocytosis or poikilocytosis or specific red cell shape abnormalities may be even more meaningful than the hemoglobin value itself in pointing to pathology.

The second hematologic stage of pregnancy encompasses the last part of the first trimester and all of the second trimester. It is significantly influenced by the expanding plasma volume of pregnancy. The hemoglobin concentration is lowered by hemodilution, which is not a true anemia. There are wide variations from one pregnant woman to the next so that precision is impossible, and an approximation of the cut-off line between normality and abnormality is necessary. The hemoglobin level of 10 g/dl has been chosen as this arbitrary level.[1] During the middle portions of pregnancy, hemoglobin values above 10 g/dl are considered "normal," although it is very likely that there are some women with true anemia included in that range. Although the diagnosis of anemia cannot be made with certainty if the hemoglobin value is above 10 g/dl in midpregnancy, support for the suspicion that a true anemia exists can be found from other laboratory assessments. The red blood cell morphology should remain normal, and if it is not, some erythroid problem exists. The iron saturation (ratio of serum iron to iron-binding capacity) should remain above 15% throughout pregnancy. If it does not, the probability that iron deficiency has arrived, or is just about to, becomes high. Last, the serum ferritin level should remain above 12 μg/L, and this is its lowest allowable point, usually occurring about the 28th week of pregnancy. It should be higher earlier in pregnancy.

Finally, during the last trimester of pregnancy plasma volume ceases to expand, and there may actually be some contraction of plasma volume as delivery approaches. The "allowable" hemoglobin value during the last stage of pregnancy rises a bit to 11 g/dl, and anemia should be diagnosed if the level falls below that point. The considerations of red cell morphology, iron saturation, and ferritin remain the same as those for the middle portion of pregnancy. At no time during pregnancy should the MCV wander into either the microcytic or macrocytic range as established by the laboratory performing the assessments. Similarly, the MCHC should not drop below 32%. If any of these events occurs, the presence of an anemia should be considered and evaluation of it carried out.

A level of the mean cell volume (MCV) of less than 80 fl has been used to detect the significant microcytic anemias, iron deficiency and thalassemia.[41] The MCV is a particularly sensitive index of thalassemia, but iron deficiency must be quite severe to produce this finding.

HEMATOLOGIC EVALUATION DURING A ROUTINE PREGNANCY

There are basic assessments of the hematologic system that should be incorporated into routine prenatal care. Ideally these should be performed before the end of the first trimester or at the first prenatal visit, whenever that is.

The admonitions and didactics offered to medical students on the proper evaluation of an anemic patient turn out to be just as appropriate for the evaluation of the hematologic status in a routine pregnancy. The history is the first part, the most important part, and not replaceable by any amount of expensive laboratory determinations. The two most important hematologic historical points in the setting of pregnancy are those which evaluate the probable iron stores of the patient and those which detect any hemorrhagic tendencies that may be present. The stores of iron can be estimated from the history of iron intake and iron loss through diet and bleeding history. The iron content of the diet approximates 6 mg/1000 calories, if there is meat included, and is less with vegetarians. Assessment of iron loss through the menstrual cycle is routinely done by physicians with an obstetric practice, and the further contributions to iron loss produced by previous pregnancies and nongynecologic bleeding should be added to this total. The historical assessment of iron loss will not lead to assurance that iron stores are adequate (as the work of Scott and Pritchard[10] cited earlier has shown), but it will alert the physician to the probability of marginal stores if the iron loss history is prominent.

The historical evaluation of a potential bleeding diasthesis includes questions of unusual bleeding with trauma, dental work, previous pregnancies or surgery, or spontaneous bleeding, including epistaxis and purpura. Family history of the same events is equally important. Additional questions concerning other blood diseases that the patient or her family may have had should be asked, particularly to detect the possibility of an anemia other than iron or folic acid deficiency. Finally, awareness of a chronic infection, particularly a chronic urinary tract infection, is important in evaluating a potential anemia, because this produces the same mild and sometimes slightly hypochromic anemia as do pregnancy and mild iron deficiency.

In addition to the history, it is advisable to obtain a complete blood count on the first visit. This will contain the hemoglobin level (whose interpretation was noted in the previous section) and the beginning elements of evaluation of an anemia. The white cell count, differential, and platelet count complete the screening of the rest of the hematopoietic system. They are sufficient for purposes of a woman with a normal pregnancy without prior history of blood disease and with a normal physical exam. If abnormality of the white cell count, differential, or platelet status is detected, this heralds the need for independent investigation beyond the considerations of anemia and erythroid values that have been discussed here. It is not likely that white blood cell or platelet abnormalities are pregnancy produced or related, and they should be investigated in the same manner as advisable for any patient. Folic acid deficiency producing megaloblastic anemia (not usually manifest until the late phases of pregnancy) has an associated white blood cell and platelet decrease, whereas iron deficiency does not.

However, there are several other explanations for white cell and platelet abnormalities besides folic acid deficiency, and the diagnosis of folic acid deficiency requires more than notation of white cell and platelet problems. Therefore, the finding of either a white cell or a platelet abnormality should not be casually attributed to folic acid deficiency but rather should be vigorously evaluated until specific conclusions are reached.

EVALUATION OF ANEMIA WHEN FOUND

When anemia as determined by hemoglobin assessment has been demonstrated or is strongly suspected, there is a logical order of events that is pertinent in pregnancy. They would not be as logical or as pertinent for anemia found in a human condition other than pregnancy, so the procedural steps recommended here should not automatically be applied to nonpregnant conditions.

To begin with, it is not altogether unscientific (and it is certainly very practical and expedient) to approach the diagnosis of anemia in pregnancy as if it is probably due to iron deficiency. Well over 90% of anemias associated with pregnancy are so caused. The reasons for the high incidence of this kind of anemia associated with a condition with a high iron demand have been previously discussed. The anemia can be considered as resulting from iron deficiency if several important provisos are accounted for: (1) there is no current or past history of blood dyscrasia; (2) the white blood cell count, differential, and platelet count are normal; (3) the possibility of hemoglobinopathy has been dealt with by sickle cell screening in the black population and "thalassemia screening" using the MCV; (4) the anemia is discovered in the first half of pregnancy when the anemia of folic acid deficiency is unusual; and (5) the red cell indices and red cell morphology are normal. If any of these conditions is not the case, a further line of investigation suggested by each is necessary. If they are all met, the anemia can be considered due to iron deficiency and so treated, particularly if historical features of heavy iron loss have been noted.

Confirmation of the presence of iron deficiency (by other than statistical inference) can be obtained in the setting of pregnancy if the hemoglobin level is less than 10 g/dl, the white cell and platelet counts are normal, and ferritin level is less than 12 ng/L. This triad will produce convincing evidence that iron deficiency is present but does not exclude the possibility that there is also anemia due to an additional cause. The diagnosis of iron deficiency can be presumed with somewhat less surety if an anemia is present, the white cell and platelet counts are normal, and there is the finding of either a decreased iron saturation (less than 15%) or of red cell morphology changes characteristic of iron deficiency or both. The mild and often hypochronic anemia of chronic infection that simulates iron deficiency can be distinguished by means of the serum ferritin level, which approaches normal when anemia is due to infection only.

It is less important to be sure that iron deficiency is present (because the treatment is inexpensive, nontoxic, and will probably be offered anyway) than it is to be sure that there is not another cause for the anemia. Other causes of anemia during pregnancy have more important implications for the pregnancy and its outcome than does iron deficiency. Included in this list of important "other" anemias are the hemoglobinopathies, folic acid deficiency, and anemias that the patient may have had prior to becoming pregnant.

The possibility that folate deficiency is responsible for the anemia is heightened by discovery of anemia during the latter part of pregnancy or in a patient at high risk for folate deficiency (see previous discussion). The diagnosis can be made by the laboratory assessment of the serum folate concentration, which is now reliable in most laboratories. Values lower than 3 ng/ml indicate folate deficiency. (It has been shown that folate levels below 3 ng are possible without anemia, but the finding of low folate levels should suggest supplementation even if anemia is not present. Folic acid deficiency anemia does not occur without low folate levels.) Hypersegmentation of the neutrophils is a classic morphologic finding in megaloblastic anemias, either the folic acid or vitamin B_{12} type, and this microscopic finding apparently precedes red cell morphologic changes, which ensue as the deficiency becomes more severe. The finding of hypersegmented neutrophils, however, depends upon accurate assessment in the laboratory and is highly subject to error. In addition, there are other conditions besides megaloblastic anemias that produce hypersegmentation. Therefore the finding of hypersegmented neutrophils may be considered a sign of folate deficiency but not proof thereof. The latter requires demonstration of an anemia by low serum folate levels. As the anemia becomes more severe, there will be macrocytosis shown in the MCV and red cell findings such as macrocytes, anisocytosis, and an ovoid shape of some of the red cells. There will also be white cell and platelet abnormalities. However, these ancillary findings are either subtle or absent in mild folic acid deficiency anemia (hemoglobin levels in the 9 to 10 g/dl range) and cannot be depended upon to point to a diagnosis unless the anemia is severe.

If the anemia is found to be iron or folic acid deficiency in type, or if infection is present, appropriate treatment can be instituted and the patient's hematologic response noted. It is as important to be sure that the patient responds to specific anemia therapy as it was to attempt the diagnosis in the first place. Deficiency anemias respond to appropriate therapy, and confirmation of the original diagnosis can be obtained from this response.

If the diagnosis of iron or folic acid deficiency or infection cannot be made, a second level of investigation of the anemia should be instituted. This includes performing a hemoglobin electrophoresis to detect abnormal hemoglobins (if this has not been previously done), a Coombs' test to screen for immune hemolytic anemias, and obtaining a serum creatinine level to exclude previously unrecognized chronic renal disease.

If the reason for the anemia has not been determined following this second level of diagnostic studies, the probability of a complex or rare cause for the anemia is present. The patient should then be managed as an adult with an anemia that has escaped explanation with basic approaches. Whether the next step requires referral to another physician depends upon the experience and interest in hematologic matters of the physician responsible for the obstetric care. The diagnostic sequence that might be undertaken is beyond the scope and intentions of this book, and the investigation of the anemia would be unrelated to the pregnant state.

REFERENCES

1. Scott, D.E., and Pritchard, J.A.: Anemia in pregnancy. Clin Perinatol *1*:491, 1974.
2. Kerr, D.N.S., and Davidson, J.: The prophylaxis of iron deficiency anemia in pregnancy. Lancet *2*:483, 1958.
3. Hibbard, B.: Anemia in pregnancy. Nursing Mirror September 9, 1981, p. 18.
4. Williams, J.W.: Am J Obstet Gynecol *80*:1, 1919.
5. Peck, T.M., and Arias, F.: Hematologic changes associated with pregnancy. Clin Obstet Gynecol *22*:785, 1979.
6. Chesley, L.C., and Duffus, G.M.: Posture and apparent plasma volume in late pregnancy. J Obstet Gynecol Br Cwlth *78*:406, 1971.
7. Chesley, L.C.: Plasma and red cell volumes during pregnancy. Am J Obstet Gynecol *112*:440, 1972.
8. Pritchard, J.A., Baldwin, R.M., and Dickey, J.C.: Blood volume changes in pregnancy and the puerperium. Am J Obstet Gynecol *84*:1271, 1962.
9. Lund, C.J., and Donovan, J.C.: Blood volume changes in pregnancy. Am J Obstet Gynecol *98*:393, 1967.
10. Scott, D.E., and Pritchard, J.A.: Iron deficiency in healthy young college women. JAMA *199*:147, 1967.
11. Scott, D.E., et al.: Iron Deficiency During Pregnancy, Iron Deficiency Pathogenesis—Clinical Aspects—Therapy. New York: Academic Press, 1970.
12. Monsen, E.R., Kuhn, J.H., and Finch, C.A.: Iron status of menstruating females. Am J Clin Nutr *20*:842, 1967.
13. Committee on Iron Deficiency, Council of Foods and Nutrition of the American Medical Association. Iron Deficiency in the United States. JAMA *203*:407, 1968.
14. Svanberg, B., et al.: Absorption of supplemental iron during pregnancy—A longitudinal study with repeated bone marrow studies and absorption measurements. Acta Obstet Gynecol Scand *48*:87, 1975.
15. Dewees, C.B.: Hematologic disorders of pregnancy. Nurs Clin North Am *17*:57, 1982.
16. McFee, J.G.: Iron metabolism and iron deficiency during pregnancy. Clin Obstet Gynecol *22*:799, 1979.
17. Messer, R.H.: Pregnancy anemias. Clin Obstet Gynecol *17*:163, 1974.
18. Herbert, V., and Bertin, J.R.: The Vitamins. 2nd Ed. New York: Academic Press, 1967.
19. Willoughby, M.L.D., and Jewell, F.J.: Folate status throughout pregnancy and the postpartum period. Br Med J *4*:356, 1968.
20. Baker, S.J., et al.: Vitamin B_{12} deficiency in pregnancy and the puerperium. Br Med J *1*:1658, 1962.
21. Lampkin, B.C., Shore, N.A., and Chadwick, D.: Megaloblastic anemia of infancy secondary to maternal pernicious anemia. N Engl J Med *274*:1168, 1966.
22. Wintrobe, M.M., et al., (eds.): Clinical Hematology. 8th Ed. Philadelphia, Lea & Febiger, 1981.
23. Chanarin, I., McFadyen, I.R., and Kyle, R.: The physiologic macrocytosis of pregnancy. Br J Obstet Gynaecol *84*:504, 1977.
24. Taylor, D.J., and Lind, T.: Haematologic changes during normal pregnancy: Iron induced macrocytosis. Br J Obstet Gynaecol *83*:760, 1976.
25. Lewis, D., Stockley, R.J., and Chanarin, J.: Changes in the mean corpuscular red cell volume in women with β-thalassemia trait during pregnancy. Br J Haematol *50*:423, 1982.
26. Fenton, V., Cavill, J., and Fisher, J.: Iron stores in pregnancy. Br J Haematol *37*:145, 1977.
27. Jacobs, A., et al.: Ferritin in the serum of normal subjects and patients with iron deficiency and iron overload. Br Med J *4*:206, 1972.
28. Puolakka, A., Janne, O, Pakarinen, A., and Vihko, R.: Serum ferritin in the diagnosis of anemia during pregnancy. Acta Obstet Gynecol Scand (Suppl) *95*:57, 1980.

29. Lipschitz, D.A., Cook, J.D., and Finch, C.A.: A clinical evaluation of serum ferritin as an index of iron stores. N Engl J Med *290*:1213, 1974.
30. deLeeuw, N.K.M., Lowenstein, L., and Hsieh, Y-S.: Iron deficiency and hydremia in normal pregnancy. Medicine *45*:291, 1966.
31. Green, R., Watson, L.R., Saab, G.A., and Crosby, W.H.: "Normal" serum ferritin—a caution. Blood *50*:545, 1977.
32. Lappin, T.R.J., Whiteley, L.A., and Murnaghan, G.A.: Reliability of serum ferritin determinations after total dose infusion of iron dextran in pregnancy. Ann Clin Biochem *16*:124, 1979.
33. Pritchard, J.A., Scott, D.E., and Whalley, P.J.: Folic acid requirements in pregnancy-induced megaloblastic anemia. JAMA *208*:1163, 1969.
34. Behera, S.K., Rao, A.S., Ahmed, B., and Patnick, B.K.: Serum iron and iron binding capacity in the newborns in relation to maternal anemia. Ind J Pediatr *16*:99, 1979.
35. Ogunbode, O.: The relationship between hematocrit levels in gravidae and their newborns. Int J Gynaecol Obstet *18*:57, 1980.
36. Sood, S.K., et al.: WHO-sponsored collaborative studies on nutritional anaemia in India. The effect of parenteral iron administration in the control of anemia of pregnancy. Br J Nutr *42*:399, 1979.
37. Hemminki, E., and Starfield, B.: Routine administration of iron and vitamins during pregnancy: Review of controlled clinical trials. Br J Obstet Gynaecol *85*:404, 1978.
38. Editorial (author unspecified): Br Med J *6148*:1317, 1978.
39. WHO Scientific Group: Nutritional Anaemias. WHO Tech Rep Ser No 405, 1968.
40. Pritchard, J.A., et al.: Infants of mothers with megaloblastic anemia due to folate deficiency. JAMA *211*:1982, 1970.
41. Alger, L.S., Golbus, M.S., and Laros, R.K.: Thalassemia and pregnancy: Results of an antenatal screening program. Am J Obstet Gynecol *134*:662, 1979.

Chapter 2

NUTRITIONAL ANEMIAS COMPLICATING PREGNANCY

Kathy S. Gookin/John C. Morrison

Anemia is one of the most frequently encountered complications related to pregnancy.[1] The relative anemia of pregnancy that occurs because of the proportionately larger increase in plasma volume relative to red cell mass is noted in most normal gestations. Nutritional deficiencies are the most frequent cause of true or absolute anemia. Because nutrition plays a major role in the etiology and management of this commonly encountered disorder, emphasis should be placed on prevention and early recognition of such deficiencies. The adverse impact of inadequate nutrition on general health and in particular on pregnancy outcome leads one to investigate various acquired anemias induced or complicated by nutritional deficiencies. This chapter includes a discussion of the effects of trace element deficiencies, vitamin depletion, and protein deprivation on the hematologic system and indirectly on the mother, fetus, and newborn (Table 2–1).

MINERAL DEFICIENCY ANEMIA

About 4% of the body's weight is composed of minerals. Many of these elements, although present in minute amounts, are essential to body functions.

CALCIUM AND PHOSPHORUS

Calcium metabolism and absorption are altered significantly during pregnancy. Increasing levels of estrogen seen during pregnancy have been associated with diminished bone resorption, but a reciprocal increase in parathryoid hormone enhances absorption of calcium as well as decreasing its excretion. This hormonal relationship prevents a significant change in serum calcium levels. The placenta actively transports calcium against a concentration gradient, making fetal levels higher than maternal levels and creating an environment that favors skeletal growth.[2] Current Recommended Daily Allowance (RDA) for calcium during pregnancy is 1200 mg/day as compared with an RDA of 800 mg/day in the nonpregnant female[3] (Table 2–2). Milk and milk products are known to be the principal sources of calcium and are an extremely important part of the pregnant woman's diet. In the case of milk intolerance or taste aversion, supplemental calcium preparations may be indicated. Blood levels are usually not adequate indicators for calcium replacement. Approximately 85% of the body's phosphorus is found in combination with calcium. The phosphorus to calcium ratio in bones is two to one. Additionally, phosphorus is necessary for the completion of many metabolic processes.[4] Nutritional deficiency of phosphorus is not appreciated

Table 2–1. Nutritional Deficiencies Causing Anemias

Mineral Deficiencies
Calcium and phosphorus
Zinc
Copper and manganese
Iron
Vitamin Deficiencies
Fat-soluble
Water-soluble
Folic acid
Vitamin B_{12}
Alcohol-Related Anemia
Protein Deficiency

in the human because of its availability in practically all natural foods. The RDA in the nonpregnant state is 800 mg. An increase of 400 mg/day is offered to ensure adequate sources for pregnancy[3] (see Table 2–2).

ZINC

This element is a constituent of numerous enzymes involved in essential metabolic pathways. Although the etiology of zinc deficiency is varied, nutritional deficiencies are a common cause and are usually related to inadequate protein intake. The increased consumption of cereal proteins has predisposed many to zinc deficiency, as has excessive ingestion of alcohol. Iatrogenic causes of zinc deficiency are associated with the use of chelating agents, diuretics, antimetabolites, and anti-anabolic drugs.[5] Animal studies have linked this mineral deficiency to various types of malformations involving all organ systems in the fetus.[6] Furthermore, central nervous system anomalies in humans have been noted with increased incidence in areas of the world where zinc deficiency is prevalent. The teratogenic effects of zinc deficiency have been related to

Table 2–2. Recommended Daily Allowances for Vitamins, Minerals, and Protein

	Nonpregnant Women	Pregnant Women
Calcium	800 mg	1200 mg
Phosphorus	800 mg	1200 mg
Zinc	15 mg	20 mg
Copper	2 mg	*
Manganese	*	*
Iron	12 mg	18 mg
Vitamin A	3750 IU	5000 IU
Vitamin E	12 IU	15 IU
Vitamin D	400 IU	600 IU
Vitamin K	*	*
Vitamin C	45 mg	60 mg
Vitamin B_6	2 mg	2.5 mg
Folic acid	0.4 mg	0.8–1.0 mg
Vitamin B_{12}	5 mg	10 mg
Protein	55 g	75 g

* RDA not established.

a reduction in DNA synthesis. Reduced serum levels of zinc in human pregnancy are related to prolonged gestations, dysfunctional labor patterns, and congenital anomalies.[7] Zinc deficiency in patients with sickle cell anemia and thalassemia has been noted, but there is no existing evidence to show that zinc deficiency causes the anemia.[8] A recent report has demonstrated reduced serum zinc levels in a group of ten pregnant women as compared with a nonpregnant control group.[9] Because both groups consumed equal amounts of zinc (16 mg/day), the authors related this decrease to a reduction in the serum albumin resulting from expanded blood volume rather than to inadequate zinc. There were no demonstrable adverse fetal effects. Zinc is found in abundance in animal protein sources; therefore, vegetarian diets are lacking in this mineral. The current RDA for zinc in pregnancy is 20 mg, an increase of 5 mg over the requirements in the nonpregnant state[3] (see Table 2–2).

COPPER AND MANGANESE

Maternal serum copper levels increase progressively throughout gestation, while fetal levels are ten times those in the mother.[10] The primary role of copper seems to be related to its effect on absorption and utilization of iron and its part in phospholipid synthesis. For this reason, severe copper deficiency in humans has been characterized by a microcytic anemia not responsive to iron supplementation.[11] Pregnancy itself has not been shown to have any adverse effects on copper metabolism. Animal studies have associated maternal deficiency of copper with fetal skeletal and neurologic abnormalities. Because copper is found in most foods and dietary deficiencies are rare, an RDA during pregnancy has not been established. In the nonpregnant state 2 mg/day seem to be adequate to prevent a negative balance (see Table 2–2).

Maternal manganese levels during pregnancy remain unchanged, and deficiency of this mineral is rarely noted in humans. On the other hand, animal studies have demonstrated maternal manganese deficiency to be associated with fetal skeletal and neurologic abnormalities.[12] Because little investigation has been performed on the requirements of manganese, no RDA has been established.

IRON

Iron deficiency anemia (IDA) accounts for 75% of all anemias diagnosed in pregnancy. Hemoglobin values <11.0 g/dl occur in as many as 80% of normal pregnant women at term if no iron supplementation is used. Increased utilization of iron, even during a normal pregnancy, dictates the need for supplementation, whether it be nutritional or exogenous.[13] This need may be further enhanced in the presence of multiple gestations, adolescent pregnancy, chronic blood loss, successive gestations less than two years apart, or poor iron absorption. In order to predict the pathophysiologic effects of inadequate iron, one must first understand the mechanisms of iron distribution, absorption, loss, and metabolism.

Iron Compartments

Multiple iron compartments have been identified that contain iron necessary for normal body function as well as reserve stores. This normal distribution includes hemoglobin iron, storage iron, myoglobin iron, labile pool iron, and transport iron. The dispersion of iron in each compartment can be affected by concurrent disease processes as well as by nutritional status.

Hemoglobin iron constitutes over 60% of total body iron and during pregnancy is increased by 20% in association with the concomitant increase in total blood volume (red cell mass). The hemoglobin molecule contains 0.34% iron by weight, and subsequently about 1 mg of iron is present in each milliliter of red blood cells. Laboratory indices, such as packed cell volume (PCV) or hemoglobin (Hgb), are generally reflective of hemoglobin iron. However, storage iron compartments must first be depleted before these laboratory values begin to decrease.

Storage iron generally accounts for 30% of total body iron. This iron compartment is equally divided between hemosiderin (found only in the cells of the reticuloendothelial system) and ferritin (found in plasma and virtually all cells of the body).[13] When iron utilization or loss exceeds the amount of available iron, depletion of the storage compartment begins. Hemosiderin contains approximately 25% iron by weight and is equally divided among the bone marrow, liver, and spleen. Prussian blue stains of bone marrow aspirates reveal the quantity of iron in this compartment and are a measure of iron balance. Ferritin exists as a complex of ferric hydroxide and the protein apolferritin. At maximum saturation, the ferritin molecule is 30% iron by weight. Ferritin has the ability to release and attach iron rapidly and therefore plays a direct role in iron absorption. Even though plasma levels of ferritin are low, these levels usually correlate with the body's iron stores and may be a useful measurement of iron stores when bone marrow aspiration is not advised, as in pregnancy.

Approximately 3% of the body's storage iron is found in myoglobin molecules. As its name indicates, myoglobin is found in most muscle cells, primarily cardiac and skeletal.[13] Its primary purpose is to serve as an oxygen reservoir when cellular hypoxia occurs. There is not evidence that pregnancy alters this compartment.

A study of kinetics has identified the iron that moves from the plasma to interstitial and intracellular fluid as the labile iron pool. It constitutes about 2% of the storage iron and contains 80 mg of iron. This "labile" iron is bound to proteins within the cellular membranes for short intervals prior to entering storage compartments or being utilized in the formation of heme compounds. "Acetate-extractable ferroprotein" has been identified as responsible for this short-term binding and subsequent release of iron.[15] Measurement of the iron-binding ability of this protein allows an indirect assessment of iron clearance rates and incorporation data based on its correlation with the labile iron pool. Previous studies have shown that the incorporation of iron in IDA is unaffected.

Parenchymal iron is composed of the cytochromes as well as a variety of oxidase enzymes such as peroxidase, catalase dehydrogenase, and acyl-CoA. It represents 0.2 to 0.5% of the body's storage iron and contains approximately 6 mg iron by weight.[14] Because of its enzymatic functions, it is an extremely vital compartment that is normally unchanged with pregnancy. Iron deficiency greatly impacts a variety of body functions by reducing the efficiency of the mitochondrial system and altering steroidogenesis as well as protein synthesis. Fortunately, iron in this compartment is reduced only when a state of very severe IDA exists.

Transport iron represents the smallest compartment of iron storage, making up less than 0.1% of the total body iron.[14] In spite of this, the turnover rate of 2.5 hours qualifies it as the most active compartment. Iron exchange from all the other compartments is mediated through this common pathway. Transport iron is bound to the protein transferrin, which has two glycoprotein moieties. Iron atoms may be bound at each end of the molecule. Once a site is occupied, the binding affinity of the molecule is increased. At any given time approximately one third of the binding sites are saturated if the patient is iron-replete; two thirds of the sites are unoccupied.

Iron Absorption

Iron absorption is a multidependent process that reflects the quantities and types of iron available for absorption as well as the status of the intestinal mucosa. Absorption of iron occurs primarily in the upper part of the small intestine.[16] It is absorbed mainly in the ferrous form (Fe^{++}) from elemental iron rather than the ferric form (Fe^{+++}) found mainly in vegetable complexes. Ferric iron must be reduced to the divalent state before it can be absorbed into the mucosal cell. Hemoglobin iron found in animal protein is readily absorbed only after it is hydrolyzed in the gut lumen. For this reason, the ferrous salts are best used for iron supplementation.

The body has a rate-limiting ability for iron absorption. Once the storage compartment is saturated with iron, the rate of absorption from the intestinal tract is reduced. This phenomenon is related to the ability of transferrin to accept iron from the mucosal cells. Once the transferrin is saturated, its ability to absorb more iron ceases. On the other hand, when iron storage compartments are depleted and most of the transferrin is free, the rate of absorption is greatly accelerated, enhancing the body's ability to restore the depleted iron supply.

The degradation of organic iron complexes is facilitated through the actions of gastric acid. Hence, the trivalent mineral found in most vegetable proteins (Fe^{+++}) is reduced to a utilizable complex (Fe^{++}) through this process. Drugs that subsequently increase gastric acid secretion have favorable effects on trivalent iron absorption and include hydroquinone and alcohol. On the other hand, absorption of hemoglobin iron is enhanced by the alkaline environment of the small bowel. For this reason agents that enhance formation of alkaline-soluble complexes subsequently promote iron absorption. Some of these agents include ascorbic acid, succinic acid, lactate, pyruvate, sorbitol, and various amino acids such as cysteine. Atropine and reserpine are also known to enhance iron absorption by decreasing intestinal motility and subsequently increasing the length or exposure to an alkaline environment. Some agents have inhibitory effects on iron absorption. Concentrations of the trivalent complexes are increased by administration of oxidants, while chelators cause formation of insoluble complexes. Agents that reduce gastric acid production or increase intestinal motility have adverse effects on iron absorption. Gastrectomy or removal of portions of the small bowel decreases surface area for absorption.[14]

Pica, the ingestion of substances with no dietary value, e.g., geophagia (clay), amylophagia (starch), and pagophagia (ice), is commonly associated with IDA. There is now clear evidence that pica is a sign of IDA rather than a cause. The current hypothesis associates pica with a decrease in iron-containing enzymes in the oral mucosa of affected patients. In pregnancy pica most often occurs after the 20th week of gestation and is associated with increased iron demands.

Transport

Once iron is absorbed from all the small intestine it is bound to transferrin and transported to the utilization pool. These complexes, or iron-bound transferrin, interact with membrane-specific receptors. The number of receptors regulates the amount of iron deposited in any particular tissue. When iron is needed by the bone marrow, trivalent iron atoms are obtained from the ferritin in the mucosal cells. The ferric iron binds to transferrin and is transported to the marrow, where it is used for the synthesis of hemoglobin. This direct transfer of iron to the normoblast is accomplished through an active process and is identified as the major pathway of iron transport. One of the minor pathways of transport is the passive acceptance of transferrin in the reticuloendothelial cells, a process known as rheopheocytosis.

Iron Homeostasis

The total amount of daily iron loss averages 0.1%. Most of this loss can be attributed to desquamation of cells in the gastrointestinal tract, blood, and bile. Epidermal cell loss and sweat amount to a daily loss of 0.2 mg, while iron loss in the urine averages 0.1 mg/day. Menstruating women usually lose 25 to 45 ml of blood with each period, which is a loss of 13 to 23 mg of iron.

Normally, compensation for iron loss occurs through consumption of a balanced diet; however, of all the required minerals, iron is the most difficult to obtain from dietary sources. The best sources are lean meats, organ meats, deep green leafy vegetables, dried fruits, and whole grain breads. Milk and milk products are poor sources of iron. Pregnancy places significant demands on iron stores, and consequently requirements for additional iron exist. Because of the lack of menses, iron-replete women require no additional iron therapy in the first half of pregnancy. However, after 20 weeks, fetal and maternal demands increase, and even increased abilities to absorb iron cannot fully compensate. Subsequently, unless supplemental iron is administered, iron stores become parasitized. For women with previously depleted iron stores, the additional requirements of pregnancy lead to a negative iron balance and subsequent IDA. The RDA for iron in nonpregnant state is 11 to 13 mg; pregnancy increases the requirements to 18 mg/day (see Table 2–2).[3]

Clinical Symptoms

Iron deficiency is a common cause of anemia during pregnancy. Decreased amounts of total body iron lead to varying degrees of iron depletion.[15] In its earliest stage, stores of iron are decreased, but no effect is reflected in the hematocrit (Hct) or serum iron (SI) level. No clinical symptoms are associated with simple iron depletion.

"Iron deficiency" indicates a state of depleted iron stores with a slight reduction in SI and transferrin saturation. Although easy fatigue and lethargy may be associated with iron deficiency, they are common complaints during normal pregnancy. Paresthesias, headaches, and a burning sensation of the tongue may be symptoms of tissue iron deficiency. Pica involving clay, dirt, ice, or starch is a classic manifestation of iron deficiency and is particularly common in some ethnic groups.

Iron deficiency anemia is the final stage of deficiency and is associated with absent iron stores, decreased Hgb and Hct values, reduced SI levels, and a decreased transferrin saturation. Because iron is the major mineral required for synthesis of the hemoglobin molecule, its absence leads to a characteristic hypochromic, microcytic erythrocyte on the peripheral blood smear. Clinical symptoms in IDA include pallor, glossitis (smooth red tongue), and cheilitis (inflammation of the lips). Nails that are ridged longitudinally and concave (koilonychia) rather than convex have been associated with chronic IDA but this is a rare finding. Retinal hemorrhages, shortness of breath, and splenomegaly have been noted in patients with Hgb <5 g/dl; however, IDA this severe is rarely seen in developed countries.

Laboratory Assessment

As discussed in the previous chapter, the hematologic changes normally associated with pregnancy make the diagnosis of anemia difficult. In order to assess the degree of iron depletion and hematologic compromise, appropriate laboratory intervention is indicated in those patients suspected of having an iron-deficient state.

In normal gestations the red blood cell (RBC) mass increases after 20 weeks and may be an indicator of the normal iron stores. If iron stores are depleted, this increase will not be observed. Since bone marrow assessment in pregnancy is only indicated when unusual hematologic disease is suspected, other laboratory indices become important markers in evaluating an iron-deficient state. A reduced Hgb or Hct value or alteration in the RBC indices should alert the clinician to monitor the hematologic status closely. Characteristically, iron stores will be reduced with chronic blood loss and nutritional anemias, including iron deficiency anemia.

Lack of the appropriate amounts of iron for hemoglobin synthesis and early red cell division during the maturation phase lead to the development of a characteristic hypochromic, microcytic erythrocyte. For this reason, peripheral blood smears frequently aid in making the diagnosis of IDA; however, other causes of hypochromic anemias must be excluded. These include (1) inflammatory processes, (2) chemical toxicity, (3) malignancy, (4) hemoglobinopathies, and (5) pyridoxine-responsive anemia. The appearance of schistocytes (red cell fragments) and basophilic stippling on the peripheral smear is also a common finding. During pregnancy, the relationship of Hgb to Hct is variable, and therefore the RBC indices are less useful. The mean corpuscular volume (MCV) is the most useful in revealing hypoproliferative anemias, with decreased values seen in iron-deficient states.[15]

Many authors have documented that SI levels decline as gestation advances. Increasing iron requirements by the fetus as well as low or exhausted iron stores in the mother help explain this phenomenon.[14] In the nonpregnant female SI values range between 50 and 110 μg/dl; however, the serum iron values are subject to many variables (Table 2–3). Serum values <60 μg/dl usually indicate an iron-deficient state, while values <30 μg/dl are indicative of IDA. Because of the diurnal, pulsatile release of iron, highest serum values are seen between 7 and 10 A.M. Many pathologic states are also related to reduced levels of serum iron and include inflammatory processes, malignancy, and hemoglobinopathies.

Decreased iron stores in the bone marrow are the earliest indicator of an iron-deficient state. Because of the discomfort and risks involved in bone marrow aspiration,

Table 2–3. Normative Laboratory Values

	Nonpregnant Women	Pregnant Women
Hemoglobin	12.5–14 g/dl	10–13 g/dl
Hematocrit	0.34–0.45 L/L	0.33–0.38 L/L
Reticulocyte count	0.5–1.0 %	1.0–2.0 %
Serum iron	50–110 μg/dl	40–100 μg/dl
Unsaturated iron-binding capacity	250–300 μg/dl	280–400 μg/dl
Transferrin saturation	25–35 %	15–30 %
Serum ferritin	75–100 μg/L	55–70 μg/L
Serum folate	6.5–19.6 μg/ml	5–10 μg/ml

this procedure is usually not indicated in pregnancy. Serum ferritin levels have been shown to be a consistent indicator of available iron stores, and this procedure yields clinically useful information. Normal serum ferritin levels during pregnancy are >30 $\mu g/L$, with values <10 $\mu g/L$ indicating reduced iron stores and anemia. (For additional information on serum ferritin, refer to Chapter 1.) An attempt to measure iron stores with nuclear magnetic resonance imaging has yielded poor results in those patients with iron depletion. However, it has proved useful in those patients with hemosiderosis. Increased levels of estrogen during pregnancy seem to have an effect on the hematologic system, resulting in increased transferrin levels. This, in association with increased iron utilization, results in reduced saturation of the transferrin molecule. Transferrin saturation during pregnancy is generally 15 to 30%. Levels $<15\%$ are seen in IDA. Since one third of the transferrin in iron-replete subjects is saturated, measurement of the unoccupied transferrin is expressed as the UIBC. During pregnancy the UIBC ranges from 280 to 400 $\mu g/dl$ (see Table 2–3). A value >400 $\mu g/dl$ is found in IDA.[13]

In iron depletion, protoporphyrin is manufactured by erythrocytes and incorporated into hemoglobin. In iron deficiency the amount of free erythrocyte protoporphyrin (FEP) is increased. Measurement of FEP has been advocated as a screen for IDA; however, the results are correlated with the duration of the anemia rather than its severity. Also, its specificity for IDA is lacking.[17] In iron-deficient states zinc may replace iron in the protoporphyrin ring. Measurement of red blood cell zinc protoporphyrin may also yield some useful information when evaluating iron deficiency. Even though this is an easily performed and inexpensive test, it is not specific for IDA.

Therapy

Most clinicians advocate the use of prophylactic iron supplementation during pregnancy. The debate involving this issue is covered in Chapter 1. The response to iron therapy is frequently diagnostic in an iron-deficient state and may obviate extensive laboratory investigations. Iron administration rarely causes problems for the low risk patient; however, close monitoring should be utilized so that an iron-unresponsive anemia will not go undetected. Reticulocytosis should be observed seven to ten days after iron supplementation if IDA is the correct diagnosis. An increase in the Hgb concentration should be seen in the nonpregnant patient in three to four weeks; however, the increased demand for iron during pregnancy and hemodilution may mask this response. After other causes of anemia have been excluded, iron supplementation should continue throughout the pregnancy.

Satisfactory iron supplementation can be accomplished by a variety of agents.[14] Oral preparations containing elemental salts are most commonly employed. Occasionally the need arises for parenteral administration of an iron-carbohydrate complex or a blood transfusion. Although an array of iron preparations is available, ferrous sulfate compounds are the least expensive and have proved efficacious for iron supplementation. Other forms of oral preparations exist but are more expensive and are not more effective than ferrous sulfate. The maximum absorption of iron from the gastrointestinal tract occurs four to six hours after the element is ingested; therefore, supplementation three to four times daily is recommended for peak absorption. Generally 30 to 60 mg of elemental iron daily are sufficient for the iron-replete woman, whereas 200 to 300 mg/day may be needed if iron deficiency exists.

Gastrointestinal complaints associated with oral iron may be nausea, vomiting, diarrhea, or constipation. Recent data demonstrate that sustained released capsules may reduce some of the intolerance and increase patient compliance. Slowly absorbed iron compounds may also be of value in reducing gastrointestinal complaints. Ferrous sulfate syrups are usually better tolerated and may be an excellent substitute if other ferrous salts cannot be taken. To avoid staining the teeth, this preparation should be diluted in water or juice and taken through a straw. Last, some clinicians have found that gastrointestinal side-effects are decreased without reduced absorption when iron is taken with meals.

Parenteral administration of iron is rarely indicated but is available as iron complexes with dextran or sorbitol. Administration of these agents is by either the intramuscular or the intravenous route and may be indicated for those patients with severe IDA who are unable to tolerate oral administration or those patients with absorptive disorders. Skin staining, discomfort at the injection site, malaise, and a metallic taste occur in fewer than 10% of patients. Some of the moderate reactions, including hyperpyrexia, lymphadenopathy, phlebitis, and leukemoid reactions, occur in 1 to 2% of patients, while severe systemic reactions such as anaphylaxis occur in 0.5% of patients. Administration of a test dose is recommended in those receiving parenteral iron supplementation.[14]

In summary, iron deficiency or depletion may be difficult to diagnose and often is not suspected until changes in the Hgb or PCV are noted. Because iron depletion is so common in most women, supplementation during pregnancy is recommended.

VITAMIN DEFICIENCY ANEMIA

An early interest in vitamins was first displayed when their role in the prevention of various diseases such as scurvy, beriberi, and pellagra was appreciated. The term vitamin is used when referring to a group of compounds other than fats, carbohydrates, and protein that are necessary for growth and maintenance of various body functions. Two groups of vitamins are identified by their solubility. The water-soluble group includes vitamin B complex, C, and folic acid and the fat-soluble group vitamins A, D, E, and K. Vitamins play a vital role in facilitating metabolism of amino acids, carbohydrates, and fats and as such are involved in anemias. Indeed, during pregnancy folic acid deficiency is second only to IDA as a cause of nutritional anemia.

FAT-SOLUBLE VITAMINS

These vitamins (A, D, E, and K) are primarily stored in the liver and the stores serve as reservoirs during times of deprivation or increased utilization. Characteristically, fetal levels of fat-soluble vitamins are lower than maternal levels.

Vitamin A

Vitamin A crosses the placenta by simple diffusion and fetal levels of this vitamin have been found to be slightly less than those of the mother. A 25% increase over RDA for nonpregnant females is recommended for gestational requirements, resulting in a daily requirement of 5000 IU[3] (see Table 2–2). Foods high in vitamin A content include liver, whole milk products, cheese, green and yellow vegetables, yellow fruit, and fortified margarine. Some investigators have shown that chronic vitamin A deficiency produces an anemia similar to IDA.[11] Various hematologic parameters, such as the MCV and MCHC, are reduced and low SI levels are noted, as seen in the iron-deficient subject. Unlike IDA, however, iron stores are increased and iron supplementation does not correct the hematologic abnormalities. Studies conducted in other countries have shown a similar correlation between serum vitamin A levels and hemoglobin concentrations. Although one case report documented renal anomalies in an infant whose mother had ingested excessive doses of vitamin A during pregnancy, moderate doses less than 1500 IU of this vitamin should not be harmful.[18]

Vitamin D

The primary role of vitamin D is facilitation of calcium absorption from the gut. During pregnancy fairly extensive changes in calcium metabolism occur in addition to increased calcium needs by the fetus. Calcium ions are transported by the placenta against a concentration gradient from the mother to the fetus in order to enhance fetal skeletal growth. Vitamin D and its metabolites also cross the placenta and play vital roles in the metabolism of calcium in the fetus as well as the newborn.[2] Since positive calcium balance in pregnancy is regulated by vitamin D, an additional 200 IU/day is advised, resulting in an RDA of 600 IU/day during pregnancy[3] (see Table 2–2). Vitamin D is found in large quantities in fish liver oils, fortified milk, and in small amounts in butter, liver, egg yolks, and salmon. Exposure to sunlight is an excellent source of vitamin D.

Vitamin E

Throughout pregnancy vitamin E levels in the mother gradually rise and actually double by term. There is only partial transfer of this vitamin across the placenta. Because of a reduced fetal need and its abundance in the diet, the RDA for vitamin E is increased only 3 IU (to 15 IU daily) during pregnancy[2] (see Table 2–2). Since vitamin E deficiency is rarely seen in this country, except in those patients with cystic fibrosis, it is generally assumed that dietary sources are adequate. Even though animal foods are poor sources of this vitamin, it is found in abundance in vegetable oils, green leafy vegetables, nuts, and legumes. One investigation has associated daily administration of 400 to 800 IU of vitamin E with lengthening the life span of erythrocytes in those patients with G6PD deficiency.[19] Furthermore, daily administration of 450 IU of vitamin E to patients with sickle cell anemia for periods of 6 to 36 weeks seemed to have a significant effect in reducing the number of sickled red cells.[20]

Vitamin K

Vitamin K is synthesized by bacteria of the lower intestinal tract and requires the presence of bile for its absorption. Because of individual variations in synthesis and dietary intake, an RDA has not been established; however, dietary deficiency is not a problem.[2] No supplementation in pregnancy is indicated; however, it remains common practice to administer this vitamin intramuscularly to the newborn because of the newborn's lack of intestinal bacteria. Newborns of mothers who have taken hydantoin derivatives need vitamin K supplementation. Plant sources of vitamin K can be found in green leafy vegetables, e.g., spinach, cabbage, and alfalfa.

WATER-SOLUBLE VITAMINS

These compounds (B group, C, folic acid) are excreted in the urine, and the lack of the body's ability to store these vitamins leaves little reserve for times of deprivation.

Unlike fat-soluble vitamins, water-soluble vitamin levels are usually higher in the fetus than in the mother.

Vitamin B

Vitamin B deficiencies are uncommon in humans. A discussion of pyridoxine (vitamin B_6), folate, and B_{12} deficiencies follows. Because other B complex vitamin deficiencies such as niacin, thiamin, riboflavin, and pantothenic acid are almost never seen during pregnancy, they will not be discussed. Most data associating any of the above nutritional deficiencies with anemia are inconclusive, and further research is warranted. Vitamin B_6 requirements during pregnancy increase in association with increased protein intake. Serum levels of B_6 fall 75% from nonpregnant levels during gestation. As with vitamin C, the placenta concentrates B_6 levels, thus enhancing fetal values two to three times those of the mother. Even though pyridoxine deficiency was at one time thought to be related to pre-eclampsia, a double blind study showed vitamin B_6 supplementation to have no effect on the subsequent development of pre-eclampsia.[21] To provide for increased protein ingestion by the mother and placental transfer, during pregnancy the RDA for vitamin B_6 is 2.5 mg (see Table 2–2). Meat, poultry, and fish are food sources rich in vitamin B_6. A relationship between pyridoxine deficiency and a hypochromic, microcytic anemia is suspected. Pyridoxine deficiency induced in infants leads to a hypochromic, microcytic type anemia.[11] There has also been one case report of a patient with a hypochromic anemia who failed to respond to iron supplementation but afterward responded to pyridoxine administration.[11] In addition to a hypochromic anemia, an increased number of ring sideroblasts are seen on the peripheral smear. Increased levels of SI and serum ferritin, in association with a low UIBC, help to differentiate pyridoxine-responsive anemia from IDA.[14]

Vitamin C

Ascorbic acid (vitamin C) is readily absorbed from the gastrointestinal tract and is held in reserve in various body and glandular tissues. It is required for the formation of collagenous substances and is responsible for many cellular functions. During pregnancy vitamin C levels decline progressively and at term reach levels half of those found in midpregnancy. Fetal levels are 50% above maternal values.[2] To date the effects of vitamin C deficiency on pregnancy and pregnancy outcome are unanswered. The association of pre-eclampsia and premature rupture of the membranes with vitamin C deficiency has arisen in the past, but at present there are no data to substantiate a relationship. Confusion also exists as to the role that vitamin C plays in hematopoiesis. Eighty percent of patients with ascorbic acid deficiency (scurvy) are anemic. However, the anemia observed is hypochromic and varies between normocytic and macrocytic. It has been proposed that the anemia is a result of the interaction of ascorbic acid and iron metabolism. The RDA for ascorbic acid during pregnancy is 60 mg, a daily increase of 15 mg over that required in the nonpregnant state (see Table 2–2).[2] Excellent food sources of vitamin C are fresh, frozen, or canned citrus fruits and virtually all fresh fruits and vegetables.

MEGALOBLASTIC ANEMIAS

Megaloblastic anemia refers to a group of hematologic disorders exhibiting impaired DNA synthesis. It is the second most common type of anemia in pregnancy and is frequently related to vitamin B_{12} or folic acid deficiency. Of women with anemia during pregnancy, 95 to 98% have either IDA or megaloblastic anemia. Vitamin B_{12} and folate deficiencies produce a common, characteristic morphology as well as functional alterations in peripheral blood and bone marrow. In all stages of development, erythrocyte precursors are morphologically larger (macrocytic) than the other cells. Since both vitamin B_{12} and folate deficiencies delay nuclear maturation, the common denominator is large cells. As hemoglobin synthesis continues, a "nuclear-cytoplasmic asynchronism" becomes more evident, and the maturity of the cytoplasm does not correspond to the immaturity of the nucleus. This abnormal nuclear-cytoplasmic appearance is diagnostic of megaloblastic anemia.[22] Although these macrocytic cells have normal oxygen-carrying abilities, their fragility leads to a shorter life span. Abnormal maturation in granulocytes and thrombocytes eventually leads to neutropenia and thrombocytopenia.

Folic acid and vitamin B_{12} deficiencies are the most common causes of megaloblastic anemia. The effect of vitamin B_{12} deficiency on hematopoiesis may either be direct or a result of its function in folate metabolism. The direct effect of B_{12} deficiency is slowing of the conversion of ribonucleotides to deoxyribonucleotides. The more important effect is the indirect one, when conversion of hemocysteine to methionine is retarded. Causes of these deficiencies may be varied and relate to decreased intake, poor absorption, impaired utilization, or increased requirements, such as pregnancy, hyperthyroidism, hyperparathyroidism, or malignancies. Other etiologies of megaloblastic anemia not related to folic acid or vitamin B_{12} deficiency are seen in patients treated with metabolic inhibitors such as chemotherapeutic agents. Pyridoxine and thiamin deficiencies and Di Guglielmo syndrome are also uncommon causes of megaloblastic anemia. Last, those patients with various inborn errors of metabolism, such as Lesch-Nyhan syndrome, orotic aciduria, or certain enzymatic deficiencies, may also present with megaloblastic anemia. Fortunately, 98% of the cases of megaloblastic anemia can be attributed to folic acid or vitamin B_{12} deficiency, with the vast majority of these related to folic acid.[14]

Laboratory Assessment

Clinical manifestations and laboratory detection of a megaloblastic anemia are variable and usually are not evident until the deficiency is severe. As with other anemias, symptoms increase with the severity of the anemia and may include pallor, malaise, weakness, dizziness, palpitations, and shortness of breath. Laboratory features may also vary with the severity of the anemia. A peripheral smear demonstrating hypersegmented granulocytes as well as RBC inclusions (particularly Howell-Jolly bodies and basophilic stippling) is usually diagnostic. The megaloblastic anemias are characteristically normochromic and macrocytic. The MCH (mean corpuscular hemoglobin) and MCHC (mean corpuscular hemoglobin concentration) are usually normal; however, the dramatically increased mean corpuscular volume (MCV) helps differentiate this anemia from IDA or physiologic changes of pregnancy. An elevated SI and increased transferrin saturation (findings opposite from those in IDA) also help differentiate this type of anemia. Ineffective erythropoiesis and intramedullary hemolysis associated with megaloblastic anemias result in an elevated serum bilirubin level and decreased survival of the red blood cell.[14]

Folic Acid Deficiency

Pteroylglutamic acid is the primary compound for a large group of chemicals called "folates." This molecule contains a pteridine derivative, a *p*-aminobenzoic acid residue, and L-glutamic acid. In order to serve its role in the synthesis of purines and thymine, it must first be converted to 7,8-dihydrofolic acid (FH_2) and subsequently to its metabolically active form, tetrahydrofolic acid (FH_4). The enzyme dihydroglycolate reductase catalyzes this final formation to FH_4. Appropriate DNA synthesis and amino acid production require formyl FH_4 derivatives. Insufficient levels of folic acid will preclude appropriate DNA synthesis and subsequently lead to the manifestations noted in megaloblastic anemia.[22]

Folic acid is absorbed primarily in the proximal jejunum and must be provided in the diet. Before folic acid can be absorbed it must be reduced to its monoglutamate form (FH_1). Pancreatic conjugases within the intestine are responsible for this metabolic process. Once this process is complete, FH_1 enters the mucosal cells. The amount absorbed is based on cellular need. The etiology of folic acid deficiency may be varied but typically relates to decreased intake associated with poor nutrition, impaired absorption, or increased folic acid requirements, as seen during pregnancy.

Under normal circumstances the minimum daily requirement of folic acid is 50 μg; however, pregnancy or increased growth states as seen during infancy and adolescence markedly increase the requirements (see Table 2–2).[2] Because most of the dietary folate is unavailable and body folate reserves are so small, deficiency can result fairly rapidly if demands are increased or intake diminishes. The RDA is 0.4 mg; pregnancy increases this allowance to 0.8 mg to 1.0 mg/day (see Table 2–2).[3] The richest sources of folate are fruits and vegetables. Spinach, lettuce, asparagus, broccoli, and lima beans are excellent sources of folate, while the best fruit sources are lemons, melons, and bananas. High concentrations of folate are found in various organs of carnivorous animals; however, the amount of usable folate is minimal. Even though many foods have high levels of folate, excessive cooking accounts for high losses of food folate. Chronic abuse of alcohol is not only known to impact negatively on nutritional intake of folate but also to interfere with metabolism of various folate derivatives. Nutritional folic acid deficiency is usually seen in association with other vitamin deficiencies.[22]

Intestinal malabsorption or impaired utilization of folate can be pathologic but is more commonly seen as the result of administration of various drugs. Anticonvulsant drugs in particular (e.g., phenytoin, phenobarbital, gluthemide, and isoniazid) inhibit absorption of folate, while the ingestion of folic acid antagonists, such as trimethoprim-sulfamethoxazole used to treat urinary tract infections or the antimalarial drug, pyrimethamine, prevents proper synthesis of folate. Prior gastrointestinal surgery also leads to reduced folate levels.

Increased demands for fetal growth and maternal erythropoiesis increase the body's requirements for folic acid during pregnancy. Additionally, increased levels of estrogen and progesterone related to pregnancy seem to have an inhibitory effect on folate absorption. Multiple gestations or short intervals between pregnancy also increase folate requirements. Maternal folate deficiency in late pregnancy is common and has been reported to affect between 60 and 95% of women at term. Although true megaloblastic anemia is uncommon, folic acid deficiency sufficient to produce megaloblastic changes is more common. Many investigators have shown folic acid deficiency, related to increased requirements and decreased reserves, to be the major cause of megaloblastic anemia in pregnancy. Even in deficient states, the fetus has the ability to continue removing folic acid from maternal stores. The effects of folic acid deficiency in the absence of anemia are controversial. Associations with prematurity, intrauterine growth retardation, and abruptio placentae have been suggested but a direct relationship with folic acid deficiency has not been proved.[22] Since the effects are still unclear, most physicians support folate supplementation for those at risk for developing deficiency states.

Patients with folic acid deficiency typically present with characteristic symptoms of general anemia plus roughness of the skin and glossitis. In addition to those findings discussed under general megaloblastic anemia, analysis of the peripheral blood smear reveals hypersegmentation of neutrophilic nuclear material even in mild folate deficiency. Furthermore, even though serum folate levels are known to decrease with pregnancy, fasting levels $<3\ \mu g/L$ are diagnostic of folate deficiency. A low erythrocyte folate activity ($<20\ \mu g/L$) is another reliable index of folate deficiency; however, the difficulty of performing the assay and of standardizing the results limits the use of this test.

Administration of folic acid is usually oral. Since 10 to 20% of the administered dose is absorbed over six to eight hours, 0.5 mg is generally administered two or three times daily. Parenteral folic acid may be indicated for those women requiring drugs known to interfere with folate synthesis or absorption. A significant reticulocytosis should be seen within 48 to 72 hours of the initiation of therapy, and platelet counts should recover within the first few days. A neutrophilic response can be observed within two weeks. SI levels may be elevated in folate deficiency because iron stores are not efficiently used for erythropoiesis. In this case low SI levels may follow the initiation of folate therapy, indicating a concomitant IDA.[23, 24]

Vitamin B_{12} Deficiency

The uniqueness of vitamin B_{12} is associated with its synthesis by specific microorganisms. The sources of vitamin B_{12} in animals are dependent on microbial synthesis, while humans obtain this vitamin from various animal sources. Its role in the formation of succinyl-CoA and in the metabolism of folate through production of active FH_4 makes its deficiency clinically important.

The absorption of vitamin B_{12} is effected in the ileum through the action of intrinsic factor. Intrinsic factor is secreted by the fundic, parietal cells and is usually synchronous with hydrochloric acid secretion. Once vitamin B_{12} sources are ingested, they are bound to those specific binding proteins containing intrinsic factor. On reaching the serum, the intrinsic factor$=B_{12}$ complex attaches to mucosal receptors. After this process is completed, the vitamin either passes into the cellular cytoplasm, leaving intrinsic factor behind, or enters a mucosal cell and dissociates. Vitamin B_{12} not bound to intrinsic factor is transferred to the portal circulation fairly rapidly by the process of simple diffusion.

As with folic acid deficiency, vitamin B_{12} deficiencies are associated primarily with decreased intake or increased requirements. Except in strict vegetarians who avoid all animal products, this deficiency is rarely related to inadequate dietary intake. The most common causes of inadequate vitamin B_{12} intake are impaired absorption of intrinsic factor associated with defects in synthesis or production and various intestinal factors associated with the malabsorption syndromes. Inadequate production of intrinsic factor by the fundic parietal cells, known as pernicious anemia, is one cause of this megaloblastic anemia. A genetic predisposition to this defect is related to the presence of autoantibodies that respond to glucocorticoid administration. The presence of anti-intrinsic factor antibodies in the serum helps confirm the diagnosis. Partial or total gastrectomy affects levels of intrinsic factor and subsequent vitamin B_{12} absorption. Some authors advocate vitamin B_{12} supplementation for such patients to avoid deficiency syndrome. Intestinal factors associated with B_{12} deficiency include ileal resections or the presence of competitive parasites. Infestation with the tapeworm *Diphyllobothrium latum* leads to competition between the parasite and the host for vitamin B_{12}. Generally, vitamin B_{12} reserves are adequate to buffer against increased requirements for short intervals, as seen in pregnancy. However, increased requirements in association with fetal demands coupled with decreased reserves may result in a B_{12} deficiency. Because of large body stores, vitamin B_{12} deficiency takes several years to develop. Under ordinary circumstances the recommended requirement for vitamin B_{12} in the adult is 5 mg; pregnancy increases these requirements twofold (see Table 2–2).[2]

The diagnosis of vitamin B_{12} deficiency can be made with laboratory assistance. The Schilling test is one method of measuring B_{12} absorption. Because this study requires the use of radioactive cobalt, it is not advocated during pregnancy. Serum vitamin B_{12} levels may be measured using a radioimmunoassay. During pregnancy these levels may fall to 80 to 120 pg/ml; findings lower than 50 pg/ml are indicative of B_{12} deficiency. Chronic, severe deficiencies are associated with neurologic abnormalities.[22] Additionally, serum bilirubin and lactic dehydrogenase levels are elevated when a deficiency exists and are reflective of a low grade hemolytic process. Unless a coexisting folate deficiency exists, serum folate levels are often elevated when serum B_{12} levels are depressed. In the presence of documented deficiency, parenteral administration at weekly intervals of 1 mg of hydroxocobalamin for five to six weeks is followed by monthly administrations for life in cases of pernicious anemia. Response to therapy is generally measured by an increase in serum B_{12} levels within six weeks of therapy. Previously elevated bilirubin and lactic dehydrogenase levels should fall promptly after parenteral administration of this vitamin. An abrupt reticulocytosis begins on the third to fifth day after therapy.

ALCOHOL-RELATED ANEMIAS

Chronic ingestion of alcohol is associated with a variety of anemias. Nutritional deficiencies in association with poor dietary intakes are common. Folate deficiency leads to the characteristic presentation of a megaloblastic anemia. Also, alcohol has been shown to have a direct effect on folate metabolism, which contributes to decreased folate levels. Red blood cell morphology is normochromic and macrocytic, with an increased number of ring sideroblasts. Iron deficiency in addition to folate deficiency is common in these patients and alters the erythrocytic structure. In conjunction with the macrocytic patterns, red cells will also exhibit a hypochromic, microcytic morphology. Furthermore, toxic doses of alcohol have an adverse effect on porphyrin synthesis, leading to a hypochromic erythrocyte. Evaluation of the peripheral smear for increased target cells and ring sideroblasts will help differentiate this condition from IDA. Characteristically, chemical toxicity results in elevated SI and increased transferrin saturation levels, findings opposite those in IDA. An increase in iron stores seen in porphyrin synthesis deficiency will yield elevated serum ferritin levels. This contrasts with IDA, in which iron stores are depleted.[11]

PROTEIN DEFICIENCY

In the United States dietary protein deficiency of any clinical significance is rare. Pregnancy, however, is known to increase protein requirements both to meet increasing needs of the mother and demands from the fetus. Thus, increased requirements combined with poor nutritional practices make protein deficiency a bit more common in pregnancy. Protein deficiency in pregnancy has been associated with mixed pattern anemias and preterm deliveries. An adverse effect on fetal growth may be related to reduced caloric intake. RDA for protein in the nonpregnant state is 55 g, while pregnancy increases this requirement to 75 g/day (see Table 2–2). Additionally, chronic diseases such as malignancies and inflammatory processes impact on protein status and confuse the hematologic picture. Patients with malignancies occasionally present with a hypochromic anemia that must be differentiated from IDA. As in IDA, low SI levels are found. These patients will characteristically have unaffected iron stores, and therefore serum ferritin levels remain unchanged, in contrast to the decreased levels found in IDA. Transferrin saturations are increased, while the UIBC is usually decreased in malignancy states. These findings are opposite those seen in IDA. One third of patients with chronic inflammatory processes will exhibit a hypochromic anemia and present laboratory profiles similar to those of IDA. Reduced serum iron levels in both disease entities require further investigation to differentiate the cause. Transferrin saturations are decreased and UIBC increased in inflammatory processes, as seen in IDA. Normal to increased serum ferritin levels help differentiate the anemia of chronic inflammation from IDA, in which serum ferritin levels are low.

Anemia associated with severe protein deficiency (kwashiorkor) has a characteristic normochromic and normocytic erythrocyte pattern.[11] This anemia is associated with decreased erythropoiesis and reduced iron uptake.[24] Because of the serious sequelae and alterations in metabolic processes, this anemia is seen only in infancy or early childhood and either it is successfully treated or death ensues.

In summary, anemias complicating pregnancy are common but rarely have serious adverse effects on the mother or fetus or newborn. Nutritional requirements increase during pregnancy, making inadequate dietary intake more common. Since the most frequent cause of anemia in pregnancy relates to nutrition, dietary problems should be recognized and corrected prior to pregnancy or early in gestation. Furthermore, subtle changes in the gestational hematologic milieu may be masked by the dilutional anemia of pregnancy. Therefore, diagnostic and therapeutic measures should be instituted as soon as an insufficiency is suspected.

REFERENCES

1. Morrison, J.C.: Anemias and hemoglobinopathies. *In* Ambulatory Care in Obstetrics and Gynecology. Edited by G.M. Ryan. New York, Grune & Stratton, 1980.
2. Pitkin, R.M.: Vitamins and minerals in pregnancy. Clin Perinatol *2*:221, 1975.
3. Food and Nutrition Board, National Research Council: Recommended Dietary Allowances. 8th Ed. Washington, D.C., National Academy of Sciences, 1974.
4. Guyton, A.C.: Textbook of Medical Physiology. 6th Ed. Philadelphia, W. B. Saunders Company, 1981.
5. Prasad, A.S.: Zinc deficiency in human subjects. Prog Clin Biol Res *77*:165, 1981.
6. Hurley, L.S.: Teratogenic aspects of manganese, zinc, and copper nutrition. Physiol Rev *61*:249, 1981.
7. Jameson, S.: Zinc and pregnancy. *In* Zinc in the Environment, Part II: Health Effects. Edited by J.O. Nriagu. New York, John Wiley & Sons, 1980.
8. Warth, J.A., Prasad, A.S., Zwas, F., et al.: Abnormal dark adaptation in sickle cell anemia. J Lab Clin Med *98*:189, 1981.
9. Swanson, C.A., and King, J.C.: Reduced serum zinc concentration during pregnancy. Obstet Gynecol *62*:313, 1983.
10. Widdowson, E.M., Chan, H., and Harrison, G.E.: Accumulation of Cu, Zn, Mn, Cr, and Co in the human liver before birth. Biol Neonate *20*:360, 1972.

11. Oski, F.A.: Anemia related to nutritional deficiencies other than vitamin B_{12} and folic acid. *In* Hematology. Edited by W.J. Williams, E. Beutler, A.J. Erslev, and M.A. Lichtman. New York, McGraw-Hill Book Company, 1983.
12. Hurley, L.S.: The roles of trace elements in foetal and neonatal development. Phil Trans R Soc Lond *294*:145, 1981.
13. Meeks, G.R., Gookin, K.S., and Morrison, J.C.: Iron deficiency anemia in pregnancy. *In* Hematologic Problems in Pregnancy. Edited by D.Z. Kitay. In press.
14. Morrison, J.C., and Gookin, K.S.: Anemia associated with pregnancy. *In* Gynecology and Obstetrics: Maternal and Fetal Medicine. Edited by R. Depp and D.A. Eschenbach. New York, Harper & Row, 1985.
15. Fairbanks, V.F., and Beutler, E.: Erythrocyte disorders—anemias related to disturbances of hemoglobin synthesis. *In* Hematology. Edited by W.J. Williams, E. Beutler, A.J. Erslev, and M.A. Lichtman. New York, McGraw-Hill Book Company, 1983.
16. Bjorn-Rasmussen, E.: Iron absorption: present knowledge and controversies. Lancet *1*:914, 1983.
17. Piomelli, S.: A micromethod for free erythrocyte porphyrins: The FEP test. J Lab Clin Med *81*:932, 1973.
18. Bernhardt, I.B., and Dorsey, D.J.: Hypervitaminosis A and congenital renal anomalies in a human infant. Obstet Gynecol *43*:750, 1974.
19. Spielberg, S.P., Boxer, L.A., Corash, L.M., et al.: Improved erythrocyte survival with high-dose vitamin E in chronic hemolyzing G6PD and glutathione synthetase deficiencies. Ann Intern Med *90*:53, 1979.
20. Natta, C.L., Machlin, L.J., and Brin, M.: A decrease in irreversibly sickled erythrocytes in sickle cell anemia patients given vitamin E. Am J Clin Nutr *33*:968, 1980.
21. Hillman, R.W., Cabaud, P.G., Nilsson, D.E., et al.: Pyridoxine supplementation during pregnancy. Clinical and laboratory observations. Am J Clin Nutr *12*:427, 1963.
22. Beck, W.S.: Erythrocyte disorders—anemias related to disturbance of DNA synthesis (megaloblastic anemias). *In* Hematology. Edited by W.J. Williams, E. Beutler, A.J. Erslev, and M.A. Lichtman. New York, McGraw-Hill Book Company, 1983.
23. Johan, E., and Magnus, E.M.: Plasma and red blood cell folate during normal pregnancy. Acta Obstet Gynecol Scand *60*:247, 1981.
24. Grasso, J.A., Myers, T.J., Hines, J.D., et al.: Energy-dispersive x-ray analysis of mitochondria of sideroblastic anaemia. Br J Haematol *46*:57, 1980.

Chapter 3
THE HEMOGLOBINOPATHIES

Russell K. Laros, Jr.

Our understanding of the molecular genetics of the hemoglobinopathies has unfolded rapidly over the past three decades. In this chapter we will review the biochemistry and genetics of the abnormal human hemoglobins and the thalassemic syndromes. Additionally, we will consider selected aspects of genetic counseling and prenatal diagnosis.

BIOCHEMISTRY AND GENETICS

NORMAL HEMOGLOBINS

The hemoglobin molecule is a conjugated protein with a molecular weight of approximately 64,500. The majority of the molecule is protein, *globin,* with only 4% being a colored prosthetic group, *heme.* The heme is a complex of iron and protoporphyrin. The structure is schematized in Figure 3–1. All the normal human hemoglobins contain two pairs of polypeptide chains with one heme-iron complex attached to each chain. The six normal, human chains are designated alpha (α), beta (β), gamma (γ), delta (δ), epsilon (ϵ), and zeta (ζ).[1]

Because the various chains differ in amino acid composition, they each possess a unique oxygen affinity, surface charge, structural configuration, and distinguishable electrophoretic mobility when placed in a charged field. This last characteristic allows electrophoresis on cellulose acetate or citrate agar to identify types of hemoglobin.[2, 3] Table 3–1 summarizes the composition of the normal hemoglobins and their relative distribution in the adult. Fetal hemoglobin (Hb F) differs from adult hemoglobin (Hb A) in its ability to release oxygen at a lower pH and oxygen tension, its lesser solubility in acid buffer, and its resistance to denaturation by alkali. Thus, a blood smear with mixed fetal and maternal cells can be washed with dilute sodium hydroxide with subsequent lysis of only maternal cells (Apt test).

The early embryonic globin chains ϵ and ζ are rapidly replaced as the fetus develops.[4] Figure 3–2 illustrates the changes in distribution of globin chains during pregnancy and in the neonate. While at birth Hb F accounts for 60 to 80% of all hemoglobin present, by 12 months to two years of age the level has decreased to under 2%. Hb A_2 is normally at a low concentration in the adult, and levels above 3.5% may be a subtle manifestation of thalassemia.

Loci for the α-globin and ζ-globin chains of embryonic hemoglobin are located on chromosome 16. Both α-globin genes have been isolated, cloned, and sequenced. Normal individuals have four α-globin genes, each of which produces nearly equal amounts of mRNA. The β-gene complex (ϵ, γ, δ, β) is located on the short arm of

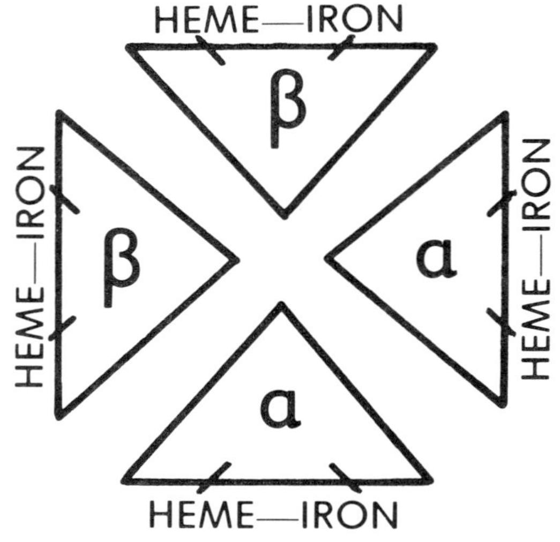

Figure 3–1. Schematized structure of the hemoglobin molecule.

chromosome 11. While β-globin genes are present in the great majority of β-thalassemias, β-globin mRNA is absent or diminished in most cases. The β and δ genes are not duplicated, that is, there are only two copies in each diploid cell. There are two structurally different gamma genes per haploid cell. They differ only in that the one ($^G\gamma$) codes for glycine at amino acid 136 while the other ($^A\gamma$) codes for alanine. The relative influence of these genes varies in different clinical situations associated with the production of fetal hemoglobin. During fetal life the $^G\gamma/^A\gamma$ is 3, while in the adult it is less than 1.[5–7]

ABNORMAL HEMOGLOBINS

The concept of structural globin abnormalities was clarified in 1956 when Ingram, using the peptide mapping or "fingerprinting" technique, showed that in hemoglobin's β polypeptide chain a glutamic acid residue, now known to be the sixth from the free amino terminal end of the molecule, was replaced by a valine residue. Since the side chain of glutamic acid is negatively charged and that of valine is neutral, it follows that the charge of the Hb S molecule is positive with respect to Hb A, thus explaining the difference in electrophoretic mobility. To date, several hundred structural variants of α, β, γ, and δ chains have been identified. Most differ from normal by only one

Table 3–1. Normal Hemoglobins

Abbreviated Name	Structure	Normal Values in Adults (%)
Hb A	$\alpha_2\beta_2$	95
Hb A_2	$\alpha_2\delta_2$	2–3.5
Hb F	$\alpha_2\gamma_2$	<2
Hb Gower 1	$\alpha_2\epsilon_2$	fetal
Hb Gower 2	$\alpha_2\epsilon_2$	fetal
Hb Portland	$\zeta_2\delta_2$	fetal

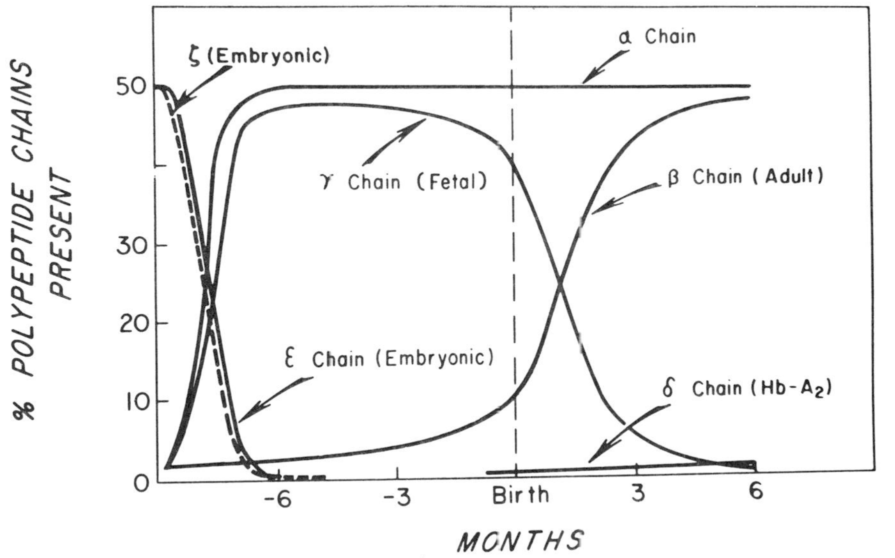

Figure 3–2. Distribution of globin chains during fetal and early neonatal life. (From Bunn, H.F., Forget, B.G., and Ranney, H.M.: Human Hemoglobins. Philadelphia, W.B. Saunders Co., 1977.)

amino acid. The molecular location of the substitution has a marked influence on the functional effect. While most substitutions are without effect, those at the sixth amino acid residue from the free amino terminal end of the molecule lead to aggregation and reduced solubility. Examples include Hb S and Hb C. Substitutions in other areas of the molecule lead to instability and reduced solubility, methemoglobinemia, and increased or decreased oxygen affinity.

The nomenclature and frequency of occurrence of the commonest hemoglobinopathies are outlined in Table 3–2.[8] An individual may be homozygous for the S or C hemoglobin gene. If so, all her adult hemoglobin will contain S (β^S) or C (β^C) globin chains instead of normal β chains. If she is heterozygous, one β^S or β^C chain will be joined with a normal β^A chain. Because of altered structure and physiology, these hemoglobins are less stable in reducing environments such as are present in conditions of hypoxia, acidosis, or infection. In these situations, the hemoglobin molecule loses flexibility and the red blood cells (RBCs) stack up in the microcir-

Table 3–2. Nomenclature and Frequency of the Commonest Hemoglobinopathies in Adult U.S. Blacks*

Hemoglobinopathy Name	Abbreviated	Frequency
Sickle cell trait	Hb SA	1:12
Sickle cell anemia	Hb SS	1:708
Sickle cell—hemoglobin C disease	Hb SC	1:757
Hemoglobin C disease	Hb CC	1:4790
Hemoglobin C trait	Hb CA	1:41
Hemoglobin S-β thalassemia	Hb Sβ-thal	1:1672
Hemoglobin S—high F	Hb S—HPFH	1:3412

* From Schneider, R.G., Hightower, B., Hasty, T.S., et al.: Abnormal hemoglobins in a quarter million people. Blood *48*:629, 1976.

culation, with consequences that will be discussed later. For the heterozygous individual, the normal hemoglobin protects the RBC, except in unusual circumstances such as extreme hypoxia or acidosis.

THALASSEMIA SYNDROMES

The thalassemia syndromes are named and classified by the type of chain that is represented inadequately. The two major groups are the α- and β-thalassemias, both of which affect the synthesis of Hb A. Reduced synthesis of γ or δ chains and combinations in which two or more globin chains are affected (e.g., $\beta\delta$, $\beta\gamma$, hereditary persistence of fetal hemoglobin [HPFH]) have been reported, but these are rare.[9, 10] In each instance, the thalassemia is a quantitative disorder of globin synthesis; structurally the chains are entirely normal. There is no single cause of these diseases. On the molecular level, a variety of defects have been demonstrated, each involving a different step along the pathway of transcription of gene DNA into messenger RNA (mRNA) and translation of mRNA into globin chains.

In the most common form of α-thalassemia, one or more structural genes are physically absent, permanently deleted from the genome.[11] In the homozygous condition when all four genes are deleted, no α chains are produced and the fetus is unable to synthesize Hb F or any of the adult hemoglobins.[12] The predominant hemoglobin is Hb Bart's (γ_4) which, owing to its high oxygen affinity, releases inadequate amounts of oxygen at the tissue level. The result is high-output cardiac failure, hydrops fetalis, and a stillborn fetus. The most severe form of α-thalassemia compatible with extrauterine life is Hb H disease, which results from the deletion of three α genes.[13] In these patients abnormal quantities of both Hb H (β_4) and Hb Bart's accumulate. Beta tetrameres precipitate during the life of the red blood cell to form inclusion bodies, and the "pitting out" of these bodies by the reticuloendothelial system causes a moderately severe hemolytic anemia. In α-thalassemia minor (α-thalassemia 1) two genes are deleted, causing a mild hypochromic, microcytic anemia that must be differentiated from iron deficiency. A single gene deletion (α-thalassemia 2) is clinically undetectable, leading to the "silent carrier" state.[5, 6] α-Thalassemia also may result from a nondeletion defect.[7] The genes are present, yet the phenotype is that of α-thalassemia 1. Apparently, only a small amount of globin can be synthesized from these genes. Still another group of defects is exemplified by a mutant hemoglobin such as Hb Constant Spring, wherein an elongated α gene product is incorporated into the hemoglobin molecule.[14]

A greatly reduced amount of this mutant product is synthesized. The various α-thalassemia genotypes are summarized in Figure 3–3.

One can see that in α-thalassemia 1, both genes may be missing on the same chromosome or one gene missing on each chromosome.[5] The cis gene deletion state is common in Orientals, while the trans state is common in blacks. This difference in gene pool is responsible for the infrequent occurrence of either hemoglobin H disease or homozygous α-thalassemia in blacks and the relatively more frequent occurrence of these disorders in Orientals.

In β-thalassemia, no gene deletions have been demonstrated. There are two forms of β-thalassemia, designated β^+ and β^0, depending upon whether β chain production is reduced or entirely absent.[14–16] In β^+ thalassemia, mRNA for β globin chains is

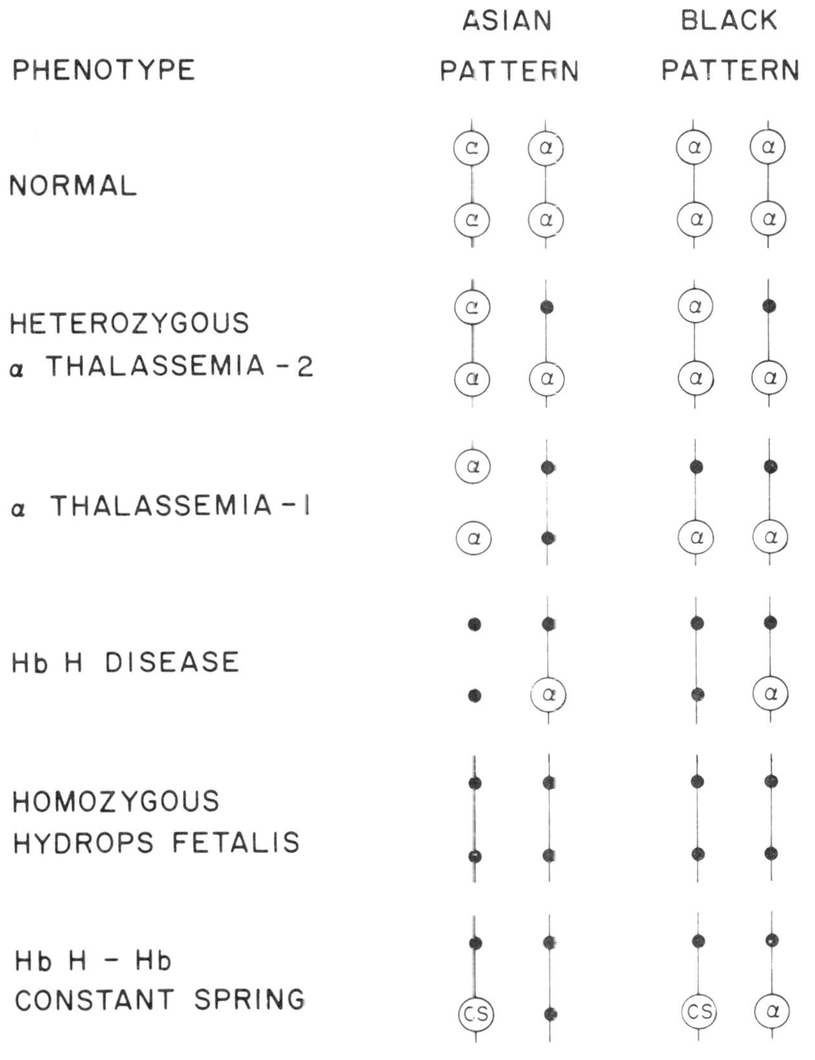

Figure 3–3. Genotypes of the various α-thalassemia syndromes.

present but is quantitatively reduced. This might be due to a particularly unstable mRNA or to a decreased rate of transcription of mRNA.[5, 6, 17] Reduced β chain synthesis may also be seen with Hb Lepore, a product of δ and β gene crossover, with HPFH, and in δβ-thalassemia. HPFH and δβ-thalassemia differ from β-thalassemia in that they both involve β gene deletions.[18]

In the homozygous β-thalassemia condition, α chain production is unimpeded, and these highly unstable chains accumulate and eventually precipitate. Markedly ineffective erythropoiesis and severe hemolysis result in a condition known as thalassemia major or Cooley's anemia,[19] the clinical manifestations of which will be discussed further on.

DIAGNOSIS AND TREATMENT

SICKLE CELL TRAIT

Approximately 10 to 12% of the American black population is heterozygous for the hemoglobin S gene; this state is referred to as sickle cell trait.[8,20] While most practitioners consider this condition in black patients, it is important to remember that the β^S gene pool stems from the Mediterranean area and that the trait also may be present in Italians, Turks, Greeks, and Caribbean natives. Although sudden death has been reported in occasional individuals with sickle cell trait,[21,22] most appear quite normal and enjoy good health.[23] They are rarely anemic, and their peripheral smear does not show sickling in most situations. Screening for the presence of Hb S may be performed inexpensively by a variety of techniques.[2]

Several investigators have contrasted the pregnancy outcome of women with normal hemoglobin and those with sickle cell trait.[24–28] They noted a comparable incidence of spontaneous abortion, low-birth-weight infants, toxemia of pregnancy, low Apgar scores in newborns, and perinatal mortality. However, gravidas with sickle cell trait did have a twofold increase in the rate of urinary tract infections.[27] Also, they may be unable to concentrate their urine (hyposthenuria), but gross hematuria is rare.[29] These women do well during pregnancy and labor, but caution must be observed when using anesthesia to assure good oxygenation. The clinical course of patients with sickle cell trait and other structural hemoglobinopathies is summarized in Figure 3-4. We have managed these patients in our regular prenatal clinic without untoward effect. The only special care required is close observation for urinary tract infections.[27] Sickle cell trait is not associated with the rapid marrow turnover characteristic of hemolysis; therefore, iron does not accumulate. Unlike the situation in sickle cell

Diagnosis	Anticipated frequency at birth[1]	Fertility	Abortions	Maternal Morbidity	Maternal mortality	Perinatal mortality	Clinical severity non-pregnant
Sickle Cell Anemia	1/708	N to ▼	N to ▲	A,▲M,▲S,▲C,▲P, Ph, Pn, T	0–11%	2–39%	+++
Sickle Trait	1/12	N	N	slight ▲ Pn	N	N	±
Sickle Cell β-thalassemia	1/1,672	N	N	▲▲ to ▲▲▲ like S/S	0–3%	0–19%	+ to ++
Sickle Cell hemoglobin C disease	1/757	N	N to	▲▲▲ like S/S Hp	0–33%	0–67%	± to ++
Hemoglobin C	1/4,790	N	N	slight ▲ A,M	N	N	+

(1)- Anticipated frequency in black Americans
A - anemia
M - megaloblastic crisis
S - sequestration
C - bone, abnormal, and cerebral crises
P - pneumonia or pulmonary embolism
Ph - antepartum hemorrhage
Pn - pyelonephritis
Hp - post-partum hemorrhage
T - toxemia

Figure 3–4. The influence of various hemoglobinopathies on reproduction.

anemia, these patients may become iron deficient, and supplementation is necessary during pregnancy.

SICKLE CELL ANEMIA

The incidence of sickle cell anemia (SCA) is 1:625 black births (0.0189%); it falls to 1:1875 by reproductive age.[20] The patient with SCA has no Hb A and may have more than 90% Hb S. Hb F is elevated in variable degrees but is usually below 14%. Females with SCA have a somewhat higher concentration of Hb F than males, and Jackson and coworkers suggest a milder course in individuals with elevated Hb F levels;[30, 31] however, others disagree.[73] Unless Hb F is distributed evenly throughout the RBCs (as in HPFH), it is not protective. Patients with SCA suffer from lifelong complications, in part due to the markedly short life span of their red blood cells. Improved blood banking techniques, better understanding of the underlying pathophysiology of the microcirculation, and prompt intervention in states of severe anemia, infection, and acidosis have led to improved survival.[32, 33] Therefore, the coexistence of pregnancy and SCA is becoming more common.

The influence of pregnancy on this illness and, reciprocally, the influence of SCA on pregnancy and its outcome have been discussed at length. The results of 667 pregnancies reported since 1969 are summarized in Table 3–3. Most observers feel that the prepregnancy course of an individual is a good index of how she will do during pregnancy. Pregnancy termination because of the risk to the patient from gestation is debatable and usually unwarranted; however, each situation must be considered on an individual basis. The spontaneous abortion rate does not appear to be increased in workers with this condition. While reports of the series followed before 1979 indicate a high perinatal mortality rate and a high incidence of infants weighing less than 2500 g, the four most recent reports show generally good fetal outcomes.

Virtually all the signs and symptoms of SCA are secondary to hemolysis, vascular occlusive disease, or an increased susceptibility to infection. Each of the pathologic events is produced by sickling of the red blood cell. The clinical manifestations of

Table 3–3. Reproductive Consequences of Sickle Cell Anemia (SCA) in 667 Pregnancies

Author	Number of Pregnancies	Spontaneous Abortion (%)	Maternal Mortality (%)	Fetal Salvage (%)	Infants < 2500 g (%)
Freeman, 1969	41	27	0	64	42
Fort, 1971	97	16	6	61	—
Perkins, 1971	50	20	0	68	—
Hendrickse, 1972	61	18	11	70	18
Horger, 1972	45	11	0	76	49
Pritchard, 1973	50	32	0	75	38
Perrine, 1974	46	—	0	80	8
Morrison, 1976	43	—	9	—	—
Cunningham, 1983	24*	—	0	96	22
Morrison, 1980	44*	7	0	98	7
Charache, 1980	43	23	2	90	27
Milner, 1981	123	17	0	89	—

* These patients were transfused prophylactically.

SCA are summarized in Table 3–4 and will not be discussed in detail; however, we do wish to stress some of these features.

Sickling of the red cell can occur without significant hypoxia whenever the concentration of Hb S is higher than 40%. Thus SCA becomes evident in early childhood as ischemic pain episodes involving the distal extremities. Dactylitis (swollen, painful dorsal surface of the hands and feet) is the presenting symptom of SCA in one third of patients. Affected children evidence significant growth retardation, and most develop classic skeletal changes that include prominence of the frontal and long bones.[41] Unfortunately, there are not yet adequate data concerning mortality rates for individuals with SCA. Diggs' data indicate that the median survival is 14.3 years, with the distribution of mortality being 20% during the first two years of life, 10% between ages 2 to 5, 50% between ages 5 to 30, and 20% after the age of 30.[42] It has recently been demonstrated that immunization with polyvalent pneumococcal polysaccharide significantly reduces the incidence of *Streptococcus pneumoniae* infections in children

Table 3–4. Clinical Manifestations of Sickle Cell Anemia

Growth and Development
- A. Retarded growth
- B. Skeletal changes
- C. Decreased life span

Sickle Cell Crisis
- A. Painful vaso-occlusive episode: bones, abdomen, chest, back

Cardiovascular—Manifestations of Hyperdynamic Circulation
- A. Cardiomegaly
- B. Systolic murmurs
- C. Failure

Pulmonary Signs
- A. Infection: pneumococcal, *Mycoplasma, Haemophilus, Salmonella*
- B. Vascular occlusion

Abdominal Involvement
- A. Painful vaso-occlusive episodes
- B. Hepatomegaly
- C. Hepatitis
- D. Cholecystitis
- E. Splenic infarction

Bone and Joint Changes
- A. Bone marrow infarction
- B. Osteomyelitis—*Salmonella*
- C. Arthritis

Genitourinary Signs
- A. Hyposthenuria
- B. Hematuria
- C. Pyelonephritis

Neurologic Manifestations
- A. Vascular occlusion
- B. Convulsions
- C. Hemorrhage
- D. Visual disturbances

Ocular Manifestations
- A. Conjunctival vessel changes
- B. Vitreous hemorrhage

and young adults.[43] It remains to be seen what impact this advance will have on mortality statistics.

A sickle cell crisis is an episode of uncomplicated, painful vaso-occlusion. The pain is described as gnawing and increases in intensity over several hours. It usually involves the extremities, especially the tibial and periarticular areas, but it may also involve the abdomen, chest, or back. The crisis usually lasts several days with gradual abatement, but it may last only a few hours. It is important not to let the diagnosis of sickle cell crisis blunt one's acuity in the search for other intercurrent disease in patients with SCA.[42]

Severe anemia subjects the cardiovascular system to repeated episodes of acute and chronic stress. Cardiomegaly, multiple murmurs, and high output failure are frequent findings. Horger described a hemoglobin concentration of less than 9.5 g/dl in 87% of his patients, and 75% required transfusion at some point during pregnancy.[34]

The major pulmonary disorders in patients with SCA are infections and vaso-occlusive episodes. Thus, the clinician must frequently differentiate between pneumonia and thrombosis and/or embolization. The organisms most commonly responsible for pneumonia are pneumococcus, *Mycoplasma, Haemophilus, Salmonella,* and *Escherichia coli.* Clinical features favoring the diagnosis of thrombosis are the absence of significant temperature elevation and of chills, the presence of associated pain in the extremities or abdomen, and the presence of "blister cells."

Chronic hemolysis leads to hepatomegaly with mildly elevated serum bilirubin levels. Barrett-Connor states that 30 to 40% of patients with SCA have gallstones, which are symptomatic in only 10%.[44] The spleen and its function are always altered. In childhood the spleen is enlarged, and splenic sequestration may occur. During sequestration the spleen enlarges rapidly, entrapping RBCs with resulting systemic hypovolemia. Over time, there are multiple episodes of splenic infarction, and the spleen becomes progressively smaller and is eventually nonfunctional. Thus, the spleen is not palpable in the majority of adults with SCA.

The individual with SCA is very susceptible to chronic leg ulcers, with subsequent scarring. Bone marrow infarctions, osteomyelitis, and joint involvement with avascular necrosis and septic arthritis are common problems. The usual offending organisms are *Salmonella* and *Staphylococcus.*

The kidneys are prone to embolic infarction, with renal papillary necrosis leading to interference with the countercurrent mechanism and subsequent hyposthenuria and impaired hydrogen ion excretion. Hematuria is common and may be prolonged and lead to significant blood loss. Recurrent pyelonephritis is also a very common problem. Although hypertension is not itself increased among nonpregnant individuals with SCA, toxemia occurs in about 33% of pregnancies associated with SCA.[35]

Because of chronic hemolysis and the body's ability to reutilize iron, the serum iron concentration is increased and these patients, when not pregnant, rarely need iron supplementation. In fact, individuals with SCA are prone to hemosiderosis because of hemolysis and multiple transfusions. However, during pregnancy iron deficiency may develop,[56] and the decision whether to give supplemental iron should be based on assessment of iron stores by serum iron studies. On the other hand, folic acid is consumed in the process of red cell synthesis, and folate supplementation is essential. Anemia may be worsened by folic acid deficiency (megaloblastic crisis), and this must not be overlooked as a cause for a falling hemoglobin level.[45] A true hemolytic crisis is rare in SCA, but painful crisis is very common.

Treatment

Therapy for patients with sickle cell anemia has been largely symptomatic, with the major objectives being aborting a painful crisis and combating infection. Despite significant gains in the understanding of the molecular pathology of sickling, a specific, nontoxic therapy has not yet been found. Agents of proven or potential benefit include those that inhibit gelation, such as urea, certain amino acids, glyceraldehyde, and cyanate salts, and those that inhibit cell-sickling, such as zinc, procaine, and cetiedil.[46–50] Unfortunately, at present all of these agents are contraindicated during pregnancy because of questionable efficacy and possible teratogenicity.

Supportive Therapy

Most authors agree that intensive and meticulous antepartum care is important in managing patients with SCA. In addition to evaluation of the hematopoietic system, careful evaluation of the renal, cardiovascular and hepatic systems is useful. Urinary tract and pulmonary infections should be promptly diagnosed and vigorously treated with appropriate antibiotics.

During the last trimester fetal surveillance with either nonstress or stress tests should be carried out regularly.[51]

Transfusions

Transfusion therapy has been widely used for years in the treatment of parturients with SCA. Hendrickse and colleagues advocate transfusion if the hemoglobin level falls below 6 g/dl,[52] while others have initiated transfusion whenever infection or crises occurred.[37] More recently, partial exchange transfusions or prophylactic transfusion or both have been advocated.[53, 54]

Partial Exchange Transfusion (PET)

The major risks to a pregnant woman with SCA occur during the third trimester, the intrapartum period, and postpartum. These risks have been detailed above and are basically those related to severe anemia and vaso-occlusion. If one were able to remove a significant amount of the patient's whole blood and replace it with fresh, carefully cross-matched, packed red blood cells at a critical time in gestation, perhaps these sequelae might be avoided. Ricks[53] and later Perkins[55] tested this hypothesis in a limited number of patients. However, the largest experience is that described by Morrison and associates.[39, 40] They utilized the protocol similar to that outlined in Table 3–5 in 60 patients with various sickle hemoglobinopathies who were admitted to the hospital during the 28th week of gestation. If the initial four-unit transfusion achieved a hematocrit (Hct) of greater than 35% and an Hb A level of greater than 40%, the patient was discharged. If not, an additional two- or four-unit exchange was performed. The patient was followed on a weekly basis and the PET repeated at 36 to 39 weeks of gestation. An early repeat PET was indicated by the occurrence of an Hct less than 25%, an Hb A level less than 20%, crisis, or labor. Their recent data indicate that repeat exchange transfusion will be required every four to six weeks. Also it is possible and safe to carry out the transfusion program on an outpatient basis.[56]

In their first series there were two cases of maternal hepatitis in 36 patients; in one of these the infant died.[39, 40] Only one patient experienced a transfusion reaction, and no premature labor was noted. There was one maternal death in a patient who received

Table 3–5. Protocol for Partial Exchange Transfusion (PET)

I. Begin at 24 to 28 weeks' gestation

II. Baseline laboratory studies:
  A. Hb, Hct, WBC, reticulocyte count
  B. Hb electrophoresis

III. Type and cross-match blood: four units of fresh, buffy coat poor, Hb S-free, washed, packed RBCs

IV. Exchange
  A. In morning:
    1. Infuse 500 ml crystalloid over 1 to 2 hours
    2. Remove 500 ml by phlebotomy over same time period
    3. Infuse two units of packed RBCs over 1 to 2 hours
  B. In afternoon: Repeat morning procedure

V. Repeat laboratory evaluation: Following morning
  A. Hb, Hct
  B. Hb electrophoresis

VI. Additional exchange (two to four units) if
  A. Hct < 35%
    or
  B. Hb A level < 40%

a single PET at 28 weeks' gestation but refused further exchange despite the occurrence of crisis. Neonatal outcome was described for the 36 pregnancies and compared with 160 gestations matched for age, race, gravidity, socioeconomic status, and length of gestation. The controls had SCA but were not treated by PET. A dramatic decrease in the perinatal death rate, reduced prematurity, and fewer low-birth-weight infants were noted in the treated group. Morrison and associates postulated that sickling in the placenta leads to vaso-occlusion and intrauterine hypoxia. If it is partial, intrauterine growth retardation may occur; if massive, spontaneous abortion or stillbirth may result.

A more recent series by the same investigators details 44 pregnancies in women with SCA.[56] There were no maternal deaths; however, morbidity included three cases of pneumonia, one of pyelonephritis, two of painful crisis, one of hepatitis, and one transfusion reaction. The pregnancies yielded three abortions, one neonatal death, and three infants weighing less than 2500 g at delivery.

Prophylactic Transfusion

Cunningham and associates have reported on an alternative approach.[54] They treated 37 pregnant women with various sickle hemoglobinopathies (16 SS, 19 SC, 2 S-thalassemia). Transfusions with packed RBCs were begun in the first trimester. The volume of RBCs to be infused was calculated to reduce the Hb S level to $\leq 50\%$ based on measurement of the patient's RBC volume, using an in vitro $Na_2\,{}^{51}CrO_4$–labeling technique.

Their data include 16 pregnancies in women with SCA. There were no maternal deaths, one abortion, and one stillbirth. One infant weighed less than 2,500 g at birth.

The exact role of aggressive transfusions in the management of the parturient with SCA is unresolved. One must balance the risks of hepatitis, transfusion reaction, and sensitization against the apparent maternal and fetal benefits. It is hoped that this issue can be resolved by a large collaborative study now under way.

Erythroblastosis Fetalis

The coexistence of maternal isoimmunization and SCA presents a particularly difficult management problem. Any maternal disorder leading to hyperbilirubinemia will lead to a parallel increase in amniotic fluid bilirubin levels.[72] While the significance of a positive antibody screen must be evaluated, as discussed in Chapter 7, the usefulness of amniotic fluid analysis is markedly hampered by the maternal contribution to amniotic fluid bilirubin. When antibody dynamics suggest fetal risk and the mother has hyperbilirubinemia, ΔOD values are useful only if they remain in Zones 1 or 2. If they are in Zone 3, the decision of transfusion versus delivery versus observation without treatment should be guided by ultrasonic evidence of placental hydrops.

Care During Labor and Delivery

Evidence in the literature does not support the practice of early elective induction of labor and, in fact, some studies have shown the use of oxytocin to be associated with decreased bone blood flow.[57, 58] Anesthesia-related hypovolemia or hypoxia or both are contraindicated; therefore, regional anesthetics should be administered with great caution. Careful fetal monitoring should be carried out throughout labor.

Patients with SCA must be watched closely for endometritis and anemia during the puerperium and if present, both should be treated aggressively. Postpartum endometritis occurs in approximately 20% of patients.[34] Pyrexia may lead to dehydration and is to be avoided. Patients with SCA also may have pregnancy-related complications not associated with their hemoglobinopathy, and sickle cell crisis may be misdiagnosed in situations in which the real problem is abruptio placentae, ectopic gestation, pyelonephritis, or pulmonary embolism.

SICKLE CELL HEMOGLOBIN C DISEASE

Women who are doubly heterozygous for both the β^S and β^C genes are referred to as having hemoglobin SC disease (Hb SCD). The incidence of Hb SCD is between 1:757 and 1:1250 in adult blacks in the United States.[8, 20] Hemoglobin electrophoresis reveals approximately 60% Hb C and 40% Hb S. The Hb C has unique properties which, unfortunately, potentiate the tendency of Hb S to sickle in reduced environments.

Patients with Hb SCD generally have a normal habitus, a healthy childhood, and a normal life span.[63] Many are diagnosed only during the latter part of pregnancy when complications occur. At the beginning of pregnancy, the woman is mildly anemic (Hct approximately 30%), and splenomegaly (present in about 50% of patients) and the appearance of target cells in the peripheral blood smear may be overlooked. Hemoglobin electrophoresis will ensure the correct diagnosis.

Hb SCD during pregnancy is more worrisome than SCA because of the high mortality rate outlined in Table 3–6. Although some investigators have reported markedly elevated maternal mortality rates,[34, 36, 39, 52] their results have not been confirmed by others.[35, 54, 56, 63, 64, 70, 71] Perhaps the high and often unanticipated mortality is related to less careful antenatal observation of previously undiagnosed patients, or to pathophysiologic problems unique to patients with Hb SCD. In contrast to patients with SCA, they frequently experience rapid and severe anemic crisis due to splenic sequestration. Also, they have a greater tendency to experience bone marrow necrosis with the release of fat or marrow emboli. Fullerton, in fact, recommends heparinization

Table 3–6. Reproductive Consequences of Hemoglobin SC Disease (Hb SCD) in 508 Pregnancies

Author	Number of Pregnancies	Spontaneous Abortion (%)	Maternal Mortality (%)	Fetal Salvage (%)	Infants <2500 g (%)
Went, 1960	17	12	0	88	—
Rivers, 1961	25	20	0	78	—
Laros, 1967	67	7	2	88	—
Freeman, 1969	34	24	9	72	—
Perkins, 1971	17	29	0	58	—
Horger, 1972	9	—	33	38	—
Pritchard, 1973	78	6	3	91	22
McCurdy, 1974	14	12	0	88	—
Morrison, 1976	18	—	6	—	—
Cunningham, 1983	26*	—	0	100	15
Morrison, 1980	26*	4	0	96	24
Charache, 1980	24	13	0	100	33
Milner, 1980	58	9	0	98	—
Ballas, 1982	34	15	0	—	—

* These patients were transfused prophylactically.

for patients with Hb SCD bone pain crises.[62] Because the efficacy of heparinization has not been documented by other studies, this practice has not been employed widely. The clinical manifestations of Hb SCD are otherwise similar to SCA but milder. The renal problems include papillary necrosis with hyposthenuria, urinary tract infections (70%), gross hematuria (30%), and pyelonephritis (21%).[60] Pulmonary infection, embolization, or infarction occur in about 50% of these patients, with aseptic necrosis of the femoral head, vitreous hemorrhage, and postpartum endometritis also being common. Pre-eclampsia occurs in about 20% of pregnant women with Hb SCD. It is important to emphasize that anemia usually is not severe until the third trimester.

The general management of symptomatic patients with Hb SCD is identical to that for patients with SCA. Both Morrison and Cunningham have reported good results using vigorous transfusion protocols.[54, 56] However, while both series indicate good fetal survival, perinatal mortality rate is almost as good in series in which prophylactic transfusion was not used. Additionally, the incidence of low-birth-weight infants remained high. We have reserved PET for patients with Hb SCD who are either symptomatic or whose Hct is less than 25%.

Considerations for the management of labor are the same as in patients with SCA. Additionally, these patients experience a high incidence of postpartum hemorrhage (12 to 22%). Thrombophlebitis occurs with increased frequency and should be watched for closely during the puerperium. Patients with Hb SCD require increased folate intake, as in SCA. Unlike gravidas with SCA, those with Hb SCD require iron supplementation and, if it is not given, they may develop a confounding iron deficiency anemia.

HEMOGLOBIN S-β-THALASSEMIA

The gene controlling the rate of β chain synthesis is intimately linked to those controlling globin chain structure. Hb S-β-thalassemia ($\alpha_2\beta^S\beta^{thal}$) is a condition in which the patient is heterozygous for the sickle cell and the β-thalassemia genes. This is an uncommon disorder believed to occur with the frequency of 1:3333 in black adults in the United States.[20] In addition to decreased β chain production, there is a variably increased production of Hb F and Hb A_2. Because of this variable production rate, hemoglobin electrophoresis reveals a spectrum of hemoglobin concentrations. Hb S may account for 70 to 95% of the hemoglobin present, with Hb F rarely exceeding 20%. Because of the thalassemia influence, Hb S exceeds Hb A concentration. This is in sharp contrast to patients with sickle cell trait, in which Hb A exceeds the concentration of Hb S. The diagnosis is made in an anemic patient by demonstrating increased Hb A_2 and Hb F levels in association with levels of Hb S exceeding those of Hb A. The peripheral smear reveals hypochromia and microcytosis with anisocytosis, poikilocytosis, basophilic stippling, and targeting. The hemoglobin electrophoresis pattern is characteristic, as noted above, and reticulocytosis is prominent.

The clinical manifestations of this disorder parallel those of SCA but are usually milder. The patient frequently is mildly anemic (hemoglobin value 9 to 11 g/dl), painful crises may occur, and chronic hemolysis is present. The hemolysis leads to hepatosplenomegaly, an elevated serum bilirubin level, and episodic jaundice. These patients have a normal body habitus and frequently enjoy an uncompromised life span. Renal complications may include hematuria, hyposthenuria, papillary necrosis, and pyelonephritis. Aseptic necrosis of the femoral head and thrombophlebitis also commonly occur.

Table 3–7 summarizes the pregnancy results in women with Hb S-β-thalassemia as being somewhat better than those seen in women with either SCA or Hb SCD. While some authors have advocated vigorous transfusion therapy for all parturients with Hb S-β-thalassemia,[54, 56] because of the inherent risks of transfusion and the lack of demonstrated benefit in this subgroup, we have reserved this treatment modality for those cases in which the mother has experienced severe crises or chronic hemolysis leading to an Hct of less than 25%.

All patients with Hb S-β-thalassemia need close supervision in the third trimester and during the intrapartum and postpartum periods for problems similar to those seen with Hb SCD. They require folic acid supplementation but not iron. The clinical severity is usually inversely proportionate to the hemoglobin S concentration.

HEMOGLOBIN C TRAIT AND DISEASE

The estimated frequency of hemoglobin C trait is 1:33 in American black adults and that of hemoglobin C disease is 1:4444. Hb C trait (Hb AC) is an asymptomatic

Table 3–7. Reproductive Consequences of Hemoglobin S-α-Thalassemia in Pregnancies

Author	Number of Pregnancies	Spontaneous Abortion (%)	Maternal Mortality (%)	Fetal Salvage (%)	Infants < 2500 g (%)
Laros, 1967	38	32	3	81	—
Fort, 1971	37	8	0	91	128
Cunningham, 1983	4	10	0	100	25
Morrison, 1980	2	0	0	100	0

state without reproductive consequences. Target cells are found in the peripheral smear, but anemia is not present. Hemoglobin C disease (Hb CC), a mild disorder usually discovered during medical evaluation for other problems, is a mild hemolytic anemia with the hematocrit in the range of 25 to 35% and a constant, mild reticulocytosis. The red blood cells are characterized by targeting, and many microspherocytes are present. Unlike SCA, there is no increased morbidity and mortality associated with pregnancy. However, these patients should receive supplementary iron and folic acid throughout pregnancy.

HEMOGLOBIN E DISEASE

The current resettlement in the United States of individuals from Southeast Asia has resulted in a significant increase in the number of cases of hemoglobin E trait and disease. Most individuals have a mild, microcytic anemia that is of no clinical significance and requires no treatment.[66–69] However, individuals homozygous for Hb E have a greater degree of microcytosis, target cells are prominently seen, and the whole blood oxygen dissociation curve is shifted slightly to the right. As in Hb C trait and disease, no special treatment is required. Reproductive outcome is normal. The various genotypes and clinical findings are summarized in Table 3–8.[69]

OTHER STRUCTURAL HEMOGLOBIN VARIANTS

There are many other hemoglobinopathies, most of which are not associated with detectable clinical manifestations. Two broad categories that do produce symptoms are the unstable hemoglobin variants and those leading to abnormal oxygen binding. In the former group, the unstable hemoglobin tends to precipitate within the RBC, leading to Heinz body formation. Individuals afflicted have a hemolytic anemia of variable clinical severity, and most patients do not require treatment. In patients with abnormal oxygen binding, the abnormal hemoglobins have an increased oxygen affinity, leading to secondary erythrocytosis. The M hemoglobins constitute a third category of unusual structural variants; they lead to methemoglobinemia and carboxyhemoglobinemia.

THE THALASSEMIA SYNDROMES

Thalassemia is found throughout the world but is concentrated in the Mediterranean coastal areas, central Africa, and parts of Asia. In these regions it is believed that the high incidence represents a balanced polymorphism due to heterozygote advantage.[12] Heterozygotes are protected against malaria when compared with the homo-

Table 3–8. Various Genotypes of Hemoglobin E and Their Phenotypic Expression

Hemoglobin Genotype	Degree of Anemia	MCV	Electrophoresis: $A + A_2$	E (%)	F	S	Phenotypic Expression
A/E	0	↓	68	30	<2	0	0
E/E	0 – +	↓↓	<4	94	<2	0	0
E/α-thal	+ – ++	↓	50	15	35	0	0
S/E	+ +	↓	0	40	0	60	0
E/β^+-thal	+ +	↓↓	10	60	30	0	splenomegaly
E/β^0-thal	+ + +	↓↓	0	60	40	0	splenomegaly

zygous normal individual. All forms of thalassemia are inherited as autosomal recessive traits. The lethal homozygous state results only when all of an individual's genes for the α or β chain are affected. Characteristics of the various thalassemias are summarized in Table 3–9.

β-Thalassemia Major (Cooley's Anemia)

β-thalassemia major is the homozygous state in which there is very little or no production of β chains. The fetus is protected from severe disease by α chain production. However, this protection disappears rapidly after birth, and the affected infant is anemic by three months of age. He or she has hepatomegaly, requires blood transfusions every three to four weeks, and dies by the third decade, usually of myocardial hemosiderosis. Those female patients surviving until puberty are usually amenorrheic with severely impaired fertility.[5, 6, 73]

As in sickle cell anemia, consideration of basic pathophysiology allows prediction of clinical events. The marrow is in a high turnover state in an effort to produce new red blood cells. This requires folate, and therefore these patients need adequate supplementation of folic acid. Failure to provide this enhances the possibility of an aplastic crisis. Because of demands for erythropoiesis, the marrow is expanded and may result in a habitus with a tower skull and long extremities. Abnormal red cells with Heinz bodies are apparent in the peripheral smear, as are very small cells with hypochromasia. Nucleated red cells reflect the degree of ineffective erythropoiesis. Hyperbilirubinemia is frequently present and may promote gallstone formation.

The clinical severity of β-thalassemia is influenced by the extent to which α chain production can compensate for deficient β chain synthesis. The rare instances of pregnancy in patients reported to have thalassemia major most likely occurred in

Table 3–9. Hematologic and Clinical Aspects of the Thalassemia Syndromes

Condition	Hemoglobin Pattern				Clinical Severity
	Hb Level	Hb A_2	Hb F	Other Hb	
Homozygotes					
α-Thalassemia	↓↓↓↓	O	O	80% Hb Bart's, remainder Hb H and Hb Portland	Hydrops fetalis
β^+-Thalassemia	↓↓↓	Variable	↑↑↑	Some Hb A	Moderately severe features of Cooley's anemia
β^0-Thalassemia	↓↓↓↓	Variable	↑↑↑	No Hb A	Severe Cooley's anemia
$\beta\delta^0$-Thalassemia	↓↓	O	100%	No Hb A	Thalassemia intermedia
Heterozygotes					
α-Thalassemia silent carrier	N	N	N	1–2% Hb Bart's in cord blood at birth	N
α-Thalassemia trait	↓	N	N	5% Hb Bart's in cord blood at birth	Very mild
Hb H disease	↓↓	N	N	4–30% Hb H in adults; 25% Hb Bart's in cord blood	Thalassemia intermedius
β^+-Thalassemia	↓–↓↓	↑	↑	none	Mild
β^0-Thalassemia	↓–↓↓	↓	↓↓↓	none	Mild

individuals who were actually heterozygous for two different β-thalassemia genes, at least one of which is a "high F" form.[36, 68]

β-Thalassemia Minor

β-thalassemia minor results in a variable degree of illness, depending upon the rate of β chain production. It is subclassified into β-thalassemia intermedius and β-thalassemia minimus. While this distinction may be of more academic than clinical importance, it should be realized that thalassemia trait may be quite subtle in clinical appearance and is frequently diagnosed by appropriate laboratory tests only after the patient fails to respond to iron therapy or delivers a child found to have the homozygous disease state.

Characteristic findings include a relatively high red blood cell count, moderate to marked microcytosis, and a peripheral smear that resembles iron deficiency, with small cells and hypochromasia. While Hb electrophoresis characteristically shows Hb A_2 to be elevated above 3.5%, Hb F may or may not be elevated. Serum iron or ferritin concentration is high and the percent saturation of iron is greater than 20%.

β-thalassemia trait does not impair fertility. The incidence of prematurity, low-birth-weight infants, and infants of abnormal size for gestational age is identical to that for normal women. Unlike previous studies,[75, 76] Alger and associates did not find an increase in placental size or an abnormal fetal-placental weight ratio.[77] The expected physiologic hemodilution of pregnancy is observed as a tendency for the Hct, Hb, and red cell count to fall after the first trimester. In Alger's series of patients, this decrease was no greater than that reported for those with normal pregnancies. These findings are in contrast to those of others, who have postulated that increasingly ineffective erythropoiesis or hypersplenism or both might contribute to the decline in hemoglobin levels seen between the first and second trimesters in pregnant thalassemic patients.[78, 79]

The double heterozygote for β-thalassemia and Hb S has been discussed above. Unfortunately, the combination is clinically more severe than either of the traits alone.

α-Thalassemia and Hemoglobin H Disease

In the most common form of α-thalassemia, the structural genes for α-globin are absent. In the homozygous condition with all four genes deleted, no α chains are produced, and the fetus is unable to synthesize Hb F or any adult hemoglobin.[80] The result is severe anemia, producing hydrops fetalis and stillbirth. The most noteworthy complication of pregnancy is that approximately 50% of women with α-thalassemia carrying a fetus will develop severe toxemia.[81]

Hemoglobin H disease results from the deletion of three α-globin genes and is recognizable as a moderate hemolytic anemia with increased reticulocytosis and an abnormal quantity of Hb H seen on electrophoresis. α-Thalassemia-1, the heterozygous state with two deleted genes, is a diagnosis by exclusion in cases of a mild hypochromic microcytic anemia in which iron deficiency and β-thalassemia trait have been excluded as etiologies. Individuals with α-thalassemia trait and hemoglobin H disease have normal pregnancy outcomes.[76]

The double heterozygote for α-thalassemia trait and hemoglobin S has little effect on either the laboratory or the clinical presentation of Hb SCD. Specifically, α-thalassemia does not beneficially influence the observed vaso-occlusive severity of the disease.[82, 83]

Hereditary Persistence of Fetal Hemoglobin (HPFH)

A rare group of disorders designated as HPFH has been described. HPFH is usually associated with deletion of β and δ genes.[84] In contrast to $\delta\ \beta^0$ thalassemia, the high levels of Hb F seen in HPFH are uniformly distributed throughout the RBCs.

In the heterozygous form the Hb F level is 10 to 35% and Hb A_2 is decreased. In the homozygous form Hb F is 100% and a mild, microcytic, hypochromic anemia is present.[1] When HPFH occurs in association with β-chain structural variants such as SCA, the clinical severity is markedly ameliorated.

γ-Thalassemia

Heterozygous γ-thalassemia causes hemolytic anemia at birth that lessens with age.[9] Homozygous γ-thalassemia is probably not compatible with life.

PRENATAL DIAGNOSIS

In all of these hemoglobinopathies, the involved genes may be considered recessive in that a heterozygous individual would have half of the genes for a particular globin chain (i.e., either one or two) functioning to make the normal protein molecule and half functioning to make an abnormal one. The individual with a hemoglobinopathy is homozygous or doubly heterozygous for the abnormal gene(s). Until very recently, the obstetrician has had little to offer patients who were α- or β-thalassemia carriers or carriers of a gene for a structurally abnormal hemoglobin. They usually had uncomplicated pregnancies, and the obstetrician's role was limited to genetic counseling and performing abortions for those couples who were fearful of delivering an affected child. The development of methods to diagnose hemoglobinopathies in utero now allows the obstetrician to give parents definite answers rather than statistical probabilities. Couples at risk can avoid having affected children without remaining childless and are spared months of anxiety awaiting the outcome of a pregnancy.

Since the homozygous state is invariably fatal, α-thalassemia does not produce the major medical and social problems associated with β-thalassemia. Even so, early diagnosis is desirable to minimize the emotional trauma of an unsuccessful pregnancy and to prevent the development of third trimester pre-eclampsia, which frequently accompanies this disease.[81]

Over the past decade there has been rapid development of techniques allowing prenatal testing for hematologic diseases. The World Health Organization (WHO) supports an International Registry for Prenatal Monitoring of Hereditary Anemias, and through December, 1982, a total of 4471 prenatal studies had been reported. Prenatal diagnosis can be accomplished by either obtaining fetal blood or fetal tissue samples for DNA analysis.[85]

FETAL BLOOD SAMPLING

During the 1960s a number of investigators demonstrated hemoglobins other than Hb F in early second trimester fetuses.[87–88] In 1972, Pataryas and Stamatoyannopoulos used peptide mapping and confirmed that Hb A first appeared at the 11th week of gestation. They also found adult hemoglobin, Hb C and Hb S, produced early in the second trimester.[89] The determination of the hemoglobin type of the fetus is most readily accomplished by examination of synthesis rather than content, and these techniques require only 10 μl (0.10 cc) of fetal blood.[90]

Fetal blood can be obtained during the second trimester by aspiration of placental blood under ultrasonic guidance or by fetoscopy.[91, 92] Regardless of the technique, sampling should be performed at 18 to 20 weeks' gestation and will be successful in 90% of patients.[92]

Method of Analysis

Both fetoscopy and placental aspiration under ultrasonic guidance will yield a mixture of fetal and maternal blood.

Since fetal red cell volume is greater than that of adult cells, the presence of fetal erythrocytes is determined by analysis of cell volume by a Coulter particle size analyzer.[93] The presence of maternal cells is not an insurmountable problem, since the overall globin synthetic rate of first trimester fetal cells is more than 500 times greater than that of maternal cells.[94] Thus, even though β chain synthesis is approximately 50% of the total in maternal cells and only 5% of the total in fetal cells, the maternal cells do not make a great contribution to the sample β chain radioactivity. Aspiration samples containing less than 50% of fetal cells can have the fetal cells separated from the mixture by differential agglutination using the antibody, anti-i. Because the i antigen is found only on fetal cells, after concentration by differential agglutination, samples will contain 75 to 100% fetal cells with no selective loss of fetal cells containing Hb A.[95] The moderate loss of fetal cells that occurs during this procedure is well compensated by the enrichment.

The fetal blood (and a maternal sample used as a control) is incubated with ^{3}H-lucine to label newly synthesized globin chains. These are then analyzed by carboxymethyl cellulose chromatography. Abnormal β-globins such as S, C, E, and Lepore are detected because they separate chromatographically from the normal β chain. A diagnosis of thalassemia is made when the normal α- and β-chain is absent or substantially reduced.

Through the end of 1982, 3959 cases of hemoglobinopathies have been reported to the WHO registry. Errors were reported in 29 cases, and 24 of these were false negative findings. The error rate appears to be slightly higher in centers that had studied only small numbers of cases. Maternal complications were rare, but leakage of amniotic fluid was reported in 1.6% of cases and most commonly occurred following fetoscopy.[85]

FETAL TISSUE SAMPLING

An alternative methodology utilizing fetal fibroblasts for prenatal diagnosis of hemoglobinopathies is now available. A specimen of amniotic fluid is obtained at 16 to 20 weeks' gestation, and fetal fibroblasts are grown in tissue cultures to provide sufficient DNA for studies of globin genes. Recently, fetal tissue has been obtained by chorionic villus biopsy, which involves aspiration of chorionic villi at 8 to 10 weeks' gestation.[85, 96–98]

Method of Analysis

The recombinant DNA technology utilizes in vitro synthesized oligonucleotides that are specific for a given globin chain mutation.[85] These probes then identify the mutant or normal globin gene and have been used for prenatal diagnosis of several varieties of β-thalassemia and for α-thalassemia.

An alternative method for prenatal diagnosis uses restriction endonucleases. Restriction endonucleases are enzymes that cleave DNA within specific base-sequence recognition sites. There is an ever-increasing repertoire of restriction endonucleases, each specific for a particular short DNA sequence. The DNA fragments are separated by agarose-gel electrophoresis, and the number and types of fragments allow genome mapping. Linked restriction fragment length polymorphism can be used to detect β^S and β^C genes, β^0 thalassemia in Sardinia and many other β-thalassemias.[98–100] Unfortunately, extensive and time-consuming family studies are usually required to establish these linkages. A few DNA point mutations that cause hemoglobinopathies occur at restriction enzyme cleavage sites and thus can be diagnosed directly. Examples include β^S with DdeI, MstII, or CvnI and a few β-thalassemia genes with their enzymes.[85, 98]

Through December 1, 1982, 170 cases of DNA studies have been reported to the WHO registry. Sixty-eight percent of the cases were sickle hemoglobinopathies and the remainder various forms of thalassemia.[85]

ANTENATAL SCREENING

The availability of prenatal diagnosis provides strong impetus for the creation of mass maternal screening programs. Since the primary aim of screening is the detection of individuals who already carry the gene and the prevention of homozygous individuals in the future, the ideal population for evaluation is reproductive age women. A good screening method should have no false negative and few false positive findings. It should be inexpensive, simple to perform, and acceptable to patients. Protocols that center upon the determination of red blood cell indices are particularly appealing since at present they afford the greatest potential for meeting the above criteria.

At our institution we have implemented a hemoglobinopathy screening program specifically designed to evaluate obstetric patients. We believe this protocol provides the information most pertinent to the pregnant patient while retaining the virtues of simplicity and low cost. Each patient registering for prenatal care at our clinic has a complete blood count with red blood cell indices performed at the time of her first prenatal visit. This includes measurement of the MCV by a Coulter electronic counter. Additionally, each black patient has a hemoglobin electrophoresis performed. If the patient is found to have an MCV less than 80 fl or if Hb S or Hb C is found on screening electrophoresis, she is further evaluated following the scheme outlined in Figure 3–5. While screening for structural hemoglobinopathies has been widely supported, screening for thalassemia traits has been neglected. This program has been very effective in identifying asymptomatic, nonanemia hemoglobinopathy carrier states, thus allowing adequate and timely genetic counseling.[77]

GYNECOLOGIC CONSIDERATIONS

CONTRACEPTION

Patients with severe hemoglobinopathies (SCA, Hb SCD) have an increased susceptibility to thromboembolic disorders. In part, this may be due to the thrombocytosis accompanying brisk hemolysis. The fact that tissue infarction and sickling are enhanced by estrogens is also important. The exact magnitude of the association between oral contraceptives, thromboembolism, and the sickling hemoglobinopathies is unclear.[101, 102] However, caution dictates that oral contraceptives are relatively contraindicated for patients with SCA, Hb SCD, and Hb S-β-thalassemia.

Although individuals with sickle hemoglobinopathies are known to have an increased susceptibility to infection, an association between Hb S and an increased

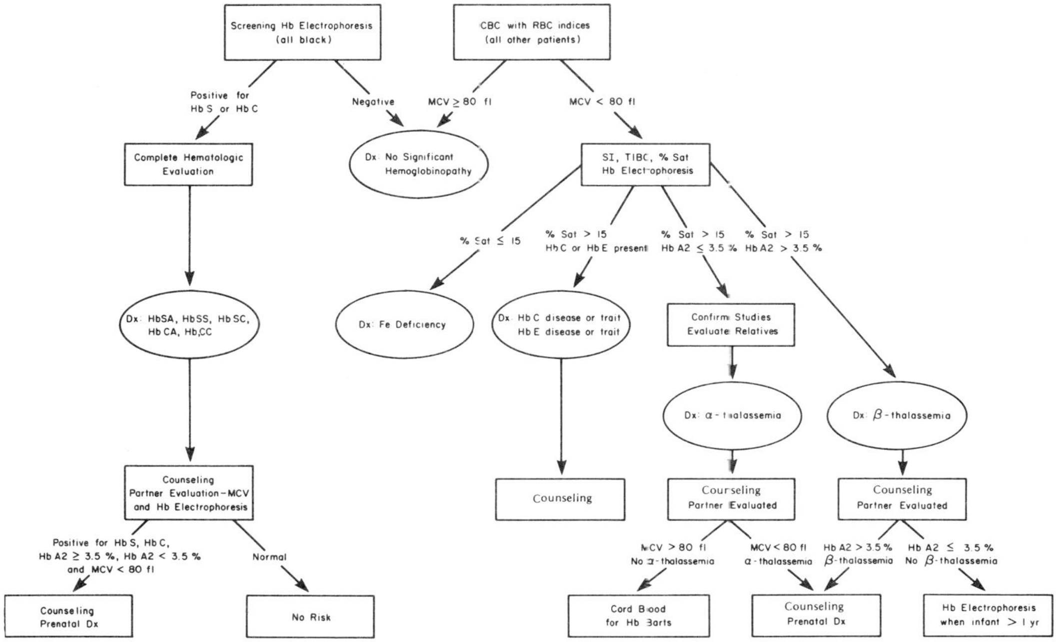

Figure 3–5. Flow chart for antenatal hemoglobinopathy screening program.

incidence of IUD–associated pelvic inflammatory disease has not been documented. Again, caution dictates that IUDs are relatively contraindicated for patients with SCA, Hb SCD, and Hb S-β-thalassemia.

The various other patients with hemoglobinopathies having no Hb S in their phenotypes can apparently use any type of contraception. This is probably also true for individuals with sickle cell trait.

PELVIC MASS

Patients with β-thalassemia intermedia often have radiologic abnormalities suggesting extramedullary hematopoiesis. Although these findings most commonly occur in the thorax and cranium, soft tissue masses may be found at any site along the vertebral column. Newton and associates recently reported extramedullary hematopoiesis presenting as a pelvic mass, and thus this possibility should be considered in the differential diagnosis of an asymptomatic pelvic mass in a patient with a known hemoglobinopathy.[104]

SURGICAL CONSIDERATIONS

Women with hemoglobinopathies may be afflicted with the whole spectrum of gynecologic disorders. Unless a woman has SCA, Hb SCD, or Hb S-β-thalassemia, operative considerations are no different than those for any woman. However, if a severe sickle hemoglobinopathy is present, great care must be taken to prevent or vigorously treat infection, to assure good tissue oxygenation, to prevent dehydration and hyperthermia, and to fully evaluate the cardiovascular, renal, and hematologic systems before surgery.

If meticulous care is exercised intraoperatively, a decrease in crisis and serious complications can be achieved.[105] However, significant morbidity still does occur. Morrison and colleagues have used partial exchange transfusion (PET) in the preoperative period.[106] Their data show significant amelioration of morbidity when PET was used. We believe that these patients also should be given prophylactic doses (minidoses) of heparin to prevent thromboembolism.

REFERENCES

1. Bunn, H.F., Forget, B.J., and Ranney, H.M.: Human Hemoglobins. Philadelphia, W. B. Saunders Company, 1977.
2. Schmidt, R.M.: Laboratory diagnosis of hemoglobinopathies. JAMA *224*:1276, 1973.
3. Schmidt, R.M.: Simple electrophoretic system for presumptive identification of abnormal hemoglobins. Blood *52*:1958, 1978.
4. Huehns, E.R., Dance, D., Beaven, G.H., et al.: Human embryonic hemoglobins. Cold Spring Harbor Symp Quant Biol *29*:327, 1964; Nature (London) *201*:1095, 1964.
5. Nienhuis, A.W., Amagnou, N.P., and Ley, T.J.: Advances in thalassemia research. Blood *63*:738, 1984.
6. Steinberg, M.H., and Adams, J.G.: Thalassemia: Recent insights into molecular mechanisms. Am J Hematol *12*:81, 1982.
7. Kan, Y.W., Dozy, A.M., Trecartin, M.S., and Todd, D.: Identification of a nondeletion defect in α-thalassemia. N Engl J Med *297*:1081, 1977.
8. Schneider, R.G., Hightower, B., Hasty, T.S., et al.: Abnormal hemoglobins in a quarter million people. Blood *48*:629, 1976.
9. Kan, Y.W., Forget, B.G., Nathan, D.G.: Gamma-beta thalassemia: A cause of hemolytic disease of the newborn. N Engl J Med *286*:129, 1972.
10. Conley, C.L., Weatherall, D.J., Richardson, S.N., et al.: Hereditary persistence of fetal hemoglobin: A study of 79 affected persons in 15 Negro families in Baltimore. Blood *21*:261, 1963.
11. Ottolenghi, S., Lanyon, W.G., Paul, J., et al.: The severe form of α-thalassemia is caused by a haemoglobin gene deletion. Nature *251*:389, 1974.
12. Weatherall, D.J., and Clegg, J.B.: The Thalassemia Syndromes. 3rd Ed. Oxford, Blackwell Scientific Publications, 1972.
13. Kan, Y.W., Dozy, A.M., Varmus, H.E., et al.: Deletion of α-globin genes in haemoglobin-H disease demonstrates multiples α-globin structural loci. Nature *255*:255, 1975.
14. Conconi, F., Rowley, P.T., Del Senno, L., Pontremoli, S., and Volpato, S.: Induction of β globin synthesis in the β thalassemia of Ferrara. Nature New Biol *238*:83, 1972.
15. Forget, B.G., Benz, E.J., Skoultchi, A., Baglioni, C., and Houseman, D.: Absence of messenger RNA for β globin chain in β^0-thalassemia. Nature *247*:379, 1974.
16. Kan, Y.W., Holland, J.P., Dozy, A.M., and Varmus, H.E.: Demonstration of nonfunctional β globin m-RNA in homozygous β^0-thalassemia. Proc Natl Acad Sci USA *72*:5140, 1975.
17. Takeshita, K., Forget, B.G., Scarpa, A., et al.: Intranuclear defect in β-globin mRNA accumulation due to a premature translation termination codon. Blood *64*:13, 1984.
18. Ramirez, F., O'Donnell, J.V., Marks, P.A., et al.: Abnormal or absent β m-RNA in β^0 Ferrara and gene deletion in β-thalassemia. Nature *263*:471, 1976.
19. Nathan, D.G., and Gunn, R.B.: Thalassemia: The consequences of unbalanced hemoglobin synthesis. Am J Med *41*:815, 1966.
20. Motulsky, A.G.: Frequency of sickling disorders in U. S. blacks. N Engl J Med *288*:31, 1973.
21. Jones, S.R., Binder, R.A., and Donowho, E.M.: Sudden death in sickle-cell trait. N Engl J Med *282*:323, 1970.
22. Dinh, T.V., Boor, P.J., and Garza, J.R.: Massive pulmonary embolism following delivery of a patient with sickle cell trait. Am J Obstet Gynecol *143*:722, 1982.
23. Kramer, M.S., Rooks, Y., and Pearson, H.A.: Growth and development in children with sickle-cell trait. N Engl J Med *299*:686, 1978.
24. Whalley, P.J., Pritchard, J.A., and Richards, J.R.: Sickle cell trait and pregnancy. JAMA *186*:1132, 1963.
25. Blattner, P., Dar, H., and Nitowsky, H.M.: Pregnancy outcome in women with sickle cell trait. JAMA *238*:1392, 1977.
26. Piomelli, S., and Corash, L.: Hereditary hemolytic anemia due to enzyme defect of glycolysis. Adv Hum Genet *6*:165, 1976.
27. Whalley, P.J., Martin, F.G., and Pritchard, J.A.: Sickle cell trait and urinary tract infections. JAMA *189*:903, 1964.

28. Pearson, H., and Vaughan, E.O.: Lack of influence of sickle cell trait on fertility and successful pregnancy. Am J Obstet Gynecol *105*:203, 1969.
29. Hatch, F.E., et al.: Nature of renal concentration defect in sickle cell disease. J Clin Invest *46*:336, 1967.
30. Jackson, J.F., Odom, J.L., and Bell, W.N.: Amelioration of sickle cell disease by persistent fetal hemoglobin. JAMA *177*:867, 1961.
31. Perrine, R.P., and John, P.: Pregnancy in sickle-cell anemia in a Caucasian group. Am J Obstet Gynecol *118*:29, 1974.
32. Henderson, A.B.: Sickle cell anemia. Am J Med *9*:757, 1950.
33. Flakpui, E.Z., and Moran, E.M.: Pregnancy in the sickle hemoglobinopathies. J Reprod Med *11*:28, 1973.
34. Horger, E.: Sickle cell and sickle cell-Hb C disease during pregnancy. Obstet Gynecol *39*:873, 1972.
35. Pritchard, J.A., Scott, D.E., Whalley, P.J., et al.: The effects of maternal sickle cell hemoglobinopathies and sickle cell trait on reproductive performance. Am J Obstet Gynecol *117*:662, 1973.
36. Fort, A.T., Morrison, J.C., Berreras, L., et al.: Counseling the patient with sickle cell disease about reproduction. Am J Obstet Gynecol *111*:324, 1971.
37. Perkins, R.P.: Inherited disorders of hemoglobin synthesis and pregnancy. Am J Obstet Gynecol *111*:120, 1971.
38. Freeman, M.G., and Ruth, G.J.: SS disease, SC disease, and CC disease—Obstetric considerations of treatment. Clin Obstet Gynecol *12*:134, 1969.
39. Morrison, J.C., and Wiser, W.L.: The effect of maternal partial exchange transfusion on the infants of parents with sickle cell anemia. J Pediatr *89*:286, 1976.
40. Morrison, J.C., and Wiser, W.L.: The use of prophylactic partial exchange transfusion in pregnancies associated with sickle cell hemoglobinopathies. Obstet Gynecol *48*:516, 1976.
41. Platt, O.S., Rosenstock, W., and Espeland, M.A.: Influence of sickle hemoglobinopathies on growth and development. N Engl J Med *311*:7, 1984.
42. Diggs, C.W.: Sickle cell crises. Am J Clin Pathol *44*:1, 1965.
43. Ammann, A.J., Addiego, J., Wara, D., et al.: Polyvalent pneumococcal-polysaccharide immunization of patients with sickle-cell anemia and patients with splenectomy. N Engl J Med *297*:897, 1977.
44. Barrett-Connor, E.: Cholelithiasis in sickle cell anemia. Am J Med *45*:889, 1968.
45. Lindenbaum, J., and Klipstein, F.A.: Folic acid deficiency in sickle cell anemia. N Engl J Med *269*:875, 1963.
46. Cerami, A.: Cyanate as an inhibitor of red-cell sickling. N Engl J Med *287*:807, 1972.
47. Kraus, A.P.: Cooperative Urea Trials Group: Clinical trials of therapy for sickle cell vaso-occlusive crises. JAMA *228*:1120, 1974.
48. Brewer, G.H.: A view of the current status of antisickling therapy. Am J Hematol *1*:121, 1976.
49. Dean, J., and Schechter, A.L.: Sickle-cell anemia: Molecular and cellular bases of therapeutic approaches. N Engl J Med *299*:752, 1978.
50. Benjamin, L.J., Kokkini, G., and Peterson, C.M.: Cetiedil: Its potential usefulness in sickle-cell disease. Blood *55*:265, 1980.
51. Morrison, J.C., Blake, P.G., McCoy, C., et al.: Fetal health assessment in pregnancies complicated by sickle hemoglobinopathies. Obstet Gynecol *61*:22, 1983.
52. Hendrickse, J.P., Harrison, K., and Watson-Williams, E.J.: Pregnancy in homozygous sickle-cell anemia. J Obstet Gynaecol Br Cwlth *79*:396, 1972.
53. Ricks, P.: Further experience with exchange transfusion in sickle cell anemia and pregnancy. Am J Obstet Gynecol *100*:1087, 1968.
54. Cunningham, F.G., Pritchard, J.A., and Mason, R.: Pregnancy and sickle cell hemoglobinopathies: Results with and without prophylactic transfusions. Obstet Gynecol *62*:419, 1983.
55. Perkins, R.P.: Partial exchange transfusion in a pregnant patient with sickle cell anemia. Obstet Gynecol *48*:22, 1976.
56. Morrison, J.C., Schneider, J.M., Whybrew, W.D., et al.: Prophylactic transfusion in pregnant patients with sickle hemoglobinopathies. Obstet Gynecol *56*:274, 1980.
57. Singer, K., Chernoff, A.L., and Singler, L.: Studies on abnormal hemoglobins. Blood *6*:429, 1951.
58. Fraser, J.L., and Watt, H.J.: Megaloblastic anemia in pregnancy and the puerperium. Am J Obstet Gynecol *89*:532, 1964.
59. Rivers, G.L., Robbans, A.S., and Schwarts, S.O.: Sickle cell hemoglobin: A clinical study. Blood *18*:385, 1961.
60. McCurdy, P.R.: Abnormal hemoglobins and pregnancy. Am J Obstet Gynecol *90*:891, 1964.
61. Went, L.N., Anderson, M., MacIver, J.E., et al.: Sickle cell disease in pregnancy. Lancet *2*:516, 1960.
62. Fullerton, W.T., and Watson-Williams, E.J.: Haemoglobin sickle cell disease and megaloblastic anemia of pregnancy. J Obstet Gynaecol Br Emp *69*:729, 1962.
63. Ballas, S.K., Lewis, C.N., Noone, A.M., et al.: Clinical, hematologic, and biochemical features of Hb SC disease. Am J Haematol *13*:37, 1982.

64. Laros, R.K.: Sickle cell hemoglobin-C disease of pregnancy. Pa Med *70*:73, 1967.
65. Laros, R.K., and Kalstone, C.: Sickle cell-β-thalassemia and pregnancy. Obstet Gynecol *37*:67, 1971.
66. Fairbanks, V.F., Gilchrist, G.S., Brimhall, B., et al.: Hemoglobin E trait reexamined: A cause of microcytosis and erythrocytosis. Blood *53*:109, 1979.
67. Frischer, H., and Bowman, J.: Hemoglobin E, an oxidatively unstable mutation. J Lab Clin Med *85*:531, 1975.
68. Wong, S.C., and Ali, M.A.M.: Hemoglobin E disease. Am J Hematol *13*:15, 1982.
69. Ferguson, J.E., and O'Reilly, R.A.: Hemoglobin E and pregnancy. Obstet Gynecol *66*:136, 1985.
70. Charache, S., Scott, J., Niebyl, J., et al.: Management of sickle cell disease in pregnant patients. Obstet Gynecol *55*:407, 1980.
71. Milner, P., Jones, B.R., and Dobler, J.: Outcome of pregnancy in sickle cell anemia and Hb SC disease. Am J Obstet Gynecol *138*:239, 1980.
72. Fort, A.T., Morrison, J.C., Ragland, J.B., et al.: Correlation of maternal serum and amniotic fluid bilirubin in gravid patients with sickle cell anemia who were actively hemolysing. Am J Obstet Gynecol *112*:227, 1972.
73. Nechelen, T.: Obstetric complications associated with haemoglobinopathies. Clin Hematol *2*:497, 1973.
74. Morrison, J.C., Whybrew, W.D., Bucovary, E.T., et al.: Fluctuation of fetal hemoglobin in sickle-cell anemia. Am J Obstet Gynecol *128*:1085, 1976.
75. Beischer, N.A., Holsman, M., and Kitchen, W.H.: Relation of various forms of anemia to placental weight. Am J Obstet Gynecol *101*:801, 1968.
76. Fleming, A.F.: Maternal anemia and fetal outcome in pregnancies complicated by thalassemia minor and "stomatocytosis." Am J Obstet Gynecol *116*:309, 1973.
77. Alger, L.S., Golbus, M.S., and Laros, R.K.: Thalassemia and pregnancy. Am J Obstet Gynecol *134*:662, 1979.
78. Fleming, A.F., and Lynch, W.: Beta-thalassemia minor during pregnancy with particular reference to iron status. J Obstet Gynaecol Brit Cwlth *76*:451, 1969.
79. Cooley, J.R., and Kitay, D.Z.: Heterozygous β-thalassemia in pregnancy. J Reprod Med *29*:141, 1984.
80. Altay, C., Gurgey, A., and Tuncbilek, E.: Hematologic evaluation of patients with various combinations of α-thalassemia. Am J Hematol *9*:261, 1980.
81. Rowley, P.T.: The diagnosis of beta-thalassemia trait: A review. Am J Hematol *1*:129, 1976.
82. Steinberg, M.H., Rosenstock, W., Coleman, M.B., et al.: Effects of thalassemia and microcytosis on the hematologic and vasoocclusive severity of sickle cell anemia. Blood *63*:1353, 1984.
83. van Enk, A., Lang, A., White, J.M., et al.: Benign obstetric history in women with sickle-cell anemia associated with α-thalassemia. Br Med J *4*:524, 1972.
84. Kan, Y.W., Holland, J.P., Dozy, A.M., et al.: Deletion of the β-globin structural gene in hereditary persistence of foetal hemoglobin. Nature *258*:162, 1973.
85. Alter, B.P.: Advances in the prenatal diagnosis of hematologic disease. Blood *64*:329, 1984.
86. Kan, Y.W., Golbus, M.S., and Dozy, A.M.: Prenatal diagnosis of α-thalassemia. N Engl J Med *295*:1165, 1976.
87. Walker, J., and Turnbull, E.P.N.: Haemoglobin and red cells in the human fetus. III. Foetal and adult haemoglobin. Arch Dis Child *30*:111, 1955.
88. Thomas, E.D., Lochte, H.L., Greenough, W.B., et al.: In vitro synthesis of foetal and adult haemoglobin by foetal haematopoietic tissues. Nature *185*:396, 1960.
89. Pataryas, H.A., and Stamatoyannopoulos, G.: Hemoglobins in human fetuses: Evidence for adult hemoglobin production after the 11th gestational week. Blood *39*:688, 1972.
90. Kan, Y.W., Dozy, A.M., Alter, B.P., et al.: Detection of the sickle cell gene in the human fetus. N Engl J Med *287*:1, 1972.
91. Hobbins, J.C., and Mahoney, M.J.: Fetal blood drawing. Lancet *2*:107, 1975.
92. Golbus, M.S., Kan, Y.W., and Naglich-Craig, M.: Fetal blood sampling in midtrimester pregnancies. Am J Obstet Gynecol *124*:653, 1976.
93. Kazazian, H.H., Kaback, M.M., Woodhead, A.P., et al.: Further studies in the antenatal detection of sickle cell anemia and other hemoglobinopathies. Adv Exp Med Biol *28*:337, 1972.
94. Nathan, D.G., Alter, B.P., and Frigoletto, F.: Antenatal diagnosis of hemoglobinopathies: Social and technical considerations. Semin Hematol *12*:305, 1975.
95. Kan, Y.W., Nathan, D.G., Cividalli, G., et al.: Concentration of fetal red blood cells from a mixture of maternal and fetal blood by anti-i serum: An aid to prenatal diagnosis of hemoglobinopathies. Blood *43*:411, 1974.
96. Alter, B.P., Modell, C.B., Fairweather, D., et al.: Prenatal diagnosis of hemoglobinopathies. N Engl J Med *295*:1437, 1976.
97. Kan, Y.W., Golbus, M.S., Trecartin, R.F., et al.: Prenatal diagnosis of β-thalassemia and sickle cell anemia. Lancet *1*:269, 1977.
98. Orkin, S.H.: Prenatal diagnosis of hemoglobin disorders by DNA analysis. Blood *63*:249, 1984.

99. Kan, Y.W., and Dozy, A.M.: Antenatal diagnosis of sickle-cell anaemia by D.N.A. analysis of amniotic fluid cells. Lancet *2*:910, 1978.
100. Kan, Y.W., Lee, K.Y., Furbetta, M., et al.: Polymorphism of DNA sequence in the β-globin gene region. N Engl J Med *302*:186, 1980.
101. Djann, J.M., and Haynes, R.L.: Sickle cell thalassemia in pregnancy. Am J Obstet Gynecol *97*:574, 1967.
102. Haynes, R.L., and Dunn, J.M.: Oral contraceptives, thrombosis and sickle cell hemoglobinopathies. JAMA *200*:994, 1967.
103. Freie, H.M.P.: Sickle cell disease and hormonal contraception. Acta Obstet Gynecol *62*:211, 1983.
104. Norton, K.L., McNeeley, G., and Novick, M.: Extramedullary hematopoiesis presenting as a pelvic mass in a patient with β-thalassemia intermedia. JAMA *250*:2178, 1983.
105. Maduska, A.L., Guinee, W.S., Heaton, A.J., et al.: Sickling dynamics of red blood cells and other physiologic studies during anesthesia. Anesth Analg *54*:361, 1975.
106. Morrison, J.C., Whybrew, W.D., and Bucovary, E. T.: Use of partial exchange transfusion preoperatively in patients with sickle cell hemoglobinopathies. Am J Obstet Gynecol *132*:59, 1978.

Chapter 4
OTHER HEMOLYTIC ANEMIAS

Russell K. Laros, Jr.

A workable definition of a hemolytic disorder is one in which the rate of red blood cell (RBC) destruction is accelerated and the bone marrow's ability to respond to anemia is unimpaired. This definition would not include disorders such as renal disease and vitamin B_{12} and folic acid deficiencies, in which increased RBC destruction is present but the marrow is unable to respond because of additional pathogenic factors.

CLASSIFICATION

In normal individuals erythrocytes survive for approximately 120 days. Thus, about 1% of the red cell mass is destroyed and replaced each day. This produces a normal reticulocyte count of 0.2 to 2.0%. In a hemolytic state the in vivo life span of the erythrocyte is shortened. Since the bone marrow is capable of a six- to eightfold increase in red cell production, anemia does not occur until the erythrocyte life span is markedly foreshortened. Hemolytic anemia may be classified as inherited or acquired (Table 4–1). The inherited forms may be on the basis of either a structural or an enzymatic defect in the red cell.

CLINICAL MANIFESTATIONS

The clinical features are shared by the large number of hemolytic disorders. The manifestations depend on both the severity of the disorder and the duration of the process.

The major features of the inherited hemolytic disorders are related to anemia, jaundice, cholelithiasis, splenomegaly, and crises. When an acquired disorder develops acutely, the symptoms may suggest an acute febrile illness. Abdominal, back, and limb pain are common and may be very severe.[1] Pallor, jaundice, tachycardia, and profound prostration may be present.

ANEMIA

The symptoms of anemia are those of cardiovascular compensation. Generally the anemia is mild or moderate because the shortened RBC survival is compensated for by increased bone marrow activity.

JAUNDICE AND CHOLELITHIASIS

In most adults icterus is either absent or very mild. However, a carefully taken history will elicit episodes of jaundice in childhood, frequently associated with mild infections. Additionally, one should inquire about any history of jaundice associated with drug usage. Because mild hyperbilirubinemia is present, the development of gallstones and symptoms of gallbladder disease are common.

Table 4–1. Classification of Hemolytic Anemias

- I. Inherited
  - A. Structural
    - 1. Spherocytosis
    - 2. Elliptocytosis
  - B. Enzymatic
    - 1. Glycolytic pathway defects
      - a. Hexokinase
      - b. Glucosephosphate isomerase
      - c. Phosphofructokinase
      - d. Triosephosphate isomerase
      - e. Phosphoglycerate kinase
      - f. Pyruvate kinase
      - g. Others
    - 2. Hexose monophosphate shunt defects
      - a. Glucose-6-phosphate dehydrogenase
      - b. 6-phosphogluconic dehydrogenase
      - c. Glutathione synthetase, reductase, and peroxidase
- II. Acquired
  - A. Autoimmune
  - B. Physical or infectious agents
  - C. Paroxysmal nocturnal hemoglobinuria
  - D. Red cell fragmentation syndromes

SPLENOMEGALY

The spleen is usually enlarged in patients with inherited hemolytic anemias. The degree of enlargement is generally only modest, but occasionally some patients are found to have massive spleens.

CRISES

The typical course for inherited hemolytic anemias is long quiescent periods of relatively asymptomatic disease interrupted by episodes of crisis. Three different sorts of crises occur: aplastic crisis, hemolytic crisis, and megaloblastic crisis.

Aplastic Crisis. In *aplastic crisis* there is a transient failure of erythropoeisis leading to a drop in the reticulocyte count. Mild leukopenia and thrombocytopenia may accompany the anemia. Crises are frequently associated with intercurrent infections.

Hemolytic Crisis. Less commonly there is an increased rate of RBC destruction or a hemolytic crisis. During these episodes the reticulocyte count and bilirubin level increase.

Megaloblastic Crisis. In *megaloblastic crisis* the marrow's decreased activity is secondary to a deficiency of folic acid. This type of crisis is commonly associated with pregnancy, which creates its own demand for increased folate. The combination of pregnancy and chronic hemolysis leads to folate deficiency, unless additional dietary intake is assured.

GENERAL DIAGNOSTIC CONSIDERATIONS

The specific diagnosis of a hemolytic anemia can be most difficult. Expert consultation usually is necessary to define the precise etiology. One must first establish that a hemolytic disorder is present and then define the specific cause.

Table 4–2 summarizes studies useful in establishing the presence of a hemolytic disorder. Other disorders associated with anemia and reticulocytosis must be excluded.

Table 4–2. Laboratory Signs of Hemolytic Disorders

Blood	
Reticulocyte count	↑
Morphology	Macrocytosis
Leukocyte and platelet counts	↑
Bone Marrow	Erythroid Hyperplasia
Heme and Iron Kinetics	
Bilirubin	↑ Serum unconjugated
Endogenous CO production	↑
LDH	↑ (LDH-2)
Hemoglobinemia	↑ In intravascular hemolysis
Haptoglobin	Absent
RBC Kinetics	↓ Life span

Common examples include hemorrhage and recovery for nutritional anemia. Individuals with compensated hemolytic anemia must be distinguished from those with the various disorders of bile metabolism. Anemia associated with marrow invasion may be associated with erythroblastosis.

The strategy for defining the specific cause of a hemolytic disorder is outlined in Figure 4–1. It should be emphasized that the specific etiologic definition can be extremely difficult to arrive at and often will require expert consultation and special laboratory studies.

SPECIFIC DISORDERS

STRUCTURAL ERYTHROCYTE DEFECTS

Hereditary Spherocytosis

The most common form of inherited hemolytic anemia is due to spherocytosis. This familial anemia is characterized by intermittent jaundice, splenomegaly, cholelithiasis, and spherocytes in the peripheral blood smear. The classic characteristic is

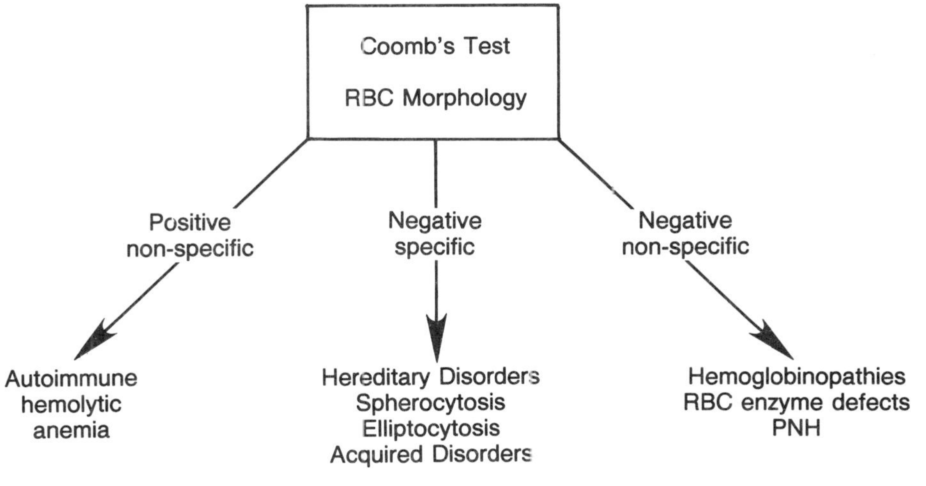

Figure 4–1. Use of the Coombs' test and red cell morphology to categorize hemolytic disorders.

an increased red cell osmotic fragility. The inheritance is as an autosomal dominant trait, and both incomplete penetrance and phenocopies have been demonstrated.[2] Approximately one fourth of the cases are sporadic, and there is a prevalence rate of 2.2×10^{-4}. This syndrome is etiologically heterogeneous, with the most commonly suggested defect being in the cell membrane.

On the basis of known prevalence, over 650 pregnancies occur annually in women with hereditary spherocytosis. A hemolytic crisis can be precipitated by many conditions, including infection, trauma, or pregnancy per se. The mechanism by which pregnancy induces hemolysis is not known. One suggestion relates the increased hemolysis to increased maternal blood volume and splenic blood flow.[3] An alternative explanation is an increase in erythrocyte osmotic fragility seen during normal pregnancy. Gottfried and associates demonstrated an increased RBC osmotic fragility during the third trimester in 32% of patients studied.[4] Prenatal care of women with spherocytosis who have not had a splenectomy should include folic acid supplementation for increased erythrocyte production and careful monitoring of the hemolytic state. A hemolytic crisis can be treated conservatively, with replacement transfusion, or with splenectomy, which will correct the shortened erythrocyte survival time.[5] Splenectomy as therapy for hemolysis in spherocytosis has been successfully performed during pregnancy in at least seven instances.[3,6] The dangers of splenectomy are the perioperative morbidity rate and thrombosis secondary to the usual postsplenectomy thrombocytosis. In the absence of a severe, untreated anemia, hereditary spherocytosis does not contribute to prenatal or neonatal morbidity.

Genetic counseling should include an explanation of autosomal dominant inheritance and of the 50% chance that each offspring will be affected. Prenatal diagnosis might be possible by examining a smear of fetal blood and determining fetal erythrocyte osmotic fragility. This would require fetal blood sampling by either fetoscopy or sonographically directed placental aspiration. The prenatal diagnosis has not yet been attempted, and in view of the moderate incapacitation caused by this disorder and the readily available therapy of splenectomy, its appropriateness is questionable.

Hereditary Elliptocytosis

Hereditary elliptocytosis is a milder hemolytic state caused by an erythrocyte structural defect. The symptoms and signs are similar to those of spherocytosis but not as severe. There are at least two genetically distinct varieties of elliptocytosis, one that is linked with the rhesus locus and one that is not. More hemolysis is seen in the "unlinked" form than in the "linked" form. Hemolysis may be precipitated by pregnancy, with the patient manifesting no symptoms or signs between pregnancies. Although splenectomy will be almost universally successful at correcting the anemia, transfusion therapy has been all that was required in the few reported cases involving pregnancy.[7,8] Hereditary elliptocytosis is inherited as an autosomal dominant trait, and the earlier comments on the genetics and prenatal diagnosis of spherocytosis also apply to this disorder.

ENZYMATIC ERYTHROCYTE DEFECTS

The reticulocyte can utilize either glucose or nonglycolytic substrates for energy metabolism, whereas the mature erythrocyte relies upon anerobic glycolysis for its energy needs. These pathways are outlined in Figures 4–2 and 4–3. This attenuation of metabolic capacity coincides with the loss of mitochondria and microsomes from

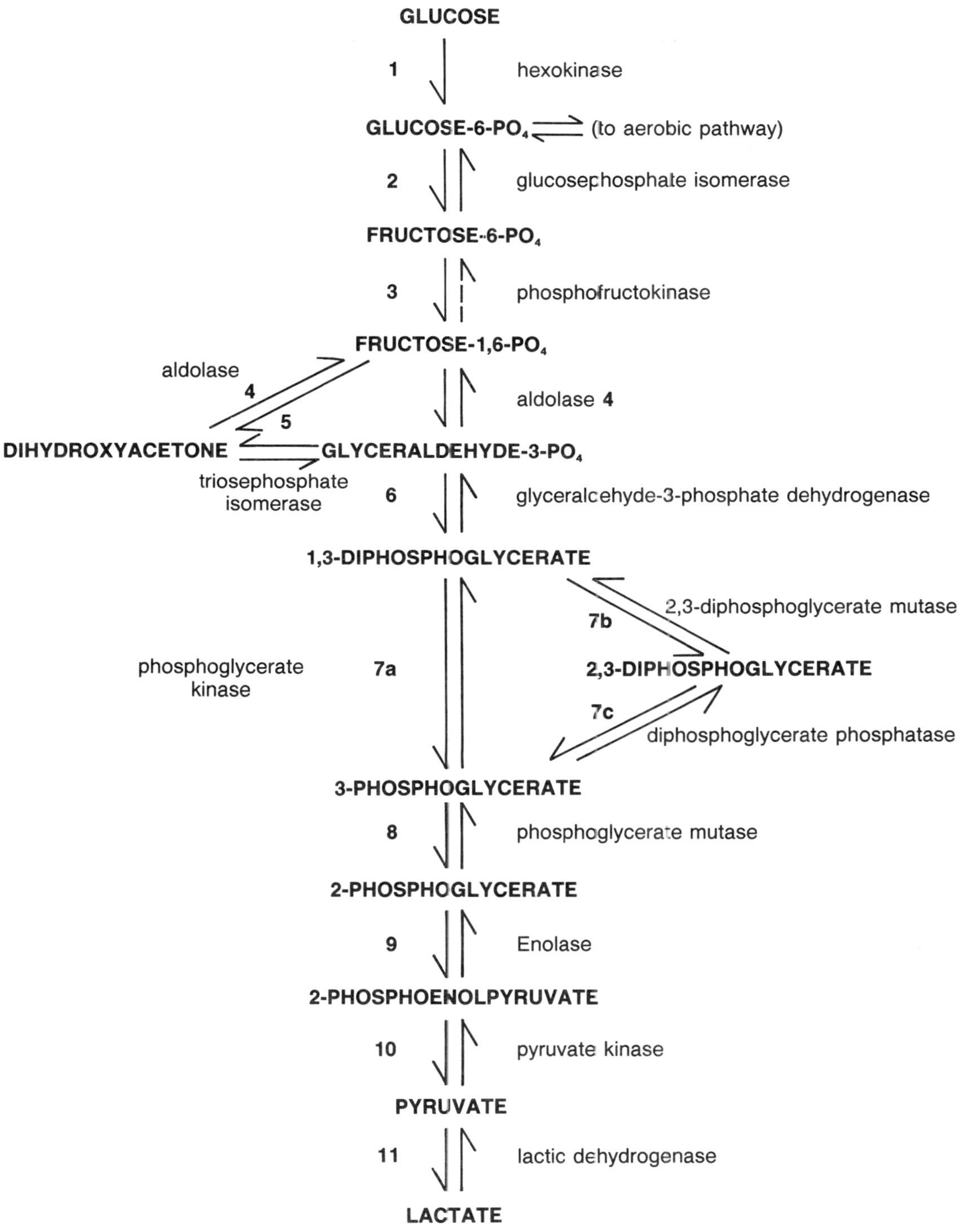

Figure 4–2. Anaerobic glycolysis in the red blood cell.

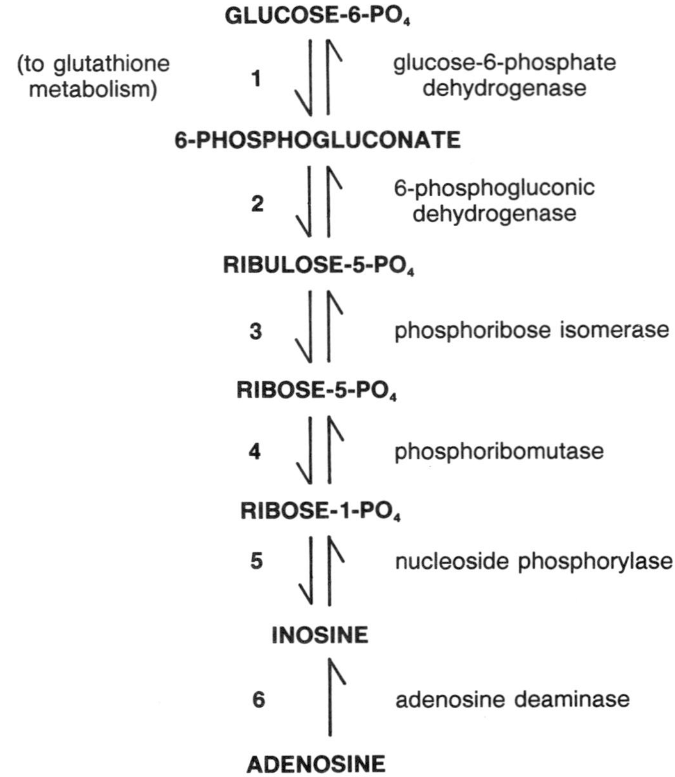

Figure 4–3. Aerobic glycolysis in the red blood cell.

the reticulocyte. Glycolysis produces only two moles of ATP per mole of glucose metabolized (**7a** and **10** in Fig. 4–2), whereas mitochondrial oxidative phosphorylation produces 36 moles of ATP per mole of glucose. The mature red cell generates 93% of its ATP via the glycolytic pathway and the remainder from the hexose monophosphate shunt. The most prevalent red cell enzyme deficiencies are those involving the hexose monophosphate shunt. Because this pathway supplies only a minor component of the cell's energy, these deficiencies are not associated with constant hemolytic anemias but rather with episodic hemolysis secondary to oxidative damage. Enzyme deficiencies in the glycolytic pathway, although rarer, are usually associated with more severe hemolysis.

Prenatal diagnosis of enzymatic defects of erythrocytes is theoretically possible; however, it has not been attempted. It would require obtaining fetal blood by fetoscopy or sonographically directed placental aspiration and determining the enzyme activities present in the fetal erythrocytes. For each disease entity the normal range of fetal erythrocyte enzyme level would have to be determined. Each disorder and each family should be considered individually, so as to provide the genetic counseling appropriate to the situation.

GLYCOLYTIC PATHWAY DEFECTS

The glycolytic pathway defects associated with hemolytic anemias will be discussed in the order in which they act in metabolizing glucose to lactic acid. The first enzyme is hexokinase (Fig. 4–2:**1**), which catalyzes the conversion of glucose to glucose-6-phosphate. The relative lethality of a deficiency of this key enzyme is reflected in the paucity of reported cases. Two clinical pictures have been reported. Four families had affected members with mild hemolysis, reticulocytosis of 4 to 21%, and decreased exercise tolerance disproportionate to the degree of anemia.[9, 10] Three other subjects had an anemia-like Fanconi's syndrome with hemolysis, pancytopenia, and chromosomal aberrations.[11] Only one of the 10 reported cases of erythrocyte hexokinase deficiency involved a woman of childbearing age, and no mention was made of the gestational history of this patient. Three of the affected neonates had hyperbilirubinemia requiring exchange transfusions.[12] This enzyme deficiency is inherited as an autosomal recessive trait.

The next enzyme in the glycolytic pathway is glucosephosphate isomerase (Fig. 4–2:**2**), which catalyzes the conversion of glucose-6-phosphate. This is the second most common glycolytic enzyme deficiency associated with a hemolytic anemia. Affected individuals have a moderately severe hemolysis and splenomegaly. Splenectomy results in marked clinical improvements. Only two of the 25 reported cases were women in their reproductive years, and no gestational histories were available.[10] At least four affected neonates had hyperbilirubinemia requiring exchange transfusion. This enzyme deficiency also is inherited as an autosomal recessive trait.

The next enzyme in the glycolytic cascade associated with a hemolytic anemia is phosphofructokinase (Fig. 4–2:**3**), which catalyzes the conversion of fructose-6-phosphate to fructose-1,6-phosphate. This enzyme deficiency is associated with mild to moderate hemolysis. Some patients also have absent muscle phosphofructokinase activity and a resultant myopathy.[13] There was no mention in the case reports as to whether the two affected females had been pregnant. This enzyme deficiency is inherited as an autosomal recessive trait.

Triosephosphate isomerase (Fig. 4–2:**5**) is the next glycolytic enzyme whose deficiency is associated with a hemolytic anemia. These patients have a severe chronic hemolysis and neurologic abnormalities. Only one reported patient survived beyond puberty, at which time her transfusion requirement ceased but her neurologic symptoms persisted.[14] This autosomal recessive trait probably could be diagnosed in utero and such a possibility should be discussed with parents of an affected child.

Phosphoglycerate kinase (Fig. 4–2:**7a**) deficiency is the next defect in the glycolytic pathway. This deficiency is associated with a severe chronic hemolysis amenable to therapy by splenectomy, and neurologic symptoms. The structural gene for phosphoglycerate kinase is on the long arm of the X chromosome.[15] Thus, only male offspring of a female carrier are at risk.

Pyruvate kinase (Fig. 4–2:**10**) deficiency is by far the most common form of red cell glycolytic defect associated with chronic hemolysis. Approximately 1:20,000 to 1:40,000 newborns have this disorder. The hemolysis is moderate to severe and preventable by splenectomy. Additional features may include cholelithiasis, jaundice, and widened bone marrow spaces with facial and roentgenographic abnormalities.[10] As with many of the inherited hemolytic anemias, a hemolytic crisis may be precipitated by biological stress states, including pregnancy.[15, 17] There are two reports of the use of oral contraceptives having intensified the hemolytic process.[17, 18] The fetal effect is evident at birth, when accentuation of hemolysis results in severe jaundice, often requiring exchange transfusion. There are at least two classes of defective red cell pyruvate kinase mutants: one with defective activity and another with kinetic abnormalities. The disorder is inherited as an autosomal recessive trait, and affected individuals may be either homozygotes for the same mutant or double heterozygotes for two different mutant genes.[19]

Deficiencies of other enzymes in the glycolytic pathway (e.g., glyceraldehyde-3-phosphate dehydrogenase [Fig. 4–2:**6**]; 2,3-diphosphoglycerate mutase [Fig. 4–2:**7b**], diphosphoglycerate phosphatase [Fig. 4–2:**7b**], and phosphopyruvate enolase [Fig. 4–2:**7c**]) also have been associated with hemolytic anemias. For each of these only a few affected individuals are known, and no information related to pregnancy or fetal effects is available. It is most likely that each is inherited as an autosomal recessive trait.

HEXOSE MONOPHOSPHATE SHUNT EFFECTS (Figure 4–3)

Glucose-6-phosphate dehydrogenase deficiency is the most common inherited form of hemolytic anemia and is found in more than 100 million persons of all races throughout the world. More than 70 variants of the enzyme have been described, with at least 20 variants associated with chronic hemolysis. This enzyme is the first step of the hexose monophosphate shunt (Fig. 4–3:**1**), which is important in maintaining the level of reduced glutathione in the red cell and thus protecting the cell against oxidants. A list of medications that are oxidants is given in Table 4–3. The severity of hemolysis is related to the specific enzyme variant, the severity of deficiency, and exposure to biological stress or certain oxidizing agents. For example, the major G6PD variant, A^+, is found in the black population, and deficiency of this variant occurs in 10% of American black males and 3% of American black females.[9] This specific deficiency is usually associated with episodic hemolysis but not a chronic

Table 4–3. Oxidants to be Avoided in Red Cell Enzyme Deficiency States

Analgesics	
Acetanilid	Acetophenetidin (phenacetin)
Acetylsalicylic acid	
Sulfonamides and Sulfones	
Sulfanilamide	Thiazolsulfone
Sulfapyridine	Salicylazosulfapyridine (Azulfidine)
Diaphenysulfone	Sulfoxone
N-Acetylsulfanilamide	Sulfamethoxypyridazine (Kynex)
Sulfisoxazole (Gantrisin)	Sulfacetamide
Antimalarials	
Primaquine	Quinocide
Pamaquine	Quinacrine (Atabrine)
Pentaquine	
Nonsulfonamide Antibacterial Agents	
Furazolidone	Para-aminosalicylic acid
Nitrofurantoin (Furandantin)	Nifuroxime
Chloramphenicol	Nitrofurazone
Miscellaneous	
Naphthalene (mothballs)	Trinitrotoluene
Methylene blue	Quinine
Nalidixic acid	Quinidine
Phenylhydrazine	Niridazole
Ascorbic acid (massive doses)	

hemolytic state. Alternatively, hemolysis induced by fava beans (favism) is seen in Caucasian and Oriental individuals with certain G6PD mutants but is unusual in the black population.[20]

Pregnancy in patients with G6PD deficiency is associated with a number of specific complications. There is decreased G6PD activity in one third of the patients during the last trimester.[21] This may predispose these women to hemolytic episodes at this time. An association with anemia is not unexpected, and a study of 180 G6PD–deficient pregnant women reported 62% had a hematocrit reading of < 30%.[22] Urinary tract infection also was suggested as being more common among the enzyme-deficient women. This infection produces an additional risk because the treatment drugs often employed are oxidants. A reasonable course would be to screen black pregnant women with urinary tract infections for G6PD deficiency prior to initiation of therapy. One report has indicated an increased incidence of low-birth-weight infants born to G6PD-deficient mothers, but no correction for the effects of anemia or urinary tract infections was made.[23]

The glucose-6-phosphate–deficient fetus is at risk both before and after delivery. Exposure to maternally ingested oxidants such as sulfisoxazole, ascorbic acid, or fava beans may produce hemolysis, hydrops fetalis, and death.[24, 25] The neonate is at risk for anemia, hyperbilirubinemia, and kernicterus.[12] The incidence of severe jaundice in randomly selected G6PD–deficient newborn males is approximately 5%. However, this incidence rises to 50% if there is a prior icteric sibling.[26]

Glucose-6-phosphate deficiency is inherited as an X-linked trait. Males are either hemizygous or unaffected. Females are homozygous, heterozygous, or unaffected. Clinical involvement may occur in heterozygous females as well as homozygous females and hemizygous males. This may be a reflection of variable X-chromosome inactivation, as there is a tremendous variation in enzyme levels among heterozygous females. Although genetic counseling and providing affected individuals with a list of oxidants to avoid are extremely important, prenatal diagnosis probably is not necessary in view of the usually benign nature of this enzyme deficiency.

A number of other enzymes in the hexose monophosphate shunt and related glutathione metabolism (Fig. 4–4) have been reported to be absent in patients with hemolytic anemias. These include 6-phosphogluconic dehydrogenase (Fig. 4–3:**2**), glutathione reductase (Fig. 4–4:**2**), glutathione peroxidase (Fig. 4–4:**3**), and glutathione synthetase. Each of these deficiencies is relatively rare, and there is no available information about maternal effects during pregnancy. Most of these may cause sufficient hemolysis in the neonate to produce hyperbilirubinemia requiring exchange transfusion.

ACQUIRED HEMOLYTIC DISORDERS

The acquired hemolytic anemias are more than twice as common as the hereditary forms. Whether this ratio holds true for hemolytic anemias during pregnancy is unknown, but it is unlikely.[27]

Autoimmune Hemolytic Anemia (AIHA)

Two broad classes of antibodies are responsible for AIHA: warm-reactive and cold-reactive. Most warm-reactive antibodies are of the IgG class[28] and are directed against some component of the Rh system.[29] Almost all cold agglutinins are IgM and usually have anti-I or anti-i specificity.[30] AIHA caused by either antibody type may be either

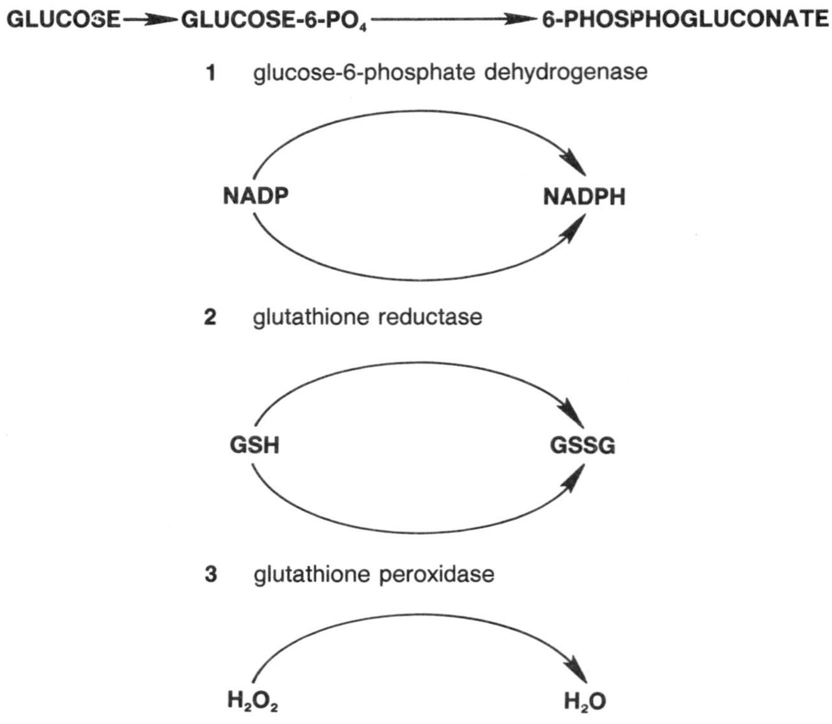

Figure 4–4. Glutathione metabolism: NADP and NADPH-oxidized and NADPH-reduced nicotinamide adenine dinucleotide; GSH-reduced glutathione; GSSG-oxidized glutathione.

primary (idiopathic) or secondary. AIHA with warm antibodies is seen in association with various hematologic malignancies (chronic lymphocytic leukemia, lymphoma), lupus erythematosus, viral infections, and drug ingestion. Penicillin, stibophen, and α-methyldopa have all been associated with AIHA. Secondary cold agglutinin disease is associated with *Mycoplasma* infections, infectious mononucleosis, and lymphoreticular neoplasm.

Autoimmune hemolytic anemia with a positive Coombs' test has been reported to be exacerbated by but not caused by pregnancy. There may be a transient hemolytic anemia in the neonate resulting from passively transferred IgG antibodies.[31, 32] One author has suggested that an increased perinatal mortality accompanies the maternal disease state,[33, 34] but others have disagreed.[35]

Acquired Hemolytic Anemia Resulting from Miscellaneous Causes

Most cases of acquired hemolytic anemia result from antibodies, fragmentation of the red cell, or paroxysmal nocturnal hemoglobinemia. However, there remains an uncommon group of disorders that are associated with exposure to certain physical or chemical agents or with infection. The infectious conditions most commonly associated with hemolysis are malaria, congenital toxoplasmosis and other TORCH (toxoplasmosis, rubella, cytomegalovirus, and herpes simplex) pathogens, bartonellosis, and infection with *Clostridum perfringens.*[36] In addition to the many drugs that have been reported to produce hemolysis, various chemicals and snake venoms also have been implicated. Last, thermal injury and ionizing radiation can also lead to a shortening of RBC survival.

Paroxysmal Nocturnal Hemoglobinuria (PNH)

Hemolysis occurs in PNH because of an unexplained structural defect in the RBC. There are distinct cohorts of long-lived and short-lived cells. The intrinsic RBC defect makes them unusually susceptible to lysis by complement.[37]

PNH usually begins insidiously, and there is no familial tendency. The disease varies considerably in severity, and the classic presentation of hemoglobinuria is found in only 25% of all patients. Exacerbations of the hemolytic process are precipitated by infections, menstruation, transfusion, operations, and ingestion of iron.[38]

The most serious complications associated with PNH are marrow aplasia, thrombosis, and infection. Thromboses account for 50% of deaths, and this is of particular concern.[39] While anemia is the most prominent hematologic feature of PNH, leukopenia and thrombocytopenia are also frequently present. The diagnosis of PNH is based on a series of special tests that demonstrate the sensitivity of the patient's cells to complement.

The ideal treatment for PNH is the replacement of the abnormal stem cell with cells capable of producing normal cellular components. This has been accomplished by bone marrow transplantation but is not an option during pregnancy. The major therapeutic modalities are iron therapy, androgen treatment, corticosteroid treatment, and transfusion therapy.

Iron can usually be administered orally to replace the considerable amount of iron lost in the urine. In a significantly iron-deficient patient, such treatment may lead to a burst of erythropoiesis, with delivery into the circulation of a cohort of cells susceptible to the lytic action of complement. If a hemolytic episode follows iron therapy, it should be treated with either suppression of erythropoiesis by transfusion or suppression of hemolysis with corticosteroids.

While androgen therapy has been useful (see Chapter 5) in the nonpregnant female and in males, it is not without side-effects and is definitely contraindicated during pregnancy. Patients with an element of marrow hypoplasia benefit most from androgen therapy.

Prednisone can be most useful in blunting hemolysis. Generally a dose of 1 mg/kg/day is used. An effective alternative is 15 to 40 mg given every other day.

When treatment of PNH with these modalities is not successful, the patient may require RBC transfusion. To limit hemolytic reactions caused by infusion of activated complement, washed or frozen reconstituted RBCs should be used.

When acute hemolytic episodes occur, treatment should be aimed at diminishing hemolysis and preventing complications. Prednisone is useful for diminishing the rate of hemolysis, as discussed above, and transfusion may ameliorate the crisis by suppressing the production of complement-sensitive cells. Because patients with PNH have frequent episodes of venous thrombosis, this must be watched for carefully. In cases of acute deep venous thrombosis (DVT) anticoagulation should be begun; however, care must be taken in the use of heparin. There have been clear-cut hemolytic episodes reported following heparin therapy. During the pregnancy itself heparin should be used; however, during the puerperium or the nonpregnant state, warfarin is the preferred agent.

Only a few pregnancies have been reported in women with PNH, and both spontaneous abortion and thrombotic complications appear to be increased.[40–45]

The Red Cell Fragmentation Syndromes

These are a variety of disorders in which the RBC is subjected to intravascular damage with production of so-called schistocytes. This is a cell that has lost a portion of its cell wall and cytoplasm but has managed to reseal its membrane. Red cell fragmentation has been observed in association with various vascular prostheses and in the broad group of disorders called the microangiopathic hemolytic anemias. Because all these disorders are usually associated with a coagulation abnormality, they will be discussed in detail in Chapter 10.

TREATMENT

Specific management depends on the diagnosis and upon whether the hemolysis is secondary to an underlying disease process.

TRANSFUSION

Blood transfusions should be used cautiously because the transfused cells may be destroyed, thus adding an additional burden on the excretory organs.

SPLENECTOMY

The spleen is the major site of RBC destruction in many hemolytic disorders. Splenectomy is clearly curative for individuals with hereditary spherocytosis and elliptocytosis. The anemia associated with deficiencies of pyruvate kinase, hexokinase, and glucose-phosphate isomerase is improved by splenectomy. The effectiveness of splenectomy for patients with AIHA is variable. In general, cases associated with warm antibodies are more likely to respond to splenectomy. When the role of splenectomy is in doubt, the role of the spleen in RBC destruction can be quantitated by radioisotope studies.

STEROIDS

Adrenocorticoid steroids are the therapy of choice for patients with AIHA due to warm antibodies. If a response is to occur, it will occur within one week of treatment. If continuous high-dose steroids are necessary to maintain remission, splenectomy should be considered.

WITHDRAWAL OF INCITING AGENTS

If the hemolytic process is secondary to some drug or other agent, it should be withdrawn. Further, oral contraceptives should be avoided in all cases of active hemolysis because of the enhanced risk of thromboembolism.

SUPPORTIVE THERAPY

Folic acid supplementation is important during active hemolysis and especially during pregnancy. Prophylactic heparin therapy should be considered for all surgical patients and in the puerperium. Prophylactic anticoagulation is particularly pertinent for patients with PNH.

REFERENCES

1. Wallerstein, R.O., and Aggler, P.M.: Acute hemolytic anemia. Am J Med *37*:92, 1964.
2. Morton, N.E., MacKinney, A.A., Kosower, N., et al.: Genetics of spherocytosis. Am J Hum Genet *14*:170, 1962.
3. Moore, A., Sherman, M.M., and Strongin, M.J.: Hereditary spherocytosis with hemolytic crisis during pregnancy. Obstet Gynecol *47*(S):19, 1976.

4. Magid, M.S., Perkins, M., and Gottfried, E.L.: Increased erythrocyte osmotic fragility in pregnancy. Am J Obstet Gynecol *144*:910, 1982.
5. Johnson, H.H.C., and McAllister, J.E.: Familial hemolytic icterus occurring during pregnancy. Can Med Assoc J *65*:377, 1951.
6. McElin, T.W., Mussey, R.D., and Watkins, C.H.: Splenectomy during pregnancy. Am J Obstet Gynecol *59*:1036, 1950.
7. Weiss, H.J.: Hereditary elliptocytosis with hemolytic anemia. Am J Med *35*:455, 1963.
8. Breckenridge, R.L., and Riggs, J.A.: Hereditary elliptocytosis with hemolytic anemia complicating pregnancy. Am J Obstet Gynecol *101*:861, 1968.
9. Nathan, D.G., and Oski, F.A.: Hematology of Infancy and Childhood. 2nd Ed. Philadelphia, W.B. Saunders Co., 1981.
10. Piomelli, S., and Corash, L.: Hereditary hemolytic anemia due to enzyme defects of glycolysis. Adv Hum Genet *6*:165, 1976.
11. Lohr, G.E., Waller, H.D., Amschutz, F., et al.: Biochemische defecte in den Blutzellen bei familiarer Poninyelopathie. Humangenetik *1*:383, 1965.
12. Gilman, P.A.: Hemolysis in the newborn infant resulting from deficiencies of red blood cell enzymes: Diagnosis and management. J Pediatr *84*:625, 1974.
13. Layzer, R.B., Rowland, L.P., and Ranney, H.M.: Muscle phosphofructokinase deficiency. Arch Neurol *17*:512, 1967.
14. Harris, S.R., Paglia, D.E., Jaffe, E.R., et al.: Triosephosphate isomerase deficiency in an adult. Clin Res *18*:529, 1970.
15. Pearson, P.L., Sanger, R., and Brown, J.A.: Report of the Commission on the Genetic Constitution of the X Chromosome. Cytogenet Cell Genet *14*:190, 1975.
16. Collier, H.B., Ashford, D.R., and Bell, R.E.: Three cases of hemolytic anemia with erythrocyte pyruvate kinase deficiency in Alberta. Can Med Assoc J *95*:1188, 1966.
17. Kendall, A.G., and Charlow, G.F.: Red cell pyruvate kinase deficiency; adverse effect of oral contraceptives. Acta Haematol *57*:116, 1977.
18. Nixon, A.D., and Buchanan, J.G.: Haemolytic anemia due to pyruvate kinase deficiency. NZ Med J *66*:859, 1967.
19. Tanaka, T.R., and Paglia, D.E.: Pyruvate kinase deficiency. Semin Hematol *8*:367, 1971.
20. Carson, P.E., and Frischer, H.: Glucose-6-phosphate dehydrogenase deficiency and related disorders of the pentose phosphate pathway. Am J Med *41*:744, 1966.
21. Vergnes, H., and Clerc, A.: Erythrocyte enzyme activity in pregnancy. Lancet *2*:834, 1968.
22. Silverstein, E., Roadman, C., Byers, R.H., et al.: Hematologic problems in pregnancy. III. Glucose-6-phosphate dehydrogenase deficiency. J Reprod Med *12*:153, 1974.
23. Perkins, R.P.: The significance of glucose-6-phosphate dehydrogenase deficiency in pregnancy. Am J Obstet Gynecol *125*:215, 1976.
24. Perkins, R.P.: Hydrops fetalis and stillbirth in a male glucose-6-phosphate dehydrogenase-deficient possibly due to a maternal ingestion of sulfisoxazole. Am J Obstet Gynecol *111*:379, 1971.
25. Mentzer, W.C., and Collier, E.: Hydrops fetalis associated with erythrocyte G-6-PD deficiency and maternal ingestion of fava beans and ascorbic acid. J Pediatr *86*:565, 1975.
26. Fessas, P.H., Doxiadis, S.A., and Valaes, T.: Neonatal jaundice in glucose-6-phosphate dehydrogenase deficient infants. Br Med J *2*:1359, 1962.
27. Bottiger, L.E., and Westerholdin, B.: Acquired hemolytic anemia. Acta Med Scand *193*:223, 1973.
28. Dacie, J.V., and Worllridge, S.M.: Autoimmune hemolytic anemias. Progr Hematol *6*:82, 1969.
29. Weiner, W., and Vos, G.H.: Serology of acquired hemolytic anemias. Blood *22*:606, 1963.
30. Worllridge, S.M., and Blajchman, H.A.: The autoimmune haemolytic anemias. Brit J Haematol *23*(S):61, 1972.
31. Bauman, R., and Rubin, H.: Autoimmune hemolytic anemia during pregnancy with hemolytic disease in the newborn. Blood *41*:293, 1973.
32. Eldor, A., Yatziv, S., and Hershko, C.: Relapsing Coombs'-negative haemolytic anemia in pregnancy with haemolytic disease in the newborn. Br Med J *1*:625, 1975.
33. MacKenzie, M.R.: Disorders of immunohematology in pregnancy Clin Haematol *211*:515, 1973.
34. Sacks, D.A., Platt, L., and Johnson, C.S.: Autoimmune hemolytic disease during pregnancy. Am J Obstet Gynecol *140*:942, 1981.
35. Fleming, A.F., and Allan, N.C.: Severe haemolytic anemia in pregnancy in Nigerians treated with prednisone. Br Med J *1*:461, 1969.
36. Wintrobe, M.M., Lee, G.R., Boggs, D.R., et al.: Hereditary hemolytic anemias associated with abnormalities of erythrocyte anaerobic glycolysis and nucleotide metabolism. *In* Clinical Haematology. Edited by Wintrobe M.M., et al. 8th Ed. Philadelphia, Lea & Febiger, 1981.
37. Wintrobe, M.M., Lee, G.R., Boggs, D.R., et al.: Glucose-6 phosphate dehydrogenase deficiency and related deficiencies involving the pentose phosphate pathway and glutathione metabolism. *In* Clinical Haematology. Edited by Wintrose M.M., et al. 8th Ed. Philadelphia, Lea & Febiger, 1981.
38. Rosse, W.F.: The complement sensitivity of PNH cells. Series Haematol *5*(3):101, 1972.

39. Dacie, J.V.: The Hemolytic Anemias, Congenital and Acquired. New York, Grune & Stratton, 1967.
40. Peyterman, R.: Thrombosis in PNH with particular reference to progressive diffuse hepatic venous thrombosis. Series Haematol *5*(3):115, 1972.
41. Frakes, J.T., Burmeister, R.E., and Giliberti, J.J.: Pregnancy in a patient with paroxysmal nocturnal hemoglobinuria. Obstet Gynecol *47*(S):22, 1976.
42. Sircha, G., and Lewis, S.M.: Paroxysmal nocturnal hemoglobinuria. Clin Haematol *4*:199, 1975.
43. Rosse, W.F.: Treatment of paroxysmal nocturnal hemoglobinuria. Blood *60*:20, 1982.
44. Hurd, W.W., Miodovnik, M., and Stys, S.J.: Pregnancy associated with paroxysmal nocturnal hemoglobinuria. Obstet Gynecol *60*:742, 1982.
45. Spencer, J.A.D.: Paroxysmal nocturnal haemoglobinuria in pregnancy. Br J Obstet Gynaecol *87*:246, 1980.

Chapter 5
APLASTIC ANEMIA

Russell K. Laros, Jr.

Aplastic anemia is characterized by a reduction in the number of circulating red blood cells (RBCs), neutrophils, and platelets and by the presence of a hypocellular bone marrow. Although bone marrow transplantation, androgen therapy, and administration of antithymocyte globulin have begun to improve the prognosis, aplastic anemia remains a serious and often fatal disorder.

PATHOGENESIS

It is clear that all blood cells originate from a single precursor. Three mechanisms have been postulated to explain the development of aplastic anemia: (1) insufficient stem cells either because of an intrinsic defect or because of a reduction in number after exposure to some noxious extrinsic agent; (2) the presence of some suppressor substance that inhibits the maturation of the myeloid precursors; and (3) the development of an autoimmune reaction that causes death of the stem cells.[1,2]

Table 5–1 lists various agents that have been reported to be associated with aplastic anemia.[3] In the first group are agents that predictably lead to marrow aplasia. This result is anticipated, and marrow activity is frequently monitored when the agents are used. However, occasionally these predictable episodes of aplasia will continue long after the agent is withdrawn.

In the second category are agents such as chloramphenicol that induce aplasia only in occasional patients.[4] The reaction is idiosyncratic and unpredictable. Finally, on occasion literally hundreds of agents of varying types have been implicated as causes of aplastic anemia.

However, in about half of all cases careful search does not reveal any possible causative agent.

HYPOPLASTIC ANEMIA OF PREGNANCY

In 1953, Holly described eight patients with hypoplastic anemia diagnosed during pregnancy that spontaneously remitted after delivery.[5] The bone marrow was described as hypocellular, with an increase in megakaryocytes. In four cases, a repeat bone marrow examination after delivery was normal. To date a total of 46 cases have been reported.[6–8] However, these cases present a spectrum of clinical and bone marrow findings that make it difficult to substantiate that a hypoplastic anemia specifically related to pregnancy does in fact exist. Support for such a hypothesis is found in those cases in which recovery occurred after delivery and relapse occurred with a subsequent pregnancy.[9,10]

Table 5–1. Agents Associated with Aplastic Anemia

Occasionally Associated
Benzene and related agents
Ionizing radiation
Nitrogen mustard and related agents
Antimetabolites (antifolic agents and purine or pyrimidine analogs)
Antimitotic agents
Certain antibiotics (e.g., daunorubicin)
Other toxic chemicals (e.g., inorganic arsenic)
Consistently Associated
Certain antibiotics (e.g., chloramphenicol)
Anticonvulsants (e.g., trimethadione)
Analgesics (phenylbutazone)
Gold salts
Rarely Associated
More than 100 described

CLINICAL FEATURES

DIAGNOSIS

The patient with aplastic anemia comes to medical attention either because of symptoms related to a profound anemia or because of bleeding or infection. A screening CBC reveals pancytopenia, and the reticulocyte count is also low. Examination of a bone marrow aspirate reveals hypoplasia but with normoblastic erythroid development. Other causes of pancytopenia are listed in Table 5–2 and must be excluded. The combination of a careful physical examination and a bone marrow examination will usually make possible this differential diagnosis between aplastic anemia and other causes of pancytopenia.[3, 34]

PROGNOSIS

Severe aplastic anemia is fatal for more than 75% of affected patients. Bone marrow transplantation is now the treatment of choice, and long-term survival of 50 to 70% of cases can be expected.[11, 12] The graft-versus-host phenomenon is the major obstacle to successful marrow transplantation. The biphasic nature of survival data has been emphasized by Lynch and associates, who document that short-term survivors differ in several ways from patients who survive past four months.[11, 12] Factors of positive

Table 5–2. Other Causes of Pancytopenia

Bone marrow infiltration
Leukemia
Multiple myeloma
Metastatic carcinoma
Myeloid metaplasia
Hypersplenism
Congestive splenomegaly
Lymphoreticular disorders
Infiltrative disorders (Gaucher's disease)
Infection (miliary tuberculosis)
Vitamin B_{12} and folate deficiencies
Lupus erythematosus
Paroxysmal nocturnal hemoglobinuria
Familial—Fanconi's pancytopenia

prognostic value were the absence of bleeding, being of the female sex, some reticulocyte response, a higher absolute neutrophil count, a higher platelet count, and a lower % of nonmyeloid cells in the marrow. Other authors have found that a high total fetal hemoglobin level (> 400 mg per dl) is also a good prognostic finding.[13]

Rovinsky summarized the results of pregnancies in women with aplastic anemia prior to the mid-1950s.[14] Table 5–3 details the more recent results available in the literature. These patients had the benefits of modern supportive therapy, including antibiotics, steroids, and platelet transfusions and bone marrow transplantation. The maternal mortality rate of only 15% is surprisingly good. Furthermore, 91% of the survivors are described as being in remission.

TREATMENT

The principles of treatment include maintenance of hemoglobin levels by periodic transfusion, prevention and treatment of infection, stimulation of hematopoiesis, and consideration of splenectomy, therapeutic abortion and premature delivery, and marrow transplantation.

The principles of RBC and platelet replacement are discussed elsewhere (see Chapter 11), and the decision to perform splenectomy requires that splenic destruction be demonstrated by radioisotope studies (see Chapter 4). Infections should be treated aggressively, keeping in mind possible adverse effects of certain therapeutic agents on the fetus.

Stimulation of Hematopoiesis

Androgen therapy was initially used because of empiric observation of positive results. However, it is clear that androgens are beneficial to those patients in the better

Table 5–3. Results of 13 Pregnancies in Women with Aplastic Anemia

Author	Number of Pregnancies	Abortion	Delivery	Infant	Mother
Rosner, 1964[15]	1	0	Induction at 37 wk	Premature, survived	Died, sepsis
King, 1966[16]	2	TAB	—	—	Died, remission
		0	Term	Survived	
Taylor, 1968[17]	1	0	Term	Survived	Remission
Evans, 1968[7]	1	SAB	—	—	Remission
Fleming, 1968[6]	2	0	Term	Survived	Remission
		0	Term	Survived	Remission
Collins, 1972[18]	1	0	Term cesarean section and splenectomy	Premature, survived	Survived, no remission
Goldstein, 1975[19]	1	0	Term	Survived	Remission
Knispel, 1976[20]	1	0	Term	Premature, survived	Remission
Perry, 1977[8]	1	0	Term	Survived	Remission
Jacobs, 1981[21]	1	0	Term	Survived	Marrow transplant 15 mo before
Deeg, 1983[22]	1	0	Term	Survived	Marrow transplant 14 mo before

prognosis group.[3, 23] It is important to remember that the granulocyte and platelet responses to anabolic steroids lag behind the RBC response. A trial of six to 10 months is required to fully assess the therapeutic efficacy.

Agents commonly used include fluoxymesterone (0.25 mg/kg—po, daily); oxymetholone (3 to 5 mg/kg—po, daily); nandrolone decanoate (3 to 5 mg/kg IM, weekly); or testosterone enanthate (1 to 3 mg/kg IM, weekly). The virilizing side-effects of all these agents are a significant disadvantage to the female patient. In addition to cosmetic problems related to hirsutism, menstrual abnormalities can also occur. These side-effects can be minimized by careful adjustment of the dose.

Anabolic steroids are contraindicated during pregnancy, especially if the woman is carrying a female fetus.

Adrenal corticosteroids also have been widely used with some benefit. However, the remission rate with corticosteroids is low (approximately 12%), and most investigators feel that the use of corticosteroids in combination with androgens is not indicated.[3, 23]

Marrow Transplantation

Bone marrow transplantation is now the treatment of choice for patients with severe aplastic anemia. Severe aplasia is defined by the presence of any two of the following three blood findings or the presence of either of the two marrow findings. The significant peripheral blood parameters are neutrophils $< 500 \times 10^6$/L; platelets $< 20 \times 10^9$/L; and reticulocytes < 1%. Marrow findings are severe hypocellularity or moderate hypocellularity, with < 30% of residual cells being hematopoietic. Because marrow transplants are far more successful when performed early in the course of the disease, one of the first decisions to be considered is whether or not a given patient is a candidate for transplant. The availability of a suitable donor obviously has a significant influence on the decision.

Recent results of marrow transplantation in nontransfused patients are excellent, with 80% of recipients being alive between 1 and 10 years after transplant. Unfortunately, most patients with aplastic anemia are not so fortunate as to have a histocompatible sibling willing to serve as a marrow donor.

Table 5–4. Management of Aplastic Anemia and Pregnancy

CHRONIC CASE RECEIVING ANABOLIC STEROIDS

- Discontinue steroids before conception
- If significant and threatening decrease in marrow activity during first trimester, perform amniocentesis for fetal sex determination:
    - If fetus is male, reinstate anabolic steroids
    - If fetus is female, give supportive therapy with transfusion or terminate pregnancy

ACUTE CASE

- Conception to approximately 24 weeks' gestation
    - Therapeutic abortion: begin therapy with anabolic steroids or marrow transplantation
- Gestational age of more than 24 weeks
    - Give supportive therapy with transfusion
    - Method and timing of delivery should be based on obstetric considerations

Pregnancy Termination

What is the role of pregnancy termination when aplastic anemia is complicated by pregnancy? Because of the anecdotal reports of complete remission following pregnancy termination, it is a tempting therapeutic step. However, a thorough examination of the available literature indicates that abortion or premature termination of pregnancy is not associated with a more favorable maternal outcome. The therapeutic approach that we follow is outlined in Table 5–4. The patient with a chronic aplastic anemia that has responded to treatment must be considered from a different point of view than the pregnant woman found to have an acute, new process.

If therapeutic abortion is chosen, it should be carried out under ideal and predictable conditions—that is, by suction curettage or dilatation and evacuation in the operating room under light, general anesthesia. Dilatation and evacuation are preferable to saline or prostaglandin induction in cases of second trimester abortion because of the lower morbidity.[24]

OTHER HYPOPROLIFERATIVE DISORDERS

Table 5–2 lists a number of specific disorders associated with pancytopenia. Additionally, there are a group of disorders in which there is interference only with the production of RBCs. These are listed in Table 5–5 and must be considered in the differential diagnosis of a hypoproliferative anemia.

GAUCHER'S DISEASE

Gaucher's disease is a rare, hereditary disorder in which there is a decreased β-glucosidase activity.[25, 26] The result of this enzymatic defect is deposition of excessive glucose-ceramide within cells. Three presentations of the disease have been described that differ in the age of onset, the amount of central nervous system involvement, and the rate of clinical deterioration.[27] The most common form and that seen by the obstetrician-gynecologist is the adult form. These patients manifest splenomegaly, anemia, thrombocytopenia, episodic bleeding, frequent fractures, yellowish skin color, and occasionally, conjunctival pingueculae. The disease appears to be inherited as an autosomal recessive trait and is most prevalent in Ashkenazic Jews.[28] The infantile and neurologic forms of Gaucher's disease are far less common.

Diagnosis

Typically, there is a moderate normochromic anemia accompanied by thrombocytopenia and leukopenia. The serum acid phosphatase activity is usually increased.[29]

Table 5–5. Other Causes of Hypoproliferative Anemia

Anemia of Chronic Disorders
Chronic infections
Chronic noninfectious inflammations
Malignant diseases
Sideroblastic Anemias
Anemia of chronic renal insufficiency
Anemia in cirrhosis
Anemia associated with endocrine disorders

The diagnosis is confirmed by finding the typical "Gaucher cell" in aspirated bone marrow.

Effects on Pregnancy. A number of pregnancies have been reported in women with Gaucher's disease.[30–32] By and large these patients have experienced unremarkable prenatal courses. The hematologic status should be assessed periodically, and folic acid supplementation should be given to avoid a superimposed megaloblastic anemia. Hemorrhagic complications have not been a problem at delivery or during the puerperium.

Treatment

Treatment is purely symptomatic. If there is significant splenomegaly, splenectomy is warranted to alleviate symptoms secondary to size or repeated infarction or if thrombocytopenia with bleeding is caused by hypersplenism.

ANEMIA OF CHRONIC DISORDERS

Chronic disorders accompanied by infection, inflammation, or neoplasia are frequently associated with a mild, normocytic anemia and a low reticulocyte count. In some instances hyperchromia will also be evident.[33] Characteristically the serum iron level and the total iron-binding capacity are decreased. Factors that have been implicated in the pathogenesis include a decreased RBC life span, impaired marrow response, and impaired release of iron from reticuloendothelial stores.[34]

Correction of the anemia requires proper identification and treatment of the primary disorder.

SIDEROBLASTIC ANEMIAS

The sideroblastic anemias are really a group of disorders characterized by excessive iron deposition within the mitochondria or normoblasts.[33] The disorder may be hereditary, idiopathic, associated with other diseases, or the result of exposure to toxic substances. Lymphoma and leukemia and exposure to certain toxins or drugs such as ethanol,[35] antituberculous drugs,[36] or lead are examples.[37, 38]

Sideroblastic anemia is usually moderately severe, with hypochromia, microcytosis, and a low or normal reticulocyte count. The leukocyte and platelet counts are normal and the RBCs exhibit prominent basophilic stippling.[33] The bone marrow evidences erythroid hyperplasia, and ringed sideroblasts constitute 10% to 40% of the normoblasts. Transferrin saturation is high. In lead intoxication an increase in Hb F and Hb A_2 has been reported in approximately 15% of patients.[37]

Treatment consists of removal of toxic causative agents when they are a factor. Pyridoxine in an oral dose of 50 to 100 mg/day should be tried; however, the response rate is disappointing, with only about 50% of patients responding. When sideroblastic anemia is secondary to antituberculous therapy, response to vitamin B_6 therapy is excellent, and the antituberculous agent can be continued in conjunction with the pyridoxine therapy.

ANEMIA OF CHRONIC RENAL DISEASE

The defect in erythropoiesis associated with chronic renal disease is in part due to a failure of the renal-erythropoietin-secretory mechanism.[39] Other factors implicated include a blunted marrow response and a shortened RBC survival. Following successful renal homograft, erythropoietic activity becomes normal.[40] There is now ample experience with pregnancy in women following kidney transplantation, and chronic anemia has not been a problem.[41, 42]

ANEMIA OF CIRRHOSIS AND OTHER CHRONIC LIVER DISEASES

Most patients with chronic liver disease will have a mild to moderate normochromic, normocytic anemia. The RBC survival time is shortened, and the reticulocyte count is frequently elevated.[33] Because of alterations in the lipid content of the RBC membrane, "spur cells" and other poikilocytes are seen.

ANEMIA ASSOCIATED WITH ENDOCRINE DISORDERS

Varying degrees of anemia have been described in association with hypothyroidism, hyperthyroidism, adrenal insufficiency, and hypopituitarism.[33] There are no specific morphologic features of the anemia, and resolution will occur after appropriate treatment of the primary endocrine disorder.

REFERENCES

1. Williams, D.M., Lynch, R.E., and Cartwright, G.E.: Drug-induced aplastic anemia. Semin Hematol *10*:195, 1973.
2. Boggs, D.R., and Boggs, S.S.: The pathogenesis of aplastic anemia. Blood *48*:71, 1976.
3. Camitta, B.M., Storb, R., and Thomas, E.D.: Aplastic anemia. N Engl J Med *306*:712, 1982.
4. Best, W.: Chloramphenicol-associated blood dyscrasias. JAMA *201*:99, 1967.
5. Holly, R.G.: Hypoplastic anemia in pregnancy. Obstet Gynecol *1*:533, 1953.
6. Fleming, A.F.: Hypoplastic anemia in pregnancy. Clin Haematol *2*:477, 1973.
7. Evans, E.L.: Aplastic anemia in pregnancy remitting after abortion. Brit Med J *2*:166, 1968.
8. Perry, C.P., and Harris, R.E.: Successful management of pregnancy-induced pancytopenia. Obstet Gynecol *50*:732, 1977.
9. Lehman, G., and Alcoff, J.: Reversible pure red cell hypoplasia in pregnancy. JAMA *247*:1170, 1982.
10. Danforth, D.N., Kyser, F.A., Boronow, R.C., et al.: Refractory anemia and thrombocytopenia due to pregnancy. JAMA *180*:629, 1962.
11. Lynch, R.E., Williams, D.M., Reading, J.C., et al.: The prognosis in aplastic anemia. Blood *45*:517, 1975.
12. O'Reilly, R.J.: Allogeneic bone marrow transplantation: Current status and future directions. Blood *62*:941, 1983.
13. Bloom, G.E., and Diamond, L.K.: Prognostic value of fetal hemoglobin levels in acquired aplastic anemia. N Engl J Med *278*:304, 1968.
14. Rovinsky, J.J.: Primary refractory anemia complicating pregnancy and delivery. Obstet Gynecol Surv *14*:149, 1959.
15. Rosner, F., and Sussman, S.N.: Aplastic anemia in pregnancy. Obstet Gynecol *23*:99, 1964.
16. King, T.M., and Todd, W.D.: Aplastic anemia in pregnancy. Bull Sloane Hosp *10*:42, 1966.
17. Taylor, J.J., and Studd, J.W.: Primary refractory anemia and pregnancy. J Obstet Gynaecol Brit Cwlth *75*:963, 1968.
18. Collins, D.J., Rosenthal, D.S., Goldstein, D.P., et al.: Aplastic anemia in pregnancy. Obstet Gynecol *39*:884, 1972.
19. Goldstein, I.M., and Coller, B.S.: Aplastic anemia in pregnancy: Recovery after normal spontaneous delivery. Ann Intern Med *82*:537, 1975.
20. Knispel, J.W., Lynch, V.A., and Viele, B.D.: Aplastic anemia in pregnancy: A case report, review of the literature, and re-evaluation of management. Obstet Gynecol Surv *31*:523, 1976.
21. Jacobs, P., and Dobovsky, D.W.: Bone marrow transplantation followed by normal pregnancy. Am J Hematol *11*:209, 1981.
22. Deeg, H.J., Kennedy, M.S., Sanders, J.R., et al.: Successful pregnancy after marrow transplantation for severe aplastic anemia and immunosuppression with cyclosporine. JAMA *250*:647, 1983.
23. Sanchez-Medal, L., Gomez-Leal, A., Duarte, L., et al.: Anabolic androgenic steroids in the treatment of acquired aplastic anemia. Blood *34*:283, 1969.
24. Grimes, D.A., Schultz, K.F., Cates, W., et al.: Mid-trimester abortion by dilatation and evacuation, a safe and practical alternative. N Engl J Med *296*:1141, 1977.
25. Beutler, E., and Kuhl, W.: The diagnosis of the adult type of Gaucher's disease and its carrier by demonstration of deficiency of β-glucosidase activity in peripheral blood leukocytes. J Lab Clin Med *76*:747, 1970.

26. Nitowsky, A.M.: Use of cell culture techniques in diagnosis and studies of inherited disease. Semin Hematol *9*:403, 1972.
27. Kolodny, E.H.: Clinical and biochemical genetics of the lipidoses. Semin Hematol *9*:251, 1972.
28. Groen, J.J.: Gaucher's disease: Hereditary transmission and racial distribution. Arch Intern Med *113*:543, 1964.
29. Matoth, Y., and Freed, K.: Chronic Gaucher's disease. Isr J Med Sci *1*:152, 1965.
30. Hoja, W.A.: Gaucher's disease in pregnancy. Am J Obstet Gynecol *79*:286, 1960.
31. Watov, S.E., and DeSandre, R.: Gaucher's disease and pregnancy. Obstet Gynecol *23*:247, 1964.
32. Mendel, E.B., and McCullough, J.A.: Gaucher's disease and pregnancy. Obstet Gynecol *32*:607, 1968.
33. Wintrobe, M.M., Lee, R.E., Boggs, D.R., et al.: Clinical Hematology. 7th Ed. Philadelphia, Lea & Febiger, 1974, p. 671.
34. Cartwright, G.E.: The anemia of chronic disorders. Semin Hematol *3*:351, 1966.
35. Eichner, E.R., and Hillman, R.S.: The evolution of anemia in alcoholic patients. Am J Med *50*:218, 1971.
36. Verwilghen, R.: Antituberculous drugs and sideroblastic anemia. Br J Haematol *11*:92, 1965.
37. Albahary, C.: Lead and hematopoiesis. Am J Med *52*:369, 1972.
38. Bottomley, S.S.: Porphyrin and iron metabolism in sideroblastic anemia. Semin Hematol *14*:169, 1977.
39. Desforges, J.F.: Anemia in uremia. Arch Intern Med *126*:808, 1970.
40. Hoffman, G.C.: Human erythropoiesis following kidney transplantation. Ann NY Acad Sci *149*:504, 1968.
41. Nolan, G.H., Sweet, R.L., Laros, R.K., et al.: Renal cadaver transplantation followed by successful pregnancies. Obstet Gynecol *43*:732, 1974.
42. Sciarra, J.J., Toledo-Pereyra, L.H., Bendel, R.P., et al.: Pregnancy following renal transplantation. Am J Obstet Gynecol *123*:411, 1975.

Chapter 6

LEUKEMIA AND LYMPHOMA

Brian J. Lewis/Russell K. Laros, Jr.

The dominant problems that arise when the obstetrician-gynecologist encounters patients with leukemia or lymphoma include (1) the coexistence of pregnancy; (2) severe, uncontrolled menorrhagia; (3) primary genital presentations; and (4) consultation regarding gonadal or fetal effects or both of chemotherapy or radiation therapy.

In this chapter we will not present a detailed discussion of the pathophysiology, diagnosis, and treatment of the various types of leukemia and lymphoma. Rather, we will review the diagnostic classifications, summarize the therapy and prognosis, and concentrate more fully on the four areas listed above.

LEUKEMIA

Leukemia is by definition an uncontrolled proliferation of leukocytes. The classification of the various types of leukemia is outlined in Table 6–1 and is based upon clinical course, cell type, and response to therapy.[1]

The cause of leukemia is unknown. However, viruses, irradiation, chromosomal defects, and chemicals have all been suggested as etiologic agents.[2] While the leukemogenic effects of large doses of radiation are indisputable,[3] the data on low levels of exposure are contradictory. Some authors find a clear association,[4, 5] while others find none.[6] Combinations of multidrug chemotherapy and radiation therapy appear to be leukemogenic in patients with Hodgkin's disease,[7] and prolonged therapy with alkylating agents has been associated with the later development of leukemia in ovarian cancer patients.[8]

ACUTE LEUKEMIA

Patients with acute leukemia usually present with symptoms of hypermetabolism, anemia, infection, or bleeding. The diagnosis is suspected from the results of a complete blood count and confirmed by examination of a bone marrow aspirate. Physical findings can include fever, petechiae, splenomegaly, hepatomegaly, and lymphadenopathy.

Although acute lymphocytic leukemia (ALL) can be seen at any age, it is predominantly a disease of childhood. In contrast, the incidence of acute nonlymphocytic leukemia (ANLL) increases with age. If the disease is untreated, the average survival for patients with acute leukemia is 2.5 months, with death being caused by infection and hemorrhage in almost equal proportions.[9]

While advances in the treatment of ANLL have led to significantly improved rates of remission (50 to 70%), the median duration of remission remains only one year.[10, 11] The principles of treatment are to induce a hematologic remission by using a com-

Table 6–1. Classification of Leukemia

ACUTE LEUKEMIA
Acute nonlymphocytic leukemia (ANLL)*
Acute lymphocytic leukemia (ALL)+
CHRONIC LEUKEMIA
Chronic myelocytic leukemia (CML)
Chronic lymphocytic leukemia (CLL)

*ANLL can be further subclassified by nuclear and cytoplasmic morphology on Wright's stain and by enzyme content of the leukemic cells after histochemical staining—e.g., acute myeloblastic leukemia with or without maturation, acute promyelocytic leukemia, acute myelomonocytic leukemia, acute monocytic leukemia, and erythroleukemia.[1]
+ Immunologic markers as well as morphologic distinctions now allow subtyping of ALL. These designations have important clinical implications.[13]

bination of drugs and then to maintain it by the cyclic administration of additional chemotherapy. Induction therapy requires ablation of all marrow elements, leukemic as well as normal, and thus exposes the patient to 3 to 6 weeks of aplasia with the attendant risks of infection and hemorrhage. Drug combinations used for induction therapy include cytosine arabinoside, 6-thioguanine, L-asparaginase, vincristine, doxorubicin, daunorubicin, cyclophosphamide, and prednisone. These agents are also used in consolidation and maintenance therapy along with methotrexate and 6-mercaptopurine. Investigational drugs with useful antileukemic activity currently include 5-azacytidine, *m*-AMSA, and VM-26.[1]

Essential improvements in the area of supportive care have paralleled the advances in cytotoxic therapy. Most important have been aggressive and early use of antibacterial antibiotics and transfusion therapy and better anticipation and treatment of fungal infections.[1] Unfortunately, the probability of long-term survival with ANLL remains low, on the order of 10 to 15%.[10] Bone marrow transplantation after the induction of a first remission may offer the hope of longer survival.[12] In contrast to those with ANLL, children with favorable forms of ALL sustain prolonged remissions and probable cures in at least 50% of cases.[13]

Pregnancy and Acute Leukemia

There are now many reports of pregnant patients with acute leukemia. McLain summarized the 256 cases of acute leukemia in pregnancy reported before 1970 and found that maternal mortality was 100% and perinatal mortality was 35%.[14] Table 6–2 details the cases reported more recently. Based on these data and the cases reviewed by McLain, there is no evidence that pregnancy has any adverse effect on the course of leukemia except if specific chemotherapy is withheld for fear of damaging the fetus. The converse is certainly not true, with the greatest risk being maternal death before delivery and fetal damage or death related to maternal chemotherapy or leukemia-induced complications during pregnancy.

The maternal and fetal outcomes in the cases summarized in Table 6–2 certainly suggest that a standard chemotherapeutic approach can produce excellent maternal and fetal results. On the other hand, review of the use of cytotoxic agents during pregnancy leads to concern about teratogenesis.[36, 37] In 164 fetuses exposed to various chemotherapeutic agents during the first trimester of pregnancy, 19 showed various malformations (12%). Aminopterin, which appears to be the most noxious agent, fortunately is no longer used therapeutically. By contrast, none of 76 fetuses exposed to chemotherapeutic agents in the second or third trimester had congenital anomalies thought to be related to the exposure. However, there has been a reported occurrence of trisomy C in a fetus exposed to cytosine arabinoside and 6-thioguanine,[38] and in Table 6–2 there is one case of a congenital malformation[33] in an infant exposed to monthly cytosine arabinoside plus 6-thioguanine throughout gestation. These data and the experience with other classes of drugs such as diethylstilbestrol indicate that the long-term well-being of fetuses exposed to chemotherapeutic agents cannot be assured, although it would appear that the fetus is most vulnerable during the first trimester.

Pregnancy Counseling

If a patient with ANLL is not pregnant when the diagnosis is made, because of the guarded long-term outlook, she should be counseled to avoid pregnancy in the future. In contrast, the good long-term results with ALL make future pregnancy a likely possibility. Siris and colleagues have reported on the reproductive function in 35 long-term survivors of ALL.[39] Normal sexual development occurred in 16 of 17 patients treated before puberty but in only 12 of 18 treated during or after menarche. It appears that agents such as cyclophosphamide cause ovarian failure more readily in adults[40] than in children.[41]

Three separate reports have noted five normal pregnancies in women with ALL and long-term remission,[19, 42, 43] and in a review of pregnancy outcome among 212 patients who received aggressive chemotherapy for various cancers at the National Cancer Institute, there were five ALL patients. One had a normal birth at 1½ years after treatment, one at five years, one at ten years, and the other two were still pregnant at the time of the report.

Control of Menorrhagia

The occurrence of menses and marked thrombocytopenia in a woman with acute leukemia can be the source of significant blood loss, control of which can be most difficult. Table 6–3 outlines both the medical and surgical approaches to therapy. Because bleeding is usually dysfunctional in nature and exacerbated by the thrombocytopenia, it is reasonable to initiate hormonal therapy without prior curettage. Possible regimens are detailed in Table 6–3 and either (a) or (b) can be used to achieve control of acute menorrhagia. Regimen (a) will produce a more rapid cessation of bleeding. Once the acute bleeding has stopped, prolonged control can be achieved with either regimen (c) or (b).[45] Regimen (d) has the advantage of avoiding intramuscular injection. The ultimate aim is to achieve an endometrium exhibiting secretory exhaustion. Estrogens are also used because the incidence of breakthrough bleeding is less than with progestin alone (38% vs. 17%).

If control cannot be achieved with medical therapy, dilatation and curettage are performed to rule out anatomic causes such as polyps or submucosal fibroids. In selective patients, hysterectomy is required to achieve control of menorrhagia. Hysterectomy should also be considered for patients with ANLL or adult onset ALL who request surgical sterilization.

CHRONIC LEUKEMIA

Chronic myelocytic leukemia (CML) is most commonly seen in young and middle-aged adults. Typical symptoms are fatigue, weight loss, and abdominal fullness. Sple-

Table 6–2. Experience with Pregnancy in 35 Cases of Acute Leukemia

Author	Diagnosis*	Therapy†	Gestational Age (wk)	Labor and Delivery	Fetal Outcome	Remission	Maternal Outcome
Pauling, 1975[15]	AML	ARA-C + 6-thioguanine + vincristine	25	induction at 39 wk	2250 g; normal infant	partial	death 7 mo post partum
Ewing, 1973[16]	APML	prednisolone	37	induction at 37 wk	2693 g; normal	none	chemotherapy started post partum; died 33 days after delivery
	APML	none	post partum	spontaneous labor and delivery	2778 g; normal		chemotherapy started post partum; died 30 days after delivery
Bhoopathi, 1973[17]	APML	none	post partum	spontaneous labor and delivery	3440 g; normal	partial	discharged
Raich, 1975[18]	AML	ARA-C + 6-thioguanine	26	spontaneous labor and delivery	3540 g; normal	complete	discharged
Wegelius, 1975[19]	ALL	6-mercaptopurine	12	spontaneous labor and delivery	2760 g; normal	complete	patient on maintenance therapy at conception; withdrawn for 3 mo
Krueger, 1976[20]	ALL	prednisone + vincristine + ARA-C + cyclophosphamide + 6-mercaptopurine; intrathecal methotrexate	26	induction at 38 wk	2970 g; normal	complete	discharged
Gokal, 1976[21]	AMML	daunorubicin + ARA-C + 6-thioguanine	20	induction at 37 wk	2880 g; normal	complete	relapse and death 6 mo after delivery
Lilleyman, 1977[22]	AML	ARA-C + 6-thioguanine; vincristine + daunorubicin + prednisone + ARA-C	10	prostaglandin abortion at 20 wk	normal fetus; normal karyotype	complete	relapse with death 2 mo after anticipated expected date of confinement
Durie, 1977[23]	AML	vincristine + ARA-C + prednisone	27	induction at 38 wk	2967 g; normal	complete	discharged

Newcomb, 1978[24]	AML	ARA-C + vincristine + prednisone	16	elective cesarean hysterectomy at term	3460 g; normal	complete	prolonged remission
	AML	doxorubicin + vincristine	12	spontaneous labor and delivery	2860 g; normal	complete	discharged
Lowenthal, 1978[25]	AML	ARA-C + daunorubicin	17	induction at 40 wk	2860 g; normal	complete	relapse 7 mo after delivery
O'Donnell, 1979[26]	AML	6-thioguanine + ARA-C + daunorubicin	27	spontaneous labor and delivery	5 kg; normal	complete	in remission at 6 mo
Doney, 1979[27]	AML	prednisone; vincristine + methotrexate + 6-mercaptopurine + prednisone	32	spontaneous delivery at 34 wk	2350 g; "cushingoid"	partial	death 13 mo after diagnosis
	AML	hydroxyurea; daunorubicin + ARA-C + vincristine + thioguanine + prednisone	17	elective abortion at 21 wk	208 g; no gross defects	complete	marrow transplant; in remission at 2 yr
	AML	daunorubicin + ARA-C + vincristine + 6-thioguanine + prednisone	27	spontaneous delivery at 31 wk	2130 g; multiple medical problems, slow growth	none	death 9 days after delivery
Hamer, 1979[28]	AML	ARA-C + 6-thioguanine	25	spontaneous delivery at 38 wk	2990 g; normal	complete	relapse, death 17 months after diagnosis
Okun, 1979[29]	ALL	vincristine, prednisone, L-asparaginase cyclophosphamide, daunomycin, 6-mercaptopurine cranial irradiation, intrathecal methotrexate	12	spontaneous labor and delivery at 31 wk	2350 g; marrow hypoplasia	complete	relapse, death 20 months after diagnosis
Tobias, 1980[30]	AML	ARA-C + 6-thioguanine + doxorubicin	24	spontaneous delivery at 32 wk	2 kg; normal	complete	discharged
Pizzuto, 1980[31]	6 ALL, 3 AML	various	1st to 3rd trimesters	spontaneous labor and cesarean at 33–41 wk	1000–3000 g; normal, stillborn	3 complete 3 partial 3 active disease	

Table 6–2. Experience with Pregnancy in 35 Cases of Acute Leukemia (Continued)

Author	Diagnosis*	Therapy†	Gestational Age (wk)	Labor and Delivery	Fetal Outcome	Remission	Maternal Outcome
Taylor, 1980[32]	AML	ARA-C + 6-thioguanine	27	vaginal delivery at 25 wk	1430 g; normal	complete	death 1 yr after diagnosis
Schafer, 1981[33]	AML	ARA-C + 6-thioguanine monthly	0 to 38 wk	cesarean at 38 wk	2212 g; absent digits	complete	became pregnant 4 mo after delivery
	AML (same patient)	same as preceding case	1st trimester	cesarean	2912 g; normal		remission for 42 mo
Alegre, 1982[34]	APML	prednisone + daunorubicin, ARA-C	9	spontaneous labor at 39 wk	3050 g; normal	complete	relapse, death 5 wk after delivery
Plows, 1982[35]	AMML	ARA-C + 6-thioguanine	22	loss of fetal movement, delivery of a macerated fetus at 25 wk	no abnormalities noted	complete	remission; conceived 1 yr later
	AMML (same patient)	ARA-C + 6-thioguanine	16	cesarean section for fetal distress at 39 wk	3133 g; normal	complete	relapse, death 14 mo after delivery

* AML = acute myelocytic leukemia; APML = acute promyelocytic leukemia; ALL = acute lymphocytic leukemia; AMML = acute myelomonocytic leukemia.
† ARA-C = cytosine arabinoside.

Table 6–3. Treatment of Menorrhagia

Hormonal Therapy
Acute control:
(a) Conjugated estrogens, IV, 20 mg every two hr until control or for six doses
or
(b) Oral medroxyprogesterone acetate, 40 mg daily
Chronic control:
(c) Depo-medroxyprogesterone acetate, 100 mg IM; repeat in one week, then 100 mg every two weeks + conjugated estrogens orally, 1.25 mg daily
or
(d) Oral medroxyprogesterone acetate, 40 mg + 1.25 mg conjugated estrogens daily
Surgical Therapy
Dilatation and curettage
Hysterectomy

nomegaly is present in almost all patients, and hepatomegaly and periperal lymphadenopathy are common findings.[1]

Laboratory features include anemia and leukocytosis, with all developmental stages of the neutrophil series being present in the peripheral blood. The platelet count is elevated in 50% of patients and may be extremely high. The Philadelphia chromosome, which is the number 22 G chromosome that has lost a portion of its long arm by translocation to chromosome 9, is present in 90% of cases.[46] The leukocyte alkaline phosphatase level is very low in CML and can be used to differentiate true CML from a leukemoid reaction.[47] Serum uric acid level is frequently elevated.

CML has two phases, one chronic and the other acute (blast crisis). The chronic phase can last from months to years (median, 3½ years). The circulating granulocytes show maturation, and therapy is relatively mild and intermittent. Daily, single-drug treatment, usually with busulfan (an alkylating agent) and less commonly with hydroxyurea (an antimetabolite), suffices to control elevated blood counts and attendant symptoms. Treatment is aimed at reducing the white count to about 8.0 to 10.0 × 10^9/L, at which time it may be stopped. The patient is observed at regular intervals, with treatment reinstituted when the count approaches 50 × 10^9/L. Usually six or more months between treatments can be anticipated. Allopurinol should be used as needed to control hyperuricemia. Several features of CML have been found to correlate with a poor prognosis. These include thrombocytopenia and the absence of Philadelphia chromosome.[48]

Blast crisis in CML is heralded by a rapid rise in the leukocyte count caused by the proliferation of blasts rather than more mature forms, as in the chronic phase. Constitutional symptoms are usually present, and prompt, intensive therapy (as in ANLL) is required. Unfortunately, sustained remissions from this phase are rare, and survival after the appearance of blast crisis is short, with a median time of two months.

Chronic lymphocytic leukemia (CLL) is characterized by the appearance of large numbers of small lymphocytes in the blood and bone marrow. It is rare in individuals younger than 30, and many patients have absolutely no symptoms attributable to CLL at the time the diagnosis is made. Lymphadenopathy is present in almost all cases, and splenomegaly is common.[49]

Mild anemia and an elevated absolute lymphocyte count above 4.5 × 10^9/L are characteristic, with the count usually about 100 × 10^9/L. Thrombocytopenia is rare. Immunoglobulin levels frequently are low.

Prolonged survival is possible with CLL, and one third of the time the cause of death will be unrelated to the leukemia.[49] The average survival after diagnosis is six years. Infection is the most common CLL-related cause of death, with complications of treatment being second most common. An abnormal immune system is evidenced by the high susceptibility to infection and by the development of autoimmune hemolytic anemia and immune thrombocytopenia. Conversion to an aggressive course (i.e., the development of an acute leukemia-like picture or to a high-grade lymphoma [Richter's syndrome]) occurs but is an infrequent event.

The principle of treatment is not to treat the leukocyte count per se but to control lymphocyte proliferation when it causes clinically significant problems (e.g., cytopenias from marrow replacement or hypersplenism), without producing undue side-effects. This can be accomplished by using an alkylating agent (most commonly chlorambucil), radiation therapy, and corticosteroids. There is no clear evidence that treatment prolongs life, but it does control symptoms. Many patients do very well without treatment for significant periods of time.[1]

Pregnancy and Chronic Leukemia

In McLain's review of 202 cases of CML in pregnancy, maternal mortality was 37% and fetal mortality was 16%[14] Because of the nature of the disease, an uneventful pregnancy can be accomplished during an inactive phase when no treatment is needed. However, patients with CML should be cautioned, as the need for chemotherapy can be unpredictable, drug effects on the oocytes are uncertain (see further on), and if blast crisis intervenes during gestation, it needs to be treated using the same principles as discussed for acute leukemia.

Chemotherapy During Pregnancy

There is no evidence that pregnancy has any adverse effect on CML; however, low-birth-weight infants and an increase in fetal mortality have been suggested.[50, 51] By contrast, Johnson found both maternal and fetal outcome reasonably good in 18 pregnancies in women with CML who were treated with cytotoxic agents.[52] Boros compared infants exposed to busulfan with those whose mothers had CML but were untreated during pregnancy and concluded that the incidence of low birth weight was greater in infants exposed to alkyating agents.[53] There is a single report of a patient with CML being treated with dibromomannitol from the 10th to the 17th week of pregnancy; the mother and child did very well.[54] It should also be remembered that busulfan therapy is frequently associated with amenorrhea in adult females.[55, 56] The amenorrhea is characterized by elevated gonadotropins and atrophic, oocyte-depleted ovaries.

CONGENITAL LEUKEMIA

More than 100 cases of congenital leukemia have been reported, and in contrast to a childhood leukemia, most have been ANLL.[1] In no instance did the mother also have leukemia. There is an interesting report of one mother who delivered at least two and probably four children with congenital leukemia[57] and another in which one twin had congenital leukemia while the other did not.[58]

Rothman's and associates' review of placental and fetal involvement by maternal malignancy contains six cases of leukemia. In the four cases in which the placenta was examined histologically, there was evidence of intervillous tumor but not intravillous malignancy. However, there were two cases in which the infants were found to have leukemia, one at nine months and one at five months of age.[59] Despite these instances, there are no well-documented cases of maternal-fetal transmission of leukemia. It should be noted that in both cases there was a delay in onset of disease in the newborn; the placenta was not examined in either case.

LYMPHOMA

The lymphomas can be broadly grouped into Hodgkin's disease and non-Hodgkin's lymphoma. The most significant advances in our understanding and treatment of these disorders have been in the development of more reliable histologic classification, a more extensive and systematic pretreatment evaluation and staging, and the more effective use of extended field radiation therapy and combination chemotherapy.

HODGKIN'S DISEASE

The diagnosis of Hodgkin's disease is a histologic one and depends upon the presence of the characteristic Reed-Sternberg cells. The morphology of the Reed-Sternberg cell and the relative proportion of other cellular elements form the basis for the Rye histologic classification outlined in Table 6–4. More recently it has become evident that the prognostic importance of each histologic subtype is secondary to the stage of the disease at presentation (Table 6–5), in contrast to the non-Hodgkin's lymphomas in which histology has a major influence on outcome.[60]

Because the choice of treatment requires that the sites of disease be carefully defined, it is necessary to employ the staging system detailed in Table 6–5.[60] Pregnancy should always be ruled out before undertaking diagnostic studies and treatment. Exact staging may require extensive testing using the following modalities: history and physical examination, complete blood count, liver function studies, chest roentgenogram, bone marrow aspirate and biopsy, computerized tomography, lymphangiography, liver biopsy, and exploratory laparotomy and splenectomy. Because of economic factors and the costs of patient discomfort and morbidity, staging procedures should be selected after discussion with the therapist who will be treating the tumor, since procedures such as laparotomy are unnecessary if they only change the stage but not the treatment plan. If a laparotomy is performed, the abdominal exploration and tissue sampling should follow a standard protocol.[61] The patient should also receive oophoropexy in anticipation of shielding the ovaries during radiation.

Treatment for Hodgkin's disease is an adequate dose of radiation therapy for patients with relatively localized disease—that is, stage IA and IIA.[62] With a proper radiation

Table 6–4. Histologic Classification of Hodgkin's Disease[60]

Histologic Type	Relative Frequency (%)	Initial Stage (%) I and II	Initial Stage (%) III and IV
Lymphocyte predominant	6	76	24
Nodular sclerosis	68	60	40
Mixed cellularity	24	44	56
Lymphocyte depleted	2	19	81

Table 6–5. Staging of Hodgkin's Disease

Stage	Characteristics
I	Involvement of a single lymph node region or of a single extranodal organ or site.
II	Involvement limited to one side of the diaphragm either ≥ two lymph node regions or localized involvement of an extralymphatic site and ≥ lymph node region.
III	Involvement of lymph node regions on both sides of the diaphragm, which may include localized involvement of an extralymphatic site or of the spleen.
IV	Diffuse or disseminated involvement of ≥ one extralymphatic organ or any liver involvement, with or without associated lymph node involvement.
Subclass	
A	If asymptomatic
B	If any of the following: unexplained weight loss of ≥ 10% of body weight in preceding six months; unexplained temperature ≥ 38°; night sweats.

dose (4000 to 4400 rad) and extended field therapy, a cure rate exceeding 90% can be anticipated. For stage IVA cases, combined chemotherapy regimens such as MOPP (nitrogen mustard + vincristine + procarbazine + prednisone) will produce a complete remission in 80 to 100% of patients and probably cure in at least 50%.[63] Stages IB and IIB are treated with total irradiation, yielding a five-year disease-free survival rate of 75 to 80%.[64] While most authorities agree that states IIIB and IVB require treatment with combination drug therapy and in some centers with radiation therapy as well, the treatment of stage IIIA remains controversial. Some centers choose total nodal irradiation therapy, while others choose chemotherapy alone or a combination of the two, depending upon the total volume of the patient's tumor.[65, 66] Two other chemotherapy regimens used successfully are ABVD (doxorubicin [Adriamycin] + bleomycin + vinblastine + decarbazine) or MVPP (in which vinblastine is used in place of vincristine).[67]

Pregnancy and Hodgkin's Disease

Hodgkin's disease is typically more indolent than acute lymphoma in its clinical course. Consequently, theoretically one has the option to consider initially delaying or attenuating staging and therapy to protect the fetus without harming the mother. However, based upon past treatment experience with the population of Hodgkin's disease patients as a whole, there has to be concern that limited staging and submaximal induction therapy or a delay in treatment will diminish the chances for long-term disease control and cure.

These issues are detailed in Table 6–6. The risks to the fetus from staging and treatment are the known or potential consequences of surgery, radiation, and cytotoxic drugs. The risks to the mother from a compromise in management are disease progression or escape from control. In the latter half of pregnancy, if the disease is limited, is causing no symptoms, and is moving at a slow pace, then one option is to delay therapy until term. If one feels compelled to treat, single-drug treatment with vinblastine could hold the line until delivery, with little apparent risk to the fetus.[68] A

Table 6–6. Risk in Mothers Diagnosed with Hodgkin's Disease Intrapartum

FIRST HALF OF PREGNANCY			
Staging			
Standard Maneuver	Fetal Risk	Option	Potential Consequence of Option
Lymphangiogram, CT scan	Radiation exposure	Avoid studies	Inadequate staging
Laparotomy	Abortion	Clinical staging	Inadequate staging
Therapeutic abortion	Fetal destruction	Maintain pregnancy	Exposure of fetus to hazards of therapy
Treatment			
Standard Maneuver	Fetal Risk	Option	Potential Consequences of Option
Radiation therapy	Teratogenesis ?Carcinogenic	Limit RT to upper hemithorax	Undertreatment of patient and scatter to fetus
Combination chemotherapy	Teratogenesis ?Carcinogenic	Single agent Rx	Undertreatment, select for drug resistance, still expose fetus to potentially toxic therapy
SECOND HALF OF PREGNANCY			
Staging			
Standard Maneuver	Fetal Risk	Option	Potential Consequences of Option
Lymphangiogram, CT scan	Radiation exposure	Avoid CT scan, limit LAG films	Inadequate staging
Laparotomy	Abortion	Clinical staging	Inadequate staging
Treatment			
Standard Maneuver	Fetal Risk	Option	Potential Consequences of Option
Radiation therapy	Teratogenesis ?Carcinogenic	Delay Rx until term	Advance in stage during delay and lose option to use RT
Combination chemotherapy	Teratogenesis ?Carcinogenic	Single agent Rx	Undertreatment; compromises later chemotherapy
		Delay Rx until term	Disease progression during delay

limited field of radiation above the diaphragm is somewhat problematic in this situation because of the unfavorable geometry and lessened ability to shield the fetus imposed by the large, gravid uterus. If the disease is rapidly progressive or immediately threatening, then aggressive therapy becomes essential, and there are reports of successful fetal outcome under these circumstances (see further on).

In the first half of pregnancy, however, a delay in treatment until term is unacceptably long. The Stanford group has recommended therapeutic abortion in this circumstance.[68] This approach will allow comprehensive staging and treatment of the mother at the time of disease presentation. It obviously moots the issue of danger to the fetus from medical maneuvers,[69, 70] and it has been criticized for ignoring anecdotal reports of the delivery of normal infants who had exposure to combination chemotherapy in utero in the first trimester or whose mothers had limited field radiation.[71–73] However, analysis of reproduction in a series of 37 patients treated on Cancer and Acute Leukemia Group B studies showed that of 14 women treated at conception or during gestation, there were four normal live births and five elective abortions but also four malformed offspring and one spontaneous abortion.[74] The latter figures represented a higher frequency of unfavorable outcome than seen either in the women in the analysis who had babies before diagnosis and treatment or after they were in remission or in the general population.

Because of the low incidence of the concurrence of Hodgkin's disease and pregnancy, the variables in disease presentation and progression, and ethical and personal considerations, there will never be prospective, randomized studies to resolve these issues. It will thus remain necessary to approach each case individually and to plan the management in light of the patient's views and the recommendation of consultants in medical oncology and radiation therapy. It is clear that pregnancy has no adverse effect on the course of Hodgkin's disease (whether the lymphoma was diagnosed and treated before or during pregnancy),[75] and it would seem prudent to advise the patient not to become pregnant for two years after treatment[76] because the risk for recurrence falls off rapidly after that time.

Effects of Treatment of Hodgkin's Disease on Ovarian Function and Reproduction

The use of oophoropexy and appropriate radiation fields and shielding can spare ovarian function in women who receive pelvic radiotherapy. In a carefully analyzed series,[77] Horning and colleagues reported that in 19 women who had total lymphoid irradiation (ages of treatment ranged from 13 to 28 years), 18 continued to have menses (nine regularly, nine irregularly). Thirteen of the 19 had periods of temporary amenorrhea varying from several months to four years, implying that one must observe patients for a sufficient length of time before drawing conclusions about fertility. Of 10 "at risk" patients—i.e., those who had menses and did not use contraception—seven became pregnant.

Patients can continue to menstruate after receiving combination chemotherapy. In the same series as above, 29 of 34 drug-treated patients (age at treatment ranged from 15 to 38 years) had regular (19 patients) or irregular (10 patients) menses. Eight of 13 of these patients "at risk" for becoming pregnant were able to conceive.

On the other hand, total irradiation therapy plus chemotherapy resulted in only 24 of 50 patients (age range at treatment was 15 to 36 years) who had menses thereafter (10 regular, 14 irregular). Five of 11 patients "at risk" became pregnant.

It would appear from this and other studies that the younger a patient is at the time of treatment and the more limited the therapy, the more likely it is that ovarian function will be preserved.[77–80] It should also be re-emphasized that, as part of proper medical management, women of childbearing age who undergo staging laparotomy should have midline oophoropexy and the placement of metallic clips next to the ovaries to allow proper location and shielding during radiation.

Even with preservation of fertility, there is still concern about the long-term impact of ionizing radiation and drugs such as the alkylating agents and procarbazine upon the ova and ultimately the children of treated patients, even when conception takes place well after treatment has ended. As Blatt and coworkers have pointed out,[44] it is known from animal studies that anomalies induced in offspring may not appear until later in life, and it is even more difficult to evaluate the risk in humans. It appears that fewer patients have children after treatment; a number of those who do not conceive may elect therapeutic abortion; aborted fetuses, infants, and children may not be adequately screened for defects; applied therapies are nonuniform from one treatment center to the next; and therapy-induced cases of mutagenesis tend to be emphasized in the literature, frustrating estimation of the true proportion of unfavorable outcomes.[44]

In the Horning study detailed earlier, in which patients were treated on protocol in a lymphoma study center,[77] there were 28 pregnancies, among which there were five therapeutic abortions, two premature and one low-birth-weight infant (all of whom developed normally), and 21 normal births. There were no birth defects or developmental abnormalities. An earlier study by Holms and Holms suggested that a history of radiation therapy alone in the mother did not increase the risk to the fetus, but the prior use of combined irradiation and chemotherapy did (nine combined therapy patients produced nine normal and five abnormal offspring).[81] However, the patients from this study were collected from a 31-year period (1944 to 1975) of nonprotocol therapy, when there had to be tremendous variation in the type and quality of the applied treatment.

NON-HODGKIN'S LYMPHOMA

The NHLs differ in several important ways from Hodgkin's disease. They tend to disseminate earlier in their course, they are less orderly and predictable in their spread, they affect older patients more frequently, and they commonly have extranodal sites of presentation. Whereas stage is the dominant factor in therapy and prognosis of Hodgkin's disease, in the NHL, histologic subtype is most important. Until recently the Rappaport classification was the standard terminology (see Table 6–7), and the reader should consult reference 83 for a review of the new Working Formulation for the Classification of the NHL. In the Rappaport system, the histologies fall into "favorable" (indolent) and "unfavorable" (aggressive) subtypes based upon the presence or absence of a nodular histologic pattern and the morphology of the malignant cells.[82]

Patients' disease is staged with the same procedures as in Hodgkin's disease, except that laparotomy is used much more sparingly because of (1) the high incidence of disseminated disease discoverable by less invasive techniques, and (2) the older age of the patients (and consequent higher risk of surgical complications).[83, 84]

Treatment options include radiation therapy for the small proportion of patients with early stage disease; single-agent or moderately aggressive combination drug therapy (chlorambucil; chlorambucil + prednisone; or cyclophosphamide, vincristine, and prednisone) for patients with more advanced favorable subtypes; or intensive

Table 6–7. Histopathologic Classification of Non-Hodgkin's Lymphoma[82, 83]

Cell Type	Pattern	Prognosis
Lymphocytic		
Well differentiated	Diffuse	Good
Poorly differentiated	Diffuse	Poor
Poorly differentiated	Nodular	Good
Histiocytic	Diffuse	Poor
	Nodular	Poor
Mixed lymphocytic and histiocytic	Diffuse	Poor
	Nodular	Good
Undifferentiated	Diffuse	Poor

combination chemotherapy (including various combinations of drugs such as cyclophosphamide, vincristine, prednisone, doxorubicin, VP16, bleomycin, and methotrexate) for patients with unfavorable subtypes.[82, 85, 86]

In patients who truly have stages I and II disease, 50 to 90% may be cured with radiation or chemotherapy or both.[85, 86] There is a paradox in the more advanced stages. Patients with favorable subtypes have a median survival of seven to eight years after diagnosis, and aggressive therapy, despite complete response rates approaching 80%, does not seem to produce durable remissions and cure and has not significantly shifted the survival curve.[85] Hence, there is a trend toward more consecutive management of these patients.

By contrast, patients with aggressive subtypes have median survival times measured in months, in the absence of effective therapies. Paradoxically, these patients can have complete response rates of 40 to 70% after intensive drug treatment, and these figures do translate into stable long-term remissions and probable cure in roughly one half to two thirds of those entering complete remission. Patients with unfavorable subtypes who do not achieve a complete remission or who relapse tend to succumb quickly. Thus, in these subtypes, initial aggressive management is the appropriate course.[86]

Pregnancy and Non-Hodgkin's Lymphoma

The coexistence of pregnancy and NHL is infrequent, reflecting in part the older ages at which patients develop these tumors (in contrast to Hodgkin's disease, which has its peak age incidence in the childbearing years). Fourteen cases have appeared in the literature.[87–89] In eleven, maternal death, prematurity, or therapeutic abortion was the outcome. In two cases, chemotherapy began in the second trimester,[87, 88] remission was obtained, and healthy infants were delivered. In the third case, the lymphoma appeared at 33 weeks and treatment was delayed to nine days post partum.[89]

As in Hodgkin's disease (see earlier), the features of the individual case (e.g., histologic subtype, extent of disease, stage of pregnancy at diagnosis, parental philosophy) will determine the options and management decisions.

GENITAL TRACT PRESENTATION OF LYMPHOMAS

Although genital tract symptoms as the primary manifestations of lymphoma are rare, genital tract involvement occurs with reasonable frequency. In series from the Armed Forces Institute of Pathology, 297 women with lymphoma presented with complaints referable to the genital tract.[90] All forms of lymphoma have been described in one location or another.[91–94] Diagnosis prior to surgery is often difficult, because patients with pelvic tumors require laparotomy to establish the exact diagnosis. When lymphoma is suspected, careful staging should be done at the time of surgery. Treatment should be based on histologic diagnosis and stage, as described previously. Excessively aggressive pelvic surgery should be avoided, as it in no way improves outcome and may significantly increase morbidity.

REFERENCES

1. Wintrobe, M.M., Lee, G.R., Boggs, D.R., et al.: Clinical Hematology. 8th Ed. Philadelphia, Lea & Febiger, 1981.
2. Ihle, J.N.: Experimental models and conceptual approaches to study of lymphomas and leukemia: Etiology, biology and control. Semin Hematol *15*:95, 1978.
3. Lillienfield, A.M.: Epidemiological studies of the leukemogenic effects of radiation. Yale J Biol Med *39*:143, 1966.
4. Stewart, A., Webb, J., and Hewitt, D.: A survey of childhood malignancies. Br Med J *1*:1495, 1958.

5. Bross, I.D.J., and Natarajan, N.: Leukemia from low-level radiation. N Engl J Med *287*:107, 1972.
6. Linos, A., Gray, J., and Orvis, A.L.: Low-dose radiation and leukemia. N Engl J Med *302*:1101, 1980.
7. Coleman, C.N., Williams, C.J., Flint, A., et al.: Hematologic neoplasia in patients treated for Hodgkin's disease. N Engl J Med *297*:1249, 1977.
8. Reimer, R.R., Hoover, R., Fraumeni, J.F., and Young, R.C.: Acute leukemia after alkylating-agent therapy of ovarian cancer. N Engl J Med *297*:177, 1977.
9. Hersh, E.M.: Causes of death in acute leukemia. JAMA *193*:105, 1965.
10. Gale, R.P.: Advances in the treatment of acute myelogenous leukemia. N Engl J Med *300*:1189, 1979.
11. Bodey, G.P., and Rodriguez, V.: Approaches to the treatment of acute leukemia and lymphoma in adults. Semin Hematol *15*:221, 1978.
12. Thomas, E.D., Clift, R.A., and Buckner, C.D.: Marrow transplantation for patients with acute non-lymphoblastic leukemia who achieve a first remission. Cancer Treat Rep *66*:1463, 1982.
13. Mauer, A.M.: Therapy of acute lymphoblastic leukemia in childhood. Blood *56*:1, 1980.
14. McLain, C.R.: Leukemia in pregnancy. Clin Obstet Gynecol *17*:185, 1974.
15. Pauling, D.F., McLean, F.W., and Noyes, W.D.: Normal fetus after cytosine arabinoside therapy. Ann Intern Med *74*:1012, 1971.
16. Ewing, P.A., and Wittaker, J.A.: Acute leukemia in pregnancy. Obstet Gynecol *42*:245, 1973.
17. Bhoopathi, B., Ostapowicz, F., and Bayley, W.: Acute promyelocytic leukemia in pregnancy. Obstet Gynecol *41*:275, 1973.
18. Raich, P.C., and Curet, L.B.: Treatment of acute leukemia during pregnancy. Cancer *36*:861, 1975.
19. Wegelius, R.: Successful pregnancy in acute leukemia. Lancet *2*:1301, 1975.
20. Krueger, J.A., Davis, R.B., and Field, C.: Multiple-drug chemotherapy in the management of acute lymphocytic leukemia during pregnancy. Obstet Gynecol *48*:324, 1976.
21. Gokal, R., Durrant, J., Baum, J.D., et al.: Successful pregnancy in acute monocytic leukemia. Br J Cancer *34*:299, 1976.
22. Lilleyman, J.S., Hill, A.S., and Anderton, K.J.: Consequences of acute myelogenous leukemia in early pregnancy. Cancer *40*:1300, 1977.
23. Durie, B.G.M., and Giles, H.R.: Successful treatment of acute leukemia during pregnancy. Arch Intern Med *137*:90, 1977.
24. Newcomb, M., Balducci, L., Thigpen, J.T., and Morrison, F.S.: Acute leukemia in pregnancy. Successful delivery after cytarabine and doxorubicin. JAMA *239*:2691, 1978.
25. Lowenthal, R.M., Marsden, K.A., Newman, N.M., et al.: Normal infant after treatment of acute myeloid leukemia in pregnancy with daunorubicin. Aust NZ J Med *8*:431, 1978.
26. O'Donnell, R., Costigan, C., and O'Connell, L.G.: Two cases of acute leukaemia in pregnancy. Acta Haematol *61*:298, 1979.
27. Doney, K.C., Kraemer, K.G., and Shepard, T.H.: Combination chemotherapy for acute myelocytic leukemia during pregnancy: Three case reports. Cancer Treat Rep *63*:369, 1979.
28. Hamer, J.W., Beard, M.E.J., and Duff, G.B.: Pregnancy complicated by acute myeloid leukaemia. NZ Med J *89*:212, 1979.
29. Okun, D.B., Groncy, P.K., Sieger, L., and Tanaka, K.R.: Acute leukemia in pregnancy: Transient neonatal myelosuppression after combination chemotherapy in the mother. Med Pediatr Oncol *7*:315, 1979.
30. Tobias, J.S., and Bloom, H.J.G.: Doxorubicin in pregnancy. Lancet *1*:776, 1980.
31. Pizzuto, J., Aviles, A., Noriega, L., et al.: Treatment of acute leukemia during pregnancy: Presentation of nine cases. Cancer Treat Rep *64*:679, 1980.
32. Taylor, G., and Bloom, J.: Acute leukemia during pregnancy. South Med J *73*:1314, 1980.
33. Schafer, A.I.: Teratogenic effects of antileukemic chemotherapy. Arch Intern Med *141*:514, 1981.
34. Alegre, A., Chunchurreta, R., Rodriguez-Alcaron, J., et al.: Successful therapy in acute promyelocytic leukemia. Cancer *49*:152, 1982.
35. Plows, C.W.: Acute myelomonocytic leukemia in pregnancy: Report of a case. Am J Obstet Gynecol *143*:41, 1982.
36. Nicholson, H.D.: Cytotoxic drugs in pregnancy. J Obstet Gynaecol Br Cwlth *75*:307, 1968.
37. Sweet, D.L., and Kinzie, J.: Consequences of radiotherapy, and antineoplastic therapy for the fetus. J Reprod Med *17*:241, 1986.
38. Maurer, L.H., Forcier, R.J., McIntyre, O.R., et al.: Fetal group C trisomy after cytosine arabinoside and thioguanine. Ann Intern Med *76*:809, 1971.
39. Siris, E.S., Leventhall, B.G., and Vaitukaitis, J.L.: Effects of childhood leukemia and chemotherapy on puberty and reproductive function in girls. N Engl J Med *294*:1143, 1976.
40. Warne, G.L., Fairley, K.F., Hobbs, J.B., et al.: Cyclophosphamide-induced ovarian failure. N Engl J Med *209*:1159, 1973.
41. DeGroot, G.W., Fairman, C., and Winter, J.S.D.: Cyclophosphamide and the prepubertal gonad. J Pediatr *84*:123, 1974.
42. Bacon, C., and Kernahan, J.: Successful pregnancy in acute leukemia. Lancet *2*:515, 1975.
43. Estiu, M.: Successful pregnancy in leukemia. Lancet *1*:433, 1977.

44. Blatt, J., Mulvihill, J.J., Ziegler, J., et al.: Pregnancy outcome following cancer chemotherapy. Am J Med *69*:828, 1980.
45. Laros, R.K.: Therapeutic amenorrhea in hematologic disorders. Obstet Gynecol *38*:589, 1971.
46. Koeffler, H.P., and Golde, D.W.: Chronic myelogenous leukemia—new concepts (first of two parts). N Engl J Med *304*:1201, 1981.
47. DeChatel, L.R.: Absence of measurable leukocyte alkaline phosphatase activity from leukocytes of patients with chronic granulocytic leukemia. Clin Chem *16*:798, 1970.
48. Koeffler, H.P., and Golde, D.W.: Chronic myelogenous leukemia—new concepts (second of two parts). N Engl J Med *304*:1269, 1981.
49. Boggs, D.R.: Factors influencing the character of survival in chronic lymphocytic leukemia. Am J Med *40*:243, 1966.
50. Miller, J.B.: Chronic myelogenous leukemia and myeloproliferative disease during the childbearing years. J Reprod Med *17*:217, 1976.
51. O'Dell, R.F.: Leukemia and lymphoma complicating pregnancy. Clin Obstet Gynecol *22*:859, 1979.
52. Johnson, F.D.: Pregnancy and concurrent chronic myelogenous leukemia. Am J Obstet Gynecol *112*:640, 1972.
53. Boros, S.J., and Reynolds, J.W.: Intrauterine growth retardation following third-trimester exposure to busulfan. Am J Obstet Gynecol *129*:111, 1977.
54. Bruder, M.L., Prager, D., and Renninger, C.W.: Dibromomannitol therapy of chronic myelogenous leukemia during pregnancy. Obstet Gynecol *43*:54, 1974.
55. Louis, J., Limarzi, L.R., and Best, W.R.: Treatment of chronic granulocytic leukemia with Myleran®. Arch Intern Med *97*:299, 1956.
56. Belohorsky, B., Sirack, J., Sandor, L., et al.: Comments on the development of amenorrhea caused by Myleran® in cases of chronic myelosis. Neoplasma *7*:397, 1960.
57. Campbell, W.A.B.: Familial neonatal leukemia. Arch Dis Child *37*:93, 1962.
58. Hogg, G.R., and Schmidt, O.A.: Myelogenous leukemia in a stillborn infant. Can Med Assoc J *78*:421, 1958.
59. Rothman, L.A., Cohen, C.J., and Astarloa, J.: Placental and fetal involvement by maternal malignancy. Am J Obstet Gynecol *116*:1023, 1973.
60. Desforges, J.F., and Rutherford, C.J.: Hodgkin's disease. N Engl J Med *301*:1212, 1979.
61. Cannon, W.B., and Nelsen, T.S.: Staging of Hodgkin's disease: A surgical perspective. Am J Surg *132*:224, 1976.
62. Kaplan, H.S.: Hodgkin's disease: Unfolding concepts concerning its nature, management, and prognosis. Cancer *45*:2439, 1980.
63. DeVita, V.T.: The consequences of the chemotherapy of Hodgkin's disease. Cancer *47*:1, 1981.
64. Hellman, S., and Mauch, P.: Role of radiation therapy in the treatment of Hodgkin's disease. Cancer Treat Rep *66*:915, 1982.
65. Stein, R.S., Golomb, H.M., Wiernik, P.H., et al.: Anatomic substages of stage III Hodgkin's disease: Follow-up of a collaborative study. Cancer Treat Rep *66*:733, 1982.
66. Hoppe, R.T., Cox, R.S., Rosenberg, S.A., and Kaplan, H.S.: Prognostic factors in pathologic stage III Hodgkin's disease. Cancer Treat Rep *66*:743, 1982.
67. Canellos, G.P., Come, S.E., and Skarin, A.T.: Chemotherapy in the treatment of Hodgkin's disease. Semin Hematol *20*:1, 1983.
68. Jacobs, C., Donaldson, S., Rosenberg, S.A., and Kaplan, H.S.: Management of the pregnant patient with Hodgkin's disease. Ann Int Med *95*:669, 1981.
69. Wells, J.H., Marshall, J.R., and Carbone, P.P.: Procarbazine therapy for Hodgkin's disease in early pregnancy. JAMA *205*:119, 1968.
70. Mennati, M.T., Shepard, T.H., and Mellman, W.J.: Fetal renal malformation following treatment of Hodgkin's disease during pregnancy. Obstet Gynecol *47*:194, 1975.
71. Manzanec, D.F., et al.: Letters to the editor. Pregnancy and Hodgkin's disease. Ann Int Med *96*:681, 1982.
72. Jones, R.T., and Weinerman, B.H.: MOPP given during pregnancy. Obstet Gynecol *54*:477, 1979.
73. Daly, H., McCann, S.R., and Temperley, I.J.: Successful pregnancy during combination chemotherapy for Hodgkin's disease. Acta Haematol *64*:154, 1980.
74. McKeen, E.A., Mulvihill, J.J., Rosner, F., and Zarrobi, M.H.: Pregnancy outcome in Hodgkin's disease. Lancet *2*:590, 1979.
75. Barry, R.M., Diamond, H.D., and Craver, L.F.: Influence of pregnancy on the course of Hodgkin's disease. Am J Obstet Gynecol *84*:445, 1962.
76. Hennessy, J.P., and Rottiono, A.: Hodgkin's disease and pregnancy. Am J Obstet Gynecol *87*:851, 1963.
77. Horning, S.J., Hoppe, R.T., Kaplan, H.S., and Rosenberg, S.A.: Female reproductive potential after treatment for Hodgkin's disease. N Engl J Med *304*:1377, 1981.
78. Chapman, R.M., Sutcliffe, S.B., and Malpas, J.S.: Cytotoxic-induced ovarian failure in Hodgkin's disease. JAMA *242*:1882, 1979.

79. Trueblood, H.W., Enright, L.P., Ray, G.R., et al.: Preservation of ovarian function in pelvic radiation for Hodgkin's disease. Arch Surg *100*:236, 1970.
80. Schilsky, R.L., Lewis, B.J., Sherins, R.J., et al.: Gonadal dysfunction in patients receiving chemotherapy for cancer. Ann Int Med *93*:109, 1980.
81. Holmes, G.E., and Holmes, F.F.: Pregnancy outcome of patients treated for Hodgkin's disease. Cancer *41*:1317, 1978.
82. Rosenberg, S.A.: Non-Hodgkin's lymphoma. N Engl J Med *301*:924, 1979.
83. The non-Hodgkin's lymphoma pathologic classification project. National Cancer Institute sponsored study of classification of non-Hodgkin's lymphoma. Summary and description of a working formulation for clinical usage. Cancer *49*:2112, 1982.
84. Chabner, B.A., Fisher, R.I., Young, R.C., et al.: Staging of non-Hodgkin's lymphoma. Semin Oncol *7*:285, 1980.
85. Portlock, C.S.: "Good risk" non-Hodgkin lymphomas: Approaches to management. Semin Hematol *20*:25, 1983.
86. Horwich, A., and Peckham, M.: "Bad risk" non-Hodgkin lymphomas. Semin Hematol *20*:35, 1983.
87. Ortega, J.: Multiple agent chemotherapy including bleomycin of non-Hodgkin's lymphoma during pregnancy. Cancer *40*:2829, 1977.
88. Falkson, H.C., Simson, I.W., and Falkson, G.: Non-Hodgkin's lymphoma in pregnancy. Cancer *45*:1679, 1980.
89. Villa Santa, U., Attar, S., and Jiji, R.: Malignant histiocytic lymphoma (reticulum cell sarcoma) in pregnancy. Gynecol Oncol *6*:383, 1978.
90. Chorlton, I., Karnei, R.F., King, F.N., et al.: Primary malignant reticuloendothelial disease involving the vagina, cervix, corpus uteri. Obstet Gynecol *44*:735, 1974.
91. Lathrop, J.C.: Malignant pelvic lymphomas. Obstet Gynecol *30*:137, 1967.
92. Buchler, D.A., and Kline, J.C.: Primary lymphoma of the vagina. Obstet Gynecol *40*:235, 1972.
93. Stransky, G.C., Acosta, A.A., Kaplan, A.L., and et al: Reticulum cell sarcoma of the cervix. Obstet Gynecol *41*:183, 1973.
94. Castaldo, T.W., Ballon, S.C., Lagasse, L.D., et al.: Reticulo-endothelial neoplasia of the female genital tract. Obstet Gynecol *54*:167, 1979.

Chapter 7

ERYTHROBLASTOSIS FETALIS

Russell K. Laros, Jr.

Erythroblastosis fetalis, or hemolytic disease of the newborn, is a condition in which the life span of the infant's red blood cells (RBCs) is shortened by the action of specific antibodies derived from the mother. These antibodies reach the fetal circulation by passive transfer across the placenta, attach themselves to antigens on the surface of the fetal red cell, and thus ultimately cause the premature destruction of the fetal RBCs in the reticuloendothelial system. In most instances, the mother becomes sensitized by foreign RBC antigens that have entered her circulation during a previous pregnancy or during abortion or blood transfusion.

HISTORY

In 400 B.C., Hippocrates described a syndrome with findings similar to what we now call hydrops fetalis. Although many individuals expounded on Hippocrates' observations, Darrow, in 1938, was the first to propose that the pathogenesis of erythroblastosis involved the formation of a maternal antibody against some component of fetal blood.[1] One year later, Levine and Stetson described an atypical agglutinin in the blood of a woman who had just delivered a stillborn infant.[2] They postulated that the maternal immunization was the result of a fetal antigen inherited from the father and absent from the surface of the maternal RBC.

During the four decades following Landsteiner and Weiner's discovery of the Rh antigen, many advances have occurred in our understanding of and treatment of erythroblastosis.[3] Some of the most significant contributions follow:

1954 Demonstration of the value of preterm delivery by Allen and associates.[4]

1956 Development of spectrophotometric analysis of amniotic fluid by Bevis.[5]

1963 Description of the first successful intrauterine transfusion used to treat erythroblastosis by Liley.[6]

1966 Development and demonstration of the efficacy of postpartum administration of Rh-immune globulin in preventing maternal sensitization by Freda, Gorman, and Pollack.[7]

1978 Development and demonstration of efficacy of a program of antenatal Rh-prophylaxis using Rh-immune globulin by Bowman and Pollack.[8]

PATHOPHYSIOLOGY

Blood groups represent systems of antigenic determinants found on the surface of RBCs. If incompatible RBCs are injected into an immunocompetent mammal, it will produce antibodies to the foreign antigens on the RBC's surface. The antibodies will then interact with the antigens, leading to the destruction of the foreign RBC and of any similar cells injected at a later time.

RED BLOOD CELL ANTIGENS

The RBC antigens are glycolipids or proteins and are always located on the surface of the cell. While the exact nature of some of these antigens has been elucidated (A, B, Lewis, I, i, P, M, N), the composition of most of the antigens is not yet known. The genes controlling the structures of the antigens in a particular blood group system occupy corresponding loci on a pair of homologous chromosomes. With the exception of the Xg^a blood group, all blood group genes are carried on autosomes. In most cases there is a direct correspondence between genes and antigens such that if an individual inherits a specific gene, the antigen will be detected on the RBCs. An exception to this rule is the interrelationship between the ABO and Lewis blood groups.

ABO Antigens

The ABO antigens are inherited as simple mendelian characters.[9] Antibodies reacting with A or B antigens are regularly found in the serum when the corresponding antigen is absent from the RBC. Additionally, there are antibodies that react preferentially with O cells, and the antigen defined by these reactions is known as H substance. Its presence is controlled by an allelic pair of genes, H-h, which are independent of the ABO system. Table 7–1 lists the various combinations possible in the ABO system.

Approximately 80% of Northern Europeans with A, B, or H antigens on their RBCs secrete the antigens into various tissues and body fluids. The capacity to secrete these substances is under the control of another pair of allelic genes, Se-se. Se is dominant, and only the homozygous se-se genotype is a "nonsecretor."[10]

Lewis Antigens

The Lewis system consists of the Le^a and Le^b antigens. Unlike their ABH counterparts, these antigens are not an integral part of the RBC membrane but are acquired from the plasma. The presence of the Le^a antigen is under the control of two allelic genes, Le-le, which are inherited independently of the ABO, H-h, and Se-se genes. A complex interrelationship among these three gene systems leads to three Lewis phenotypes: $Le(a^+b^-)$, $Le(a^-b^-)$, and $Le(a^-b^+)$.[11]

Rh Antigens

The Rh system is the most complex of the blood group systems and is currently characterized by more than 30 known antigens and a far larger number of complex alleles. According to the Fisher-Race system, the inheritance of the Rh antigens is determined by three pairs of allelic genes, C-c, D-d, and E-e, acting at three very

Table 7–1. The ABO Blood Groups

Phenotype Group	Genotype	Red Cell Antigens	Antibodies in Serum
O	OO	None	Anti-A and Anti-B
A	AA or AO	A	Anti-B
B	BB or BO	B	Anti-A
AB	AB	AB	None

closely linked loci.[11] The Wiener system, by contrast, assumes that the Rh phenotype is determined by a single genetic locus with many alleles.[12] Despite expansion over the years, the Fisher-Race system has not been adequate to account for all the reactions that have been observed within the Rh system. However, because the CDE-cde nomenclature is readily remembered and enables one to see immediately how a given sample of cells will react with the available antisera, the World Health Organization has recently recommended that the Fisher-Race system be adopted.[13] Table 7–2 details the observed frequency of the common Rh genes in a British population.[11]

A number of variants exist for each of the common Rh antigens. Examples include D^u, C^w, C^x, and E^w. These antigens are thought to be missing various components of the usual antigen and thus are rather weak in their ability to excite antibody production. The D^u antigen is of particular importance because it is common in the black population. In most individuals the D^u antigen differs from the normal D only in that there are fewer antigenic sites per RBC. In other subjects, however, D^u variants have both a qualitative and quantitative defect. These latter individuals can also make an antibody against D^u antigen. The heterogenicity of the D^u antigen is evidenced by the fact that some are detectable only by indirect antiglobulin (Coombs') techniques; some are detectable only by absorption and elution of anti-D; while others are distinguishable from D antigen only in that their agglutination is brought about by some but not all anti-D sera. Because antisera capable of distinguishing between normal D^u (quantitative defect) and D^u variants (qualitative defect) are not widely available, some argue that it is safest to consider all D^u subjects as D-negative if they are to receive a blood transfusion. However, the likelihood of exciting anti-D formation in a D^u subject by transfusion of D-positive cells is exceedingly small. Similarly, D^u individuals are not considered candidates for Rh-immunoglobulin prophylaxis following delivery. To date, only 18 cases of hemolytic disease of the newborn caused by anti-D produced by D^u-positive women have been reported.[14]

Other Blood Group Antigens

There are many other blood group systems that will not be discussed in detail. The interested reader is referred to an excellent review by Weinstein for additional material.[15] However, because they are capable of causing erythroblastosis fetalis, the genotypes and gene frequencies for the Kell, MNSs, Kidd, and Duffy blood group systems are summarized in Table 7–3.

The antigens of the Rh, Kell, Duffy, Kidd, and MNSs systems are all fully developed

Table 7–2. Frequency of the Common Rh Genes

Fisher-Race	Wiener	Frequency* (%)
cde	r	38.0
Cde	r′	0.6
cdE	r″	0.5
CdE	r^y	0.01
cDe	R^0	2.7
CDe	R^1	41.0
cDE	R^2	15.0
CDE	R^z	0.2

* Frequencies for an English population.[11]

Table 7–3. Frequencies of Kell, MNSs, Kidd, and Duffy Blood Group Genes

Blood Group System	Genotype	Frequency[11] Blacks (%)	Caucasians (%)
Kell	KK	—*	0.2
	Kk	—	8.7
	kk	—	91.1
MNSs	MS	—*	24.7
	Ms	—	28.3
	NS	—	8.0
	Ns	—	39.0
Kidd	Jk^aJk^a	57.0	26.0
	Jk^aJk^b	34.0	50.0
	Jk^bJk^b	9.0	24.0
	Jk^-Jk^-	rare	rare
Duffy	Fy^{a+b-}	5.0	17.0
	Fy^{a-b+}	12.0	34.0
	Fy^{a+b+}	1.0	49.0
	Fy^{a-b-}	82.0	0.03

* Separate data not available.

and present on the surface of the human RBC at birth.[11] In contrast, the newborn's RBCs react weakly with antibodies to the ABO, Lutheran, and Lewis antigens. The I antigen, present on some adult RBCs, is very weakly expressed on fetal RBCs. Conversely, fetal RBCs react far more strongly than do adult cells with anti-i.

RED BLOOD CELL ANTIBODIES

In humans, the immunoglobulins most commonly associated with RBC antigen-antibody reactions are of the IgM and IgG classes. These antibodies may be either naturally occurring or arise in response to sensitization by foreign RBC antigens. Anti-A and anti-B are the most common, naturally occurring antibodies, and their relationship to the ABO phenotypes is summarized in Table 7–1. Naturally occurring antibodies also exist in the MNSs system for some 2 to 3% of the population but are otherwise exceedingly rare.

The immune response to the first exposure to foreign RBC antigens is called the primary response and consists of relatively slow production of first IgM and then IgG antibody. Subsequent exposure to the same antigen invokes the secondary response, which is characterized by a more rapid production of relatively larger amounts of antibody.

A detailed discussion of the mechanism of antigen-antibody interaction is beyond the scope of this text; however, in general, IgM antibodies lead to in vivo intravascular hemolysis, whereas IgG antibodies lead to a slower destruction of RBCs in the reticuloendothelial system. Of great clinical importance is the fact that only IgG antibodies are able to cross the placenta and thus have the potential for causing erythroblastosis fetalis. This information is summarized in Table 7–4. In the laboratory, antibodies are characterized on the basis of their serologic behavior. Table 7–5 summarizes these characteristics. Most naturally occurring antibodies are saline agglutinins. In contrast, immune antibodies developing in response to transfusion or

Table 7–4. Immunoglobulin Class and Specificity

Class of Immunoglobulin	Able to Cross Placenta	Specific Antibody	
IgG	Yes	anti-AB anti-D anti-C anti-E anti-K anti-k anti-Fy^a	anti-Fy^b anti-Jk^a anti-Jk^b anti-S anti-s anti-Lu^b Public and private antigens
IgM	No	anti-A anti-B anti-H anti-I anti-Le^a anti-Le^b	anti-E anti-M anti-S anti-P anti-Lu^a Public and private antigens

pregnancy usually do not agglutinate RBCs in saline but are more likely to be albumin agglutinins or may react only in the antiglobulin (Coombs') test.

MECHANISMS OF SENSITIZATION

Table 7–6 summarizes the various mechanisms thought to be responsible for maternal sensitization. As a result of careful blood banking techniques, donor-recipeint incompatibility is now an unusual cause of either Rh or ABO sensitization. However, a recent survey of 2286 transfusion facilities discovered 44 women of childbearing age who had received blood of an inappropriate type. Because blood banks do not routinely check for donor-recipient compatibility except for A, B, and D antigens, transfusion will continue to be a source of maternal sensitization for all the other blood group systems.[16]

As recently as the 1950s it was common practice to treat children suffering from recurrent respiratory infections with a small volume injection of parental whole blood. These intramuscular injections were thought to enhance the child's resistance to further infections. Fortunately, this cause of sensitization to maternal antigens has ended.

Taylor proposed the passage of Rh-positive maternal cells into an Rh-negative fetus just before or at the time of delivery to explain the development of Rh sensitization (in an otherwise unexposed individual).[17] While this so-called "grandmother theory" of sensitization is possible, two large, prospective studies indicate that it occurs rarely and conclude that routine administration of Rh-immune globulin to Rh-negative neonates is not indicated.[18, 19]

Table 7–5. Physical and Serologic Characteristics of Antibodies

Class of Immunoglobulin	Sedimentation Constant	Serologic Reactivity
IgM	19S	Saline agglutinins
IgG	7S	Albumin agglutinins Coombs' reactive antibodies

Table 7–6. Mechanisms of Maternal Sensitization

Nonobstetric
Incompatible blood transfusion
Whole blood injections
In utero maternal to fetal tranfusion
Obstetric
Transplacental hemorrhage
Abortion
Ectopic pregnancy
Prenatal
Spontaneous
Traumatic
Postpartum

The most common cause of maternal sensitization is transplacental hemorrhage. Approximately 50% of women show evidence of transplacental hemorrhage at some time during the course of pregnancy or immediately following delivery.[20] Both the likelihood and volume of transplacental hemorrhage are increased in association with cesarean section, manual removal of the placenta, external version, and amniocentesis.[21]

Abortion and ectopic pregnancy are also associated with a significant incidence of transplacental hemorrhage. Bowman reports that transplacental hemorrhage occurs in 20% of cases undergoing therapeutic abortion, 4% of which are associated with a transfusion volume of greater than 0.2 ml. In contrast, the transfusion volume following spontaneous abortion is usually less than 0.1 ml.[21]

FETAL PATHOLOGY

The basic pathogenesis of erythroblastosis in utero is destruction of fetal RBCs by maternal antibody passively transferred across the placenta. If the rate of RBC destruction exceeds the marrow's productive capacity, progressive anemia ensues. When the normal marrow reserves are insufficient, extramedullary hematopoiesis begins and occurs primarily in the fetal liver and spleen. Thus hepato- and splenomegaly are common physical findings in erythroblastosis.

When rapid hemolysis leads to extensive hepatic extramedullary hematopoiesis, there is marked physical and functional liver impairment. Portal and umbilical venous hypertension develop, leading to ascites and placental edema. The functional liver impairment is evidenced by decreased protein synthesis, which leads to fetal hypoalbuminemia. Progressive hypoproteinemia accentuates the development of increased ascites and ultimately leads to the development of anasarca. These stages of severe edema and ascites are the findings of hydrops fetalis. In the end stage of hydrops, hydrothorax and pulmonary edema occur. Hydrops fetalis is attended by an extremely high mortality rate with or without medical intervention. Although the above pathophysiologic events are in part hypothetical, there is significant clinical and experimental evidence substantiating many of the steps.[22, 23]

MATERNAL PATHOLOGY

In 1900 Ballantyne described a syndrome of fetal hydrops, placental swelling, and maternal edema that he termed "triple edema." In the mid-20th century this entity was described as the "maternal syndrome" and is characterized by the coexistence of fetal hydrops and symptoms simulating toxemia of pregnancy.[24, 25] The maternal syndrome is rarely seen today because of early diagnosis and treatment of isoimmunization; however, its existence should be kept in mind.

DIAGNOSIS

Approximately 1% of deliveries in the United States result in an infant affected by erythroblastosis fetalis. Three quarters of these cases are related to ABO incompatibility. Although responsible for far fewer cases of erythroblastosis, the Rh system and other blood group systems producing IgG antibodies lead to more severe erythroblastosis.

SEROLOGY AND HISTORY

Obviously the history of a previously affected infant alerts the obstetrician to the risk of erythroblastosis in each subsequent pregnancy. However, if all cases of isoimmunization are to be detected and properly managed, all prenatal patients must have ABO typing, Rh typing, and a screen for the presence of atypical antibodies (other than anti-A, anti-B, or anti-D). Knowledge of a given patient's Rh and ABO blood types will tell the physician which cases are at risk for Rh or ABO isoimmunization. The antibody screen will detect actual Rh sensitization and also the presence of various atypical antibodies that also may lead to erythroblastosis.

In a study of 18,378 prenatal patients, Queenan and colleagues found evidence of isoimmunization in 574 (3.12%).[26] In this series, 53% of the antibodies were anti-D; the data are summarized in Table 7–7. Similar data reinforcing the importance of screening for atypical antibodies have been reported by both Pirofsky and Polesky.[27, 28] In contrast to Queenan's data, these studies reported a significant occurrence of anti-ABH antibodies (9.2% and 18.3%, respectively).

Table 7–7. Antibodies Found in Sera of 18,378 Prenatal Patients

Antibody	Number	Frequency (% of Positive Sera)
anti-D	304	48.3
nonspecific	84	13.3
anti-C	34	5.4
anti-E	34	5.4
anti-K	30	4.8
anti-Le^b	29	4.6
anti-Le^a	22	3.5
anti-I	15	2.4
anti-P	15	2.4
anti-M	14	2.2
anti-c	12	1.9
anti-Fy^a	11	1.7
anti-Jk^a	6	1.0
anti-S	6	1.0
anti-V	5	0.7
anti-Lu^a	3	0.4
anti-e	3	0.4
anti-Fy^b	1	0.2
anti-Go^a	1	0.2
anti-Jk^b	1	0.2
Total	630	100.0

ABO-ERYTHROBLASTOSIS FETALIS

ABO incompatibility rarely causes serious in utero erythroblastosis. Rather, it manifests itself as jaundice in the newborn, which rarely is severe enough to require exchange transfusion. ABO-erythroblastosis essentially never causes severe fetal anemia and thus does not require early delivery or intrauterine transfusion as part of its management.

A and B antigens are ubiquitous in nature and are present on many gram-negative bacteria. Thus immunization to A and B antigen does not require prior exposure to foreign RBCs. Exposure to gut bacteria stimulates the production of isoagglutinins within the first year of life, which remain thereafter. Thus the presence of naturally occurring anti-A and anti-B antibodies explains why 40% of ABO-erythroblastosis cases occur in firstborn infants.

Because A and B antigens occur on all somatic cells and 80% of individuals also secrete the antigens into body fluids, there is a large amount of antigen to compete with fetal RBCs for any passively transferred maternal antibody. This fact, as well as the relatively low affinity of maternal isoagglutinins for fetal A and B antigen, probably accounts for the mild nature of ABO-erythroblastosis.

Serologic evaluation of the mother has not been useful in defining a population at risk. Rather, a cord blood specimen should be obtained for each infant delivered from blood type O mothers. If the newborn's type is either A or B, a direct Coombs' test will usually be positive if erythroblastosis is present, and this mandates careful observation of the newborn's bilirubin levels.

Rh AND OTHER BLOOD GROUP ERYTHROBLASTOSIS FETALIS

The key feature of Rh and other blood groups is the unique character of their antigens. The antigens do not appear on other somatic cells, and sensitization occurs only as a consequence of exposure to RBCs.

Rho(D) SENSITIZATION

Rho(D) is a potent antigen and may lead to severe erythroblastosis in the first sensitized pregnancy. The probability of sensitization during a first Rh-incompatible pregnancy is approximately 17%. This incidence is reduced if the pregnancy is also ABO-incompatible.[30] It is hypothesized that the maternal isoagglutinins lead to rapid removal of fetal cells and thus lessen the risk of sensitization.

Although the first affected infant is often only mildly involved, 6% to 8% will be hydropic.[31, 32] In a series of patients not treated with early delivery or intrauterine transfusion, previous history had a profound effect on prognosis for the current pregnancy. Data collected by Walker and associates is summarized in Table 7–8 and clearly indicates that each affected infant has a progressively worse prognosis.[32]

Carefully performed anti-D titers using the same technique and the same Rh-positive test cells are of some prognostic significance. Because techniques of antibody determination vary greatly from laboratory to laboratory, it is essential for the obstetrician to become familiar with the methodology and reliability of the laboratory he or she uses. Most laboratories find no occurrences of intrauterine fetal deaths if the indirect antiglobulin titer (Coombs') is less than 1:8 or 4 IU/ml.[33] To determine if anti-D is present, it is necessary to repeat the antibody titers at regular intervals. A typical regimen is every two to four months prior to 20 weeks and then monthly to term.

Table 7–8. The Effect of Previous History on Current Risk for an Rh-Positive Fetus in an Rh-Sensitized Pregnancy*

Previous History	Risk of Stillbirth in Present Pregnancy (%)
No previously affected infant	7
Mildly affected infant	2
Moderately or severely affected infant	20
Very severely affected infant	55
One previous stillbirth	70
More than one previous stillbirth	80

* From Walker W, Murray R, Sherlagh V, et al.: Stillbirth due to haemolytic disease of the newborn. J Obstet Gynaecol Br Emp *64*:573, 1957.

Irregular Blood Group Sensitization

While primary sensitization to one of the other blood group antigens is a relatively rare occurrence, a second response will occur in an immunized individual upon re-exposure to only minute amounts of antigen. The various irregular antibodies are detected by antibody screening. The antibody screen consists of mixing the patient's serum with a mixture of human group O RBCs that possess all or most of the blood group antigens associated with either erythroblastosis or transfusion reactions or both. The study is carried out using antiglobulin serum (Coombs'). To adequately test for irregular antibodies, antibody screen should be performed on the first prenatal visit regardless of the mother's Rh type. If the screen is positive, the specific antibody(ies) are identified and the titer determined. In contrast to the situation with anti-D, virtually no laboratories have sufficient experience with the other blood group systems to allow choice of a titer level below which intrauterine hydrops or death do not occur.

Based on Weinstein's review and other reports, Table 7–9 lists situations in which amniocentesis may not be required to assess the degree of fetal anemia.[15, 34, 35]

AMNIOTIC FLUID ANALYSIS

The introduction of spectrophotometric analysis of amniotic fluid by Bevis[5] and later refinement by Liley[36] revolutionized the management of sensitized pregnancies. Many other investigators have confirmed these observations and support the concept

Table 7–9. Mild Hemolytic Disease Requiring Only Expectant Management

Blood Group System	Antigens
Kell	k, ko, kp^a, Kp^b, Js^a, Js^b
MNSs	Vw
Lutheran	Lu^a, Lu^b
Diego	Di^b
Xg	Xg^a
Public antigens	Lan, Ge
Private antigens	Batty, Becker, Berrens, Evans, Gonzales, Hunt, Jobbins, Rm, Ven

that spectrophotometric analysis of amniotic fluid provides a great deal of information concerning the status of the fetus. The amount of bilirubin pigment in amniotic fluid is directly proportional to the absorbance of monochromatic light at a wavelength of 450 mμ. Figure 7–1 is a spectrophotometric scan of normal amniotic fluid. The scan is made by a recording spectrophotometer, which plots light absorbance (optical density) against wavelength. A straight line tangent to the plot at 375 and 525 mμ is projected as representative of bilirubin-free fluid. Figure 7–2 is a spectrophotometric plot of amniotic fluid with a moderate-sized bilirubin peak at 450 mμ.

When amniotic fluid is collected by amniocentesis, it must be protected from light, which will cause a decrease in bilirubin pigment. Epithelial cells, vernix, meconium, and RBCs can also markedly alter spectrophotometric properties. Figure 7–3 shows the effects of hemoglobin contamination. Oxyhemoglobin produces peaks at 415 mμ, 540 mμ, and 580 mμ, which destroys the validity of the 450 mμ bilirubin peak. The interested reader is referred to Queenan's detailed discussion of amniotic fluid analysis.[37]

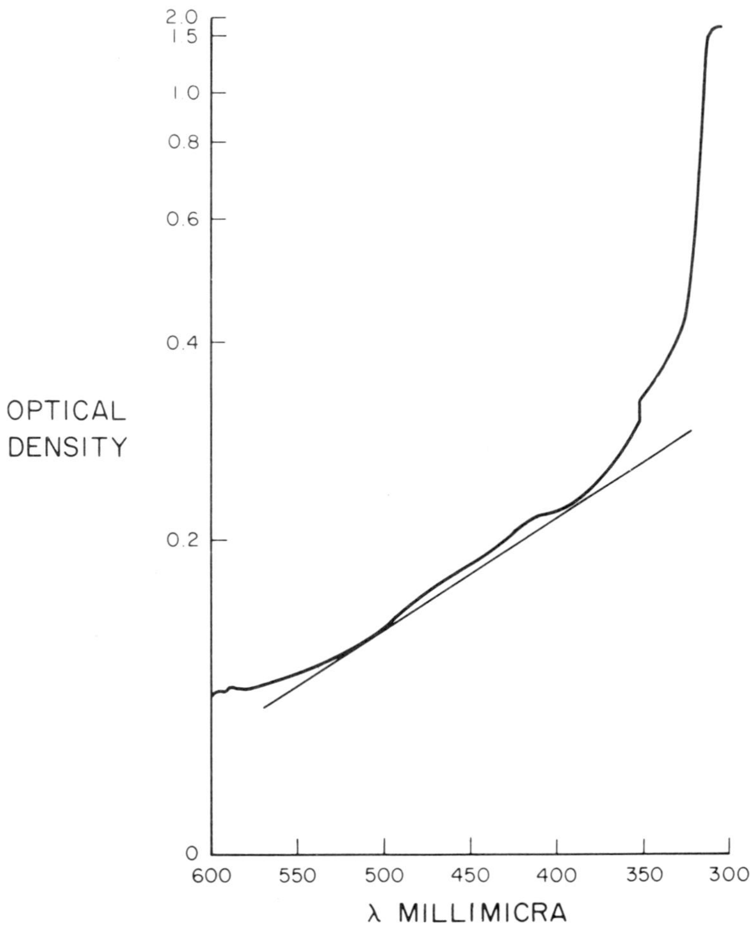

Figure 7–1. A spectrophotometric scan of normal amniotic fluid.

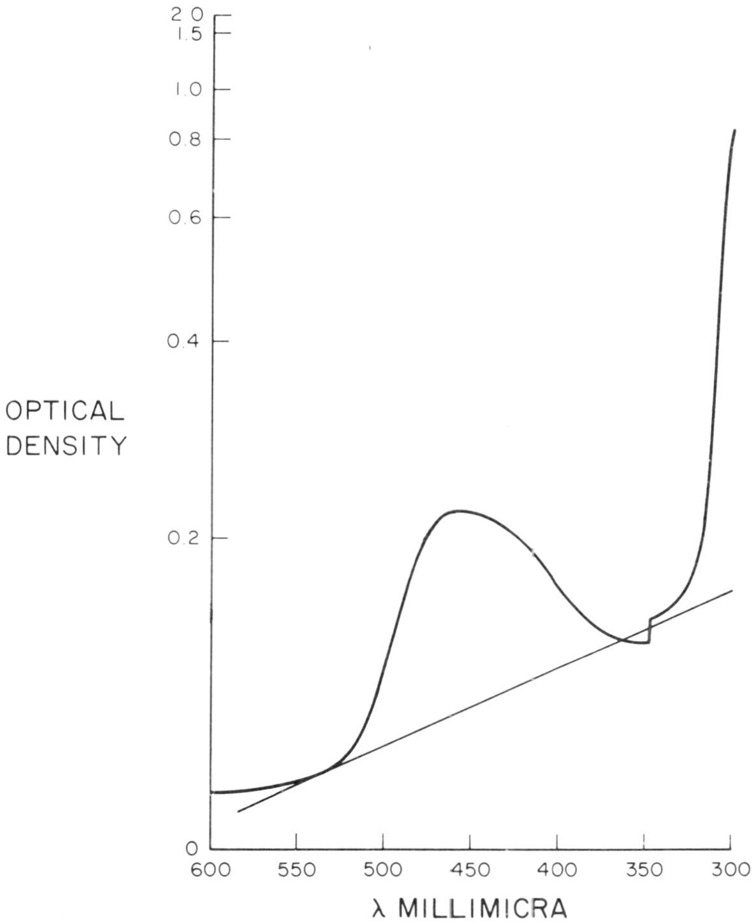

Figure 7–2. A spectrophotometric scan of amniotic fluid with a moderate ΔOD.

Liley Method of Prediction

In 1961, Liley described an empiric method of correlating the optical density determination with fetal status.[36] Recognizing that the size of the ΔOD (optical density of 450 mμ peak) in normal pregnancies decreases with increasing gestational age, he described three zones when ΔOD is plotted against gestational age on semilogarithmic paper. Figure 7–4 is a modification of Liley's original graph. The lower zone includes Rh-negative or mildly affected Rh-positive fetuses. The upper zone includes severely affected fetuses that require either prompt delivery or intrauterine transfusion if they are to survive. The middle zone is a gray area containing both types of fetuses with both mild and severe disease.

Figure 7–5 depicts the flow chart that we use in managing patients with erythroblastosis. The key steps are (1) antibody screening; (2) if positive, identification of the antibody; (3) determining if the antibody crosses the placenta (see Table 7–4); (4) if yes, initiating amniocentesis to determine the severity of fetal disease; (5) obtaining

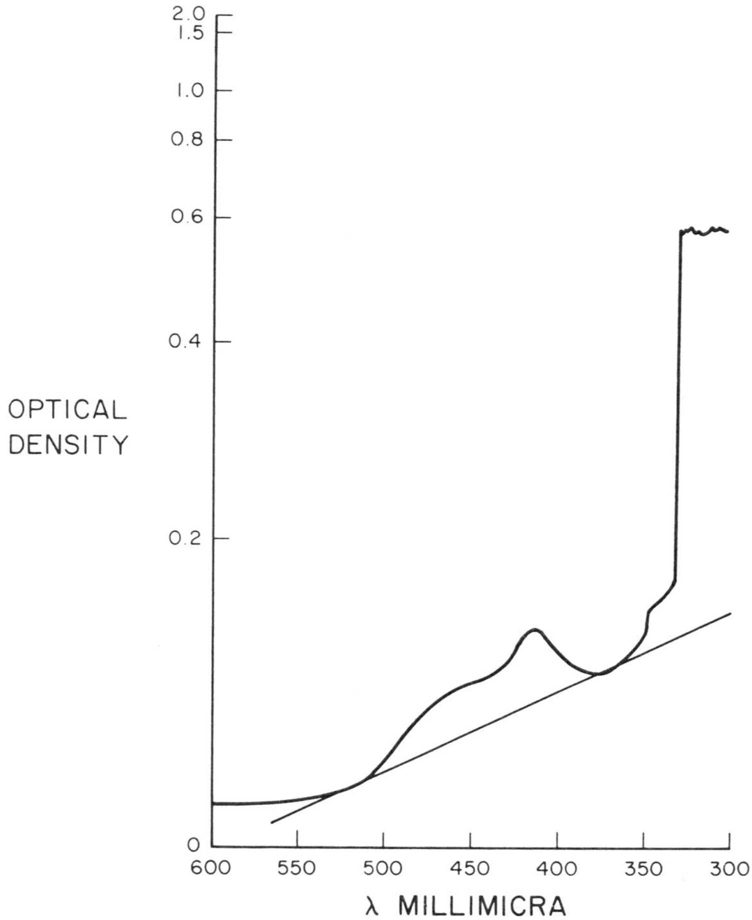

Figure 7–3. A spectrophotometric scan of amniotic fluid contaminated by blood. Note the oxyhemoglobin peak at 415 μm, 540 μm, and 580 μm.

serial observations; and (6) determining what treatment is required using the Liley zones.

Special Considerations

When Should First Amniocentesis Be Performed? The overriding consideration is not to perform the first tap after hydrops is already present. On the other hand, because there are minor risks associated with amniocentesis (infection, rupture of membranes, and fetal injury), one wishes to minimize the total number of taps required. Liley recommended that the first tap be performed between 29 and 32 weeks' gestation.[36] While this recommendation may be valid for a first sensitized pregnancy, in many situations the first amniocentesis should be performed at 20 to 22 weeks. Such situations include a high Coombs' titer, a rapidly rising titer, or a history of a previous hydropic or stillborn fetus.[21]

How Often Should Amniocentesis Be Repeated? Here the basic premise is that the ΔOD should be determined at intervals sufficiently close together to assure that

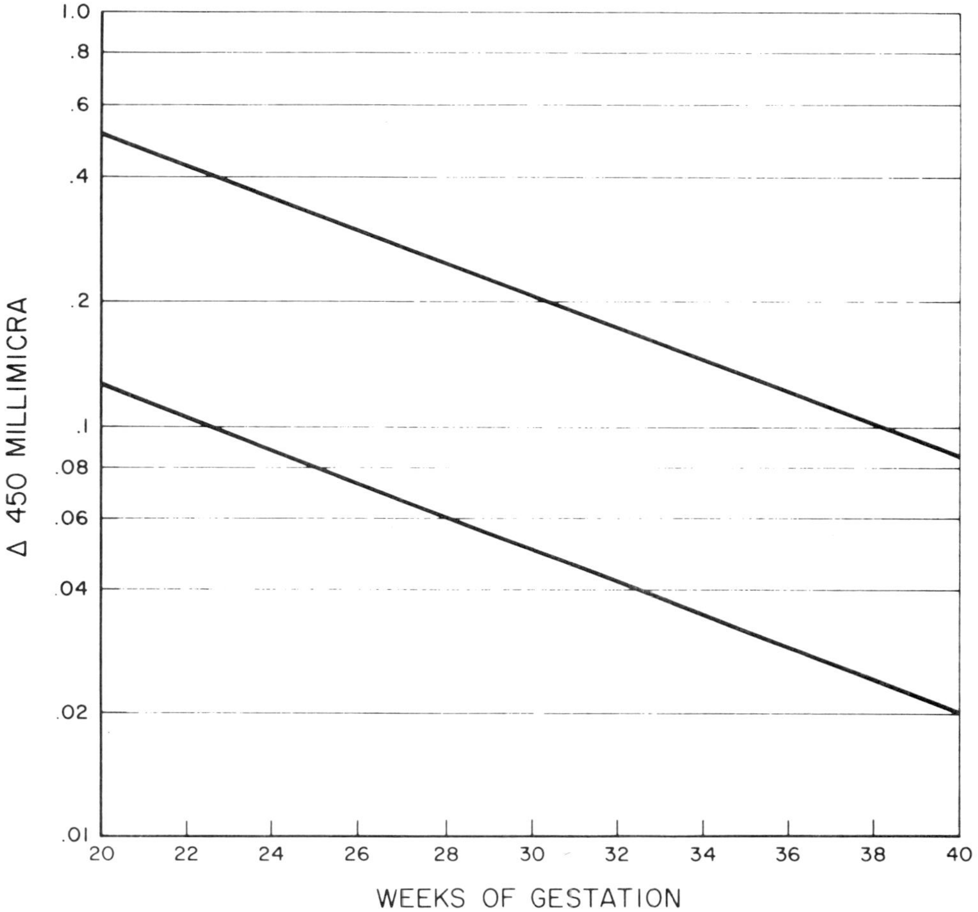

Figure 7–4. Modified Liley graph for plotting serial ΔODs against gestational age.

the value will not be in zone 3 for more than a few days before action is taken. If the first ΔOD value is in zone 1, repeat in two to four weeks; if in zone 2, repeat in one week or sooner if near the top. If in zone 3, repeat immediately and undertake treatment. Bowman's data indicate that properly timed serial amniocentesis will accurately predict the severity of erythroblastosis in 95% of cases.[21] However, to achieve this degree of accuracy one must be sure to eliminate inaccuracies caused by contamination of fluid by blood and meconium and to protect the specimen from light. Congenital anomalies that interfere with swallowing or the integrity of the gastrointestinal tract may produce misleading data. Similarly, maternal hyperbilirubinemia will also produce an elevation in the ΔOD that does not correlate with fetal status.

What About Multiple Gestations? Because there may be a marked disparity in the degree of fetal involvement even with monozygotic twins, the clinician must tap each sac in a multiple gestation. Usually this can be accomplished simply by performing amniocentesis under ultrasonic guidance. Occasionally, it may also be necessary to inject contrast medium to delineate the confines of each sac.

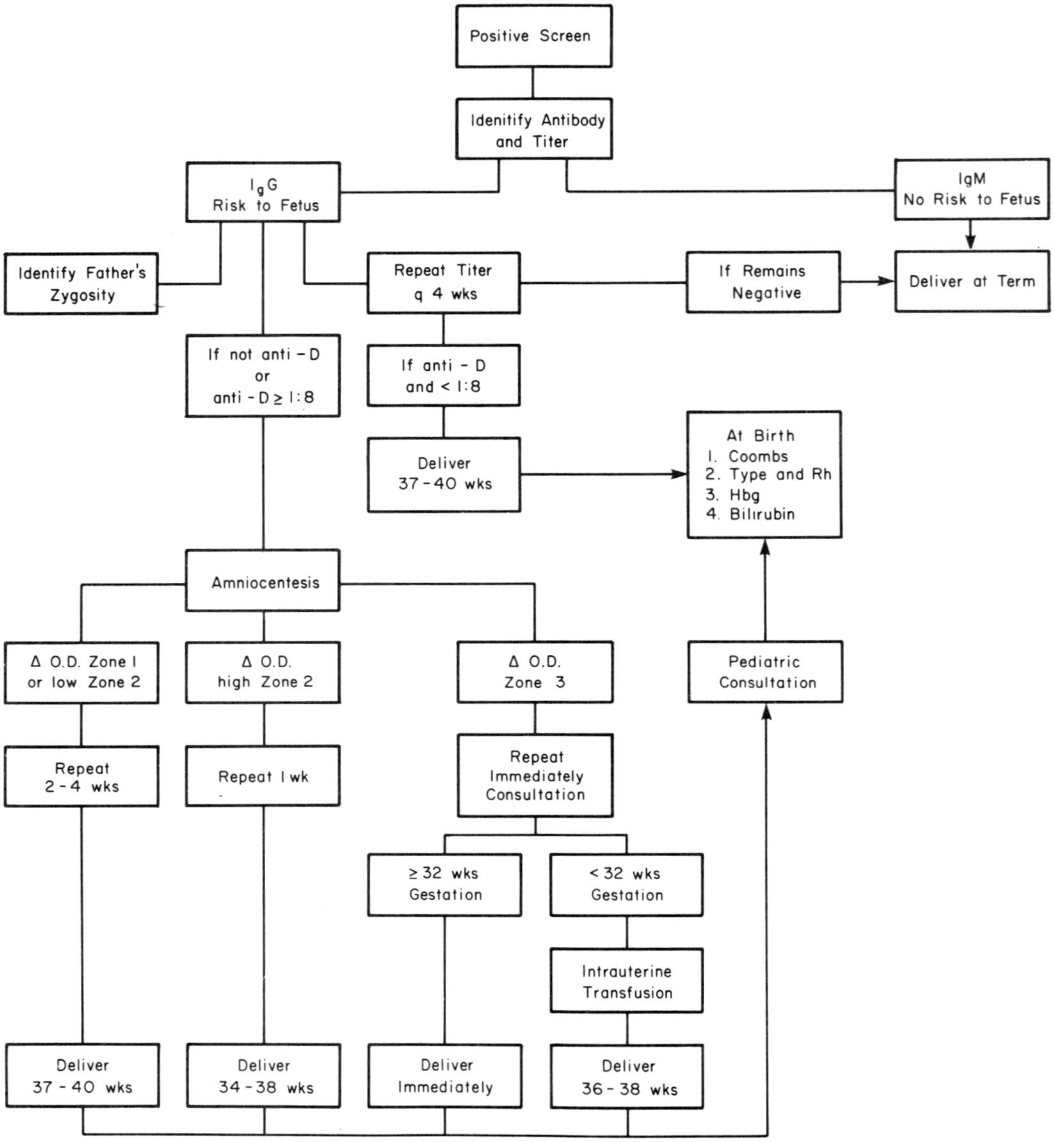

Figure 7–5. Flow chart for the management of patients found to have a positive antibody screen.

TREATMENT

As outlined in Figure 7–5, if the antibody type or titer or both preclude the need for amniocentesis, the patient is allowed to go into spontaneous labor at term. Also, if serial spectrophotometric readings remain in or fall into zone 1 or low zone 2, the mother should be allowed to go into spontaneous labor at term. If the ΔOD falls into or remains in the midportion of zone 2, induction should be carried out at 37 to 38 weeks' gestation after documenting fetal lung maturity either by a foam test[38] or by measuring the lecithin-sphingomyelin ratio.[39, 40]

EARLY DELIVERY

When the ΔOD rises into zone 3 or the initial reading falls into zone 3 after 32 weeks' gestation, delivery by induction or cesarean section should be carried out. If the fetal lung is not mature, delivery can be delayed for 24 to 48 hours and betamethasone administered to induce lung maturity.[41] Available data indicate that lung maturation in affected pregnancies is neither delayed nor accelerated as compared with that of controls.[40]

INTRAUTERINE TRANSFUSION

The introduction of intrauterine transfusion by Liley completely changed the outlook for the most severe cases of erythroblastosis.[6] The injected red cells are absorbed intact via the subdiaphragmatic lymphatics and, in the absence of ascites, complete absorption occurs in seven to nine days.[37] Studies in fetal sheep, however, suggest that absorption is far more rapid, with an average time to 99% absorption of 76 hours.[44]

Technique

We will not discuss the technique of intrauterine transfusion in detail; rather, only general principles will be reviewed. The interested reader is referred to several recent reviews for a more detailed discussion.[37, 43, 45–47]

The purpose of fetal transfusion is to maintain the fetal hemoglobin level above 10 to 11 g/dl and thus prevent the development of hydrops. Unfortunately, some fetuses will already be hydropic at the time of the first transfusion. Although the hydropic fetus does absorb red cells quite well, the rate is reduced and the likelihood of survival is reduced to 60 to 75%.[47, 48] However, this is better than certain death, and thus intrauterine transfusion is not contraindicated by hydrops.

Intrauterine transfusion is indicated when the ΔOD is in zone 3 and if the gestational age is less than 32 weeks. The steps are outlined in Table 7–10. The presence of an anterior placenta can be a problem that triples the risks associated with intrauterine transfusion. Efforts should be made to avoid the placenta; if this is not possible, it should be traversed as peripherally as possible.

Table 7–10. Outline of Intrauterine Transfusion Technique

1. Transfusion team performing at least five procedures each year
2. Demonstration of maternal and fetal anatomy with either
   a. Amniography or
   b. Ultrasound
3. Sedation—to reduce fetal movement
4. Placement of large bore needle or catheter. Guidance with
   a. Fluoroscopy using CO_2 or contrast medium, or
   b. Ultrasound
5. Use of fresh, leukocyte-poor, packed red cells either
   a. Maternal blood or
   b. O-negative donor blood
6. Slow injection of 30 to 130 ml according to formula: volume = 100 ± 10 ml for each week above or below 30 weeks' gestation
7. Repeat transfusions
   a. First repeat in 7–10 days
   b. Repeat every 2–4 weeks thereafter
   c. Last transfusion at 32–33 weeks
8. Delivery at 37–38 weeks' gestation

Delivery

As a general rule, all fetuses who have undergone intrauterine transfusion should be delivered between 37 and 38 weeks' gestation regardless of lung maturity. Fetal well-being should be monitored with weekly nonstress tests in the weeks prior to delivery. Delivery may be by induction of labor or cesarean section. Fetal well-being should be carefully monitored using electronic fetal heart rate monitoring and fetal scalp blood pH determinations if evidence of fetal distress occurs. If good labor has not been achieved after 10 to 12 hours of induction, cesarean section should be performed.

At delivery the cord should be clamped promptly. A cord blood specimen should be sent for blood typing, hemoglobin electrophoresis, and a direct Coombs' test. Frequently, the cord blood of infants who have had intrauterine transfusions will consist entirely of donor cells.

Results

Intrauterine transfusion does carry slight maternal risk such as infection and abruption. However, the fetal hazards are far greater and include puncture of a fetal vessel, injury to a fetal organ, infection, and precipitation of premature labor. Late sequelae include graft-versus-host disease[49] and leukemia,[50] but these are very rare.

The outcome of intrauterine transfusion has improved significantly from the 34% survival rate reported in 1969 by Queenan.[51] Recent reports detail survival rates as high as 75% for hydropic fetuses and 100% for these without hydrops.[46, 47]

There are now several reports detailing the long-term development of individuals undergoing intrauterine transfusions. Hardyment and colleagues collected 450 cases of which 78.2% were normal, 16.7% had minor neurologic abnormalities, and 5.1% major abnormalities.[52] In Bowman's series of 89 children, 83.1% were entirely normal, 12.4% had mild developmental delays, and 5.5% were grossly abnormal.[21] By contrast, all 15 children reported by Knobbi and associates were normal with respect to their intellectual, visual-motor, and social development.[53] All in all, if consideration is given to the effects of prematurity, the long-term development of infants undergoing intrauterine transfusion appears to be normal.

PLASMA EXCHANGE TO REDUCE ANTIBODY TITER

In 1968 Bowman and associates described plasmapheresis as a therapeutic modality for severe maternal sensitization. Sixty liters of plasma were exchanged before pregnancy and 46 L between 15 and 24 weeks' gestation. The anti-D titer fluctuated between 256 and 512, and three intrauterine transfusions were then performed.[54] Since this report, three other groups have described their experience with plasmapheresis.[55–57] Unfortunately, none of these studies is very convincing because the changes in antibody titer are not very dramatic and the outcomes are not compared with any suitable control group.[65]

IMMUNOSUPPRESSION

Walker failed to find any benefit from the administration of large doses of corticosteroids to four women with severe Rh sensitization. Although the steroids were begun at 14 weeks' gestation, all pregnancies ended with fetal death before the 30th week.[58]

Gusdon and Witherow reported a possible ameliorating effect on fetuses with erythroblastosis when their mothers were treated with large doses of promethazine hydrochloride.[59] Unfortunately, a prospective study of 21 mothers treated with 150 mg of promethazine per day showed no beneficial effect of the drug.[60]

ORAL DESENSITIZATION

Oral antigen loading has been shown to stimulate both local and circulating antibody production.[76] Although an early report in humans was encouraging,[77] a study of four pregnant women with severe Rh disease did not show any benefit from oral therapy.[78]

PREVENTION

For many years it had been hypothesized that passive immunization might prevent Rh sensitization. Preliminary studies with Rh-negative male volunteers[61] confirmed the hypothesis, and prospective trials were begun.[62–64]

Three possible mechanisms by which passive immunization prevents sensitization have been proposed:

1. Rh antibody may block or bind Rh antigenic sites on RBCs, thus preventing the antigens from making contact with surface receptors of immunocytes.
2. Rh antibody may prevent the Rh antigen from reaching the sites in the reticuloendothelial centers where sensitization occurs.
3. Rh antibody may have a direct suppressive effect on potential immunocytes.

The weight of evidence favors a central inhibition mechanism whereby IgG interacts with specific receptors for the Fc portion of IgG or IgM antibody. The former acts as a suppressor, while the latter acts as a stimulator.[65] Whatever the mechanism, a series of prospective studies showed four cases of sensitization among 2523 treated subjects as compared with 160 cases of sensitization among 2299 control subjects.[66]

POST PARTUM

Based on these data, it is recommended that every Rh-negative woman delivered (after 20 weeks' gestation) of an Rh-positive infant should receive Rh-immune globulin. After delivery a specimen of cord blood and a postpartum maternal specimen should be drawn. Rh-immune globulin should be injected intramuscularly within 72 hours of delivery. The standard dose is 300 μg, which should be given if the following conditions are met:[67]

1. The mother is Rho(D)-negative and D^u-negative.
2. The mother has no anti-D antibodies in her serum.
3. The infant is D- or D^u-positive.
4. Results of the direct Coombs' test on the infant cord blood are negative, or, if positive, this is due to an atypical antibody (such as anti-Kell or anti-Duffy).

It is essential that the Rh-immune globulin show a compatible cross-match with the postpartum blood specimen. An incompatible cross-match, if the above conditions have been met, is an indication of a large fetal-maternal bleed requiring a higher dose of Rh-immune globulin.

Large Fetal-Maternal Bleeds

Ten micrograms (10 μg) of Rh-immunoglobulin will prevent sensitization by 1 ml of fetal blood.[68] Thus the standard 300 μg dose is sufficient to cover a transfusion of up to 30 ml of fetal blood. When a larger transfusion is suspected either on the basis of a positive cross-match or the occurrence of a clinical condition known to be associated with a large fetal-maternal transfusion, a Kleihauer acid elution test should be done. The Kleihauer and Bitke test will quantitate the number of fetal cells in the maternal circulation and should be done whenever an Rh-negative mother is delivered of an Rh-positive infant by a traumatic procedure, when there is a manual removal of the placenta, there is a placenta previa, or the infant shows significant anemia. The dose of Rh-immune globulin can be calculated according to the formula:[69]

$$\mu\text{g Rh-immune globulin required} = \frac{\text{no of fetal cells} \times 50{,}000}{\text{no of maternal cells}}$$

The formula assumes a maternal blood volume of 5 L. When additional Rh-immune globulin is given or the possible need is raised, the adequacy of the dose can be established by obtaining an indirect Coombs' titer for anti-D on a maternal specimen obtained 12 hours after each dose. If the titer is negative, additional doses are given until it becomes positive.

POST ABORTION AND AFTER ECTOPIC PREGNANCY

The D-antigen is present on fetal red blood cells as early as 38 days after conception.[65, 70] Thus, Rh-immune globulin should always be administered to Rh-negative women undergoing spontaneous abortion, induced abortion, or ectopic pregnancy. Because of the much smaller fetal blood volume, a lower dose of globulin can be used. Doses of both 50 and 150 μg have been shown to be effective.[71, 72]

TRANSFUSION ERROR

Unfortunately, Rh-negative women occasionally still receive Rh-positive blood by mistake.[15] When such an error is recognized, the recipient should be given 1 vial (300 μg) of Rh-immune globulin for every 30 ml of whole blood transfused (17 vials per unit of whole blood). The total dose of Rh-immune globulin can be divided and administered over 72 hours.

AMNIOCENTESIS AND CHORIONIC VILLUS BIOPSY

Amniocentesis in either the second or third trimester is always attended by the possible risk of placental trauma and transplacental hemorrhage. While most have recommended administration of Rh-immune globulin,[67, 74] others have questioned the necessity for its use.[73, 75] A 300 μg dose should be used. These patients then become candidates for the standard antepartum prophylaxis regimen, as discussed below. At present there are no data indicating whether or not Rh-immune globulin prophylaxis is required after chorionic villus biopsy. However, the prudent course would seem to be to administer 50 μg.

ANTEPARTUM SENSITIZATION

As the use of postpartum Rh prophylaxis has grown, the occurrence of antepartum sensitization has increased in relative frequency. Bowman reports that 41% of Rh-immunized women developed their antibodies during pregnancy.[79] Because of this finding, his group initiated a trial using 300 μg of Rh-immune globulin given at 23 weeks' gestation in all Rh-negative, unsensitized women. A further dose is given after delivery if the infant is Rh-positive. Their results in 1357 cases show a significant reduction in antepartum sensitization.[8] As more data have become available confirming these findings, antepartum Rh prophylaxis has become standard therapy.[67]

Current practice is to administer 300 μg of Rh-immune globulin at approximately 28 weeks of gestation. In cases in which the father of the fetus is known to be Rh-negative, antepartum prophylaxis should be admitted. Because it is exceedingly unlikely that a patient will become sensitized after receiving antepartum prophylaxis at 28 weeks, further antibody studies are not required. At the time of delivery, the patient should again receive a 300 μg dose of Rh-immune globulin if her newborn is found to be V- or V_u-positive. It is important to remember that a small % of patients will still have a positive antibody screen caused by passive immunization. This can be differentiated from active sensitization by the absence of demonstrable IgM in the maternal blood. This weakly positive Coombs' test is not a contraindication to the administration of an additional dose of Rh-immune globulin. On the contrary, failure to administer another dose may in fact enhance the patient's risk of becoming sensitized.[65]

REFERENCES

1. Darrow, R.R.: Icterus gravis neonatorum: Examination of etiologic considerations. Arch Pathol *25*:378, 1938.
2. Levine, P, and Stetson, R.E.: Unusual cases of intragroup agglutination. JAMA *113*:126, 1939.
3. Landsteiner, K., and Weiner, A.S.: Agglutinable factor in human blood recognized by immune sera for rhesus blood. Proc Soc Exp Biol Med *43*:223, 1940.
4. Allen, F.H., Jr, Diamond, L.K., and Jones, A.R.: Erythroblastosis fetalis. IX, Problems of stillbirth. N Engl J Med *251*:453, 1954.
5. Bevis, D.C.A.: Blood pigments in hemolytic disease of the newborn. J Obstet Gynaecol Br Commonw *63*:68, 1956.
6. Liley, A.W.: Intrauterine transfusion of foetus in haemolytic disease. Br Med J *2*:1107, 1963.
7. Freda, V.J., Gorman, J.G., and Pollack, W.: Rh factor: Prevention of isoimmunization and clinical trial on mothers. Science *151*:828, 1966.
8. Bowman, J.M., and Pollack, J.M.: Antenatal Rh prophylaxis: 28-week gestation service program. Can Med Assoc J *118*:622, 1978.
9. Marcus, D.M.: The ABO and Lewis blood group system. N Engl J Med *280*:994, 1969.
10. NIH: Manual of Tissue Typing Techniques. Compiled by Transplantation Immunology Branch, NIAID, National Institutes of Health, Bethesda, MD, 1969.
11. Race, R.R., and Sanger, R.: Blood Groups in Man. 6th Ed. Oxford, Blackwell Scientific Publications, 1975.
12. Wiener, A.S.: Fundamentals of immunogenetics with special reference to human blood groups. Med Proc *10*:559, 1964.
13. WHO: Twenty-Eighth Report of WHO Expert Committee on Biological Standardization. Technical Report Series, 610, Geneva, 1977.
14. White, C.A., Stockman, C.M., and Frank, S.: Anti-D antibodies in D- and D^u-positive women: A cause of hemolytic disease of the newborn. Am J Obstet Gynecol *145*:1069, 1983.
15. Weinstein, L.: Irregular antibodies causing hemolytic disease of the newborn. Obstet Gynecol Surv *31*:581, 1976.
16. Keith, L., Berger, G., and Pollack, W.: The transfusion of Rh-positive blood into Rh-negative women. Am J Obstet Gynecol *125*:502, 1976.
17. Taylor, J.F.: Sensitization of Rh-negative daughters by their Rh-positive mothers. N Engl J Med *276*:547, 1967.
18. Bowman, J.M., Chown, B, Lewis, M., et al.: Rh-immunization during pregnancy: Antenatal prophylaxis. Can Med Assoc J *118*:623, 1978.
19. Jennings, E.R., and Clauss, B.: Maternal-fetal hemorrhage: Its incidence and sensitizing effects. Am J Obstet Gynecol *131*:725, 1978.

20. Woodrow, J.C.: Rh immunization and its prevention. Ser Haematol III *3*:16, 1970.
21. Bowman, J.: Rh-isoimmunization. Obstet Gynecol *52*:1, 1978.
22. James, L.S.: Shock in the newborn in relation to hydrops. Ann Obstet Gynecol *92*:599, 1971.
23. Phibbs, R.H., Johnson, P., and Tooley, W.H.: Cardiorespiratory status of erythroblastotic newborn infants. Pediatrics *53*:13, 1974.
24. Kaiser, I.H.: Ballantyne and triple edema. Am J Obstet Gynecol *110*:115, 1971.
25. Goodlin, R.C.: Impending fetal death in utero due to isoimmunization. Obstet Gynecol *10*:299, 1957.
26. Queenan, J.T., Smith, B.D., Haber, J.M., et al.: Irregular antibodies in the obstetric patient. Obstet Gynecol *34*:767, 1969.
27. Pirofsky, B.: Erythroblastosis—a changing serologic problem. Am J Obstet Gynecol *92*:720, 1965.
28. Polesky, H.F.: Blood group antibodies in prenatal sera. Minn Med *50*:601, 1967.
29. Springer, G.F., Williamson, P., and Readler, B.L.: Blood group active gram-negative bacteria and higher plants. Ann NY Acad Sci *97*:104, 1962.
30. Ascari, W.Q., Levine, P., and Pollack, W.: Incidence of maternal Rh immunization by ABO compatible and incompatible pregnancies. Br Med J *1*:399, 1969.
31. Bowman, J.M., and Pollack, J.M.: Amniotic fluid spectrophotometry and early delivery in the management of erythroblastosis fetalis. Pediatrics *35*:815, 1965.
32. Walker, W., Murray, R., Sherlagh, V., et al.: Stillbirth due to haemolytic disease of the newborn. J Obstet Gynaecol Br Emp *64*:573, 1957.
33. Bowell, P., Wainscoat, J.S., Peto, T.E.A., et al.: Maternal anti-D concentrations and outcome in rhesus haemolytic disease of the newborn. Br Med J *285*:327, 1982.
34. American College of Obstetricians and Gynecologists: Management of erythroblastosis. ACOG Technical Bulletin #80. Washington, D.C., September, 1984.
35. Purohit, D.M., Taylor, H.L., and Spivey, M.A.: Hemolytic disease of the newborn due to anti-Js^b. Am J Obstet Gynecol *131*:755, 1978.
36. Liley, A.W.: Liquor amnii analysis in the management of the pregnancy complicated by rhesus sensitization. Am J Obstet Gynecol *83*:1359, 1961.
37. Queenan, J.T.: Modern Management of the Rh Problem. New York, Harper & Row, 1977.
38. Schuleter, M.A., Phibbs, R.H., and Creasy, R.K.: Antenatal prediction of graduated risk of hyaline membrane disease by amniotic fluid foam test. Am J Obstet Gynecol *134*:761, 1979.
39. Hallman, M., Kulovich, M., Kirkpatrick, E., et al.: Phosphatidylinositol and phosphatidylglycerol in amniotic fluid. Am J Obstet Gynecol *125*:613, 1976.
40. Gluck, L., Kulovich, M, and Borer, R.C.: The diagnosis of the respiratory distress syndrome by amniocentesis. Am J Obstet Gynecol *109*:440, 1971.
41. Liggins, G.C., and Lowie, R.N.: A controlled trial of antepartum glucocorticoid treatment for prevention of the respiratory distress syndrome in premature infants. Pediatrics *50*:515, 1973.
42. Quinlan, R.W., Buhi, W.C., and Cruz, A.C.: Fetal pulmonary maturity in isoimmunized pregnancies. Am J Obstet Gynecol *148*:787, 1984.
43. Bowman, J.M., Friesen, R.F., Bowman, W.D., et al.: Fetal transfusion in severe RH isoimmunization. JAMA *207*:1101, 1969.
44. Harman, C.R., Biehl, D.R., Pollack, J.M., et al.: Intrauterine transfusion: Kinetics of absorption of donor cells in fetal lamb. Am J Obstet Gynecol *145*:830, 1983.
45. Bowman, J., and Manning, F.: Intrauterine fetal transfusions: Winnipeg 1982. Obstet Gynecol *61*:203, 1083.
46. Harman, C.R., Manning, F.A., Bowman, J.M., et al.: Severe Rh disease—Poor outcome is not inevitable. Am J Obstet Gynecol *145*:823, 1983.
47. Scott, J.R., Kochenhour, N.K., Larkin, R.M., et al.: Changes in the management of severely Rh-immunized patients. Am J Obstet Gynecol *149*:336, 1984.
48. Hamilton, E.G.: Intrauterine transfusion. Obstet Gynecol *50*:255, 1977.
49. Parkman, R., Mosier, D, Umansky, I., et al.: Graft-versus-host disease after intrauterine and exchange transfusions for hemolytic disease of the newborn. N Engl J Med *290*:359, 1974.
50. Turner, J.H., Hutchinson, D.L., and Petricciani, J.C.: Chimerism following fetal transfusion. Scand J Haematol *10*:358, 1974.
51. Queenan, J.T.: Intrauterine transfusion: A cooperative study. Am J Obstet Gynecol *104*:397, 1969.
52. Hardyment, A.F., Salvador, H.S., Towell, M.E., et al.: Follow-up of intrauterine transfused surviving children. Am J Obstet Gynecol *133*:235, 1979.
53. Knobbi, T., Meier, P., Wenar, C., et al.: Psychological development of children who received intrauterine transfusions. Am J Obstet Gynecol *133*:877, 1979.
54. Bowman, J.M., Peddle, L.J., and Anderson, C.: Plasmapheresis in severe Rh iso-immunization. Vox Sang *15*:272, 1968.
55. Powell, L.C.: Intense plasmapheresis in the pregnant Rh-sensitized woman. Am J Obstet Gynecol *101*:153, 1968.
56. Clark, C.A., Bradley, J., Elson, C.J., et al.: Intensive plasmapheresis as a therapeutic measure in rhesus-immunized women. Lancet *1*:794, 1970.

57. Fraser, I.D., Bothamley, J.E., Bennet, M.O., et al.: Intensive antenatal plasmapheresis in severe rhesus isoimmunisation. Lancet *1*:6, 1976.
58. Walker, W.: The changing pattern of haemolytic disease of the newborn. Vox Sang *3*:225, 1958.
59. Gusdon, J.P., and Witherow, P.C.: Possible ameliorating effects of erythroblastosis by promethazine hydrochloride. Am J Obstet Gynecol *117*:1101, 1973.
60. Stenchever, M.A.: Promethazine hydrochloride: Use in patients with Rh isoimmunization. Am J Obstet Gynecol *130*:665, 1978.
61. Stern, K., Goodman, H.S., and Berger, M.: Experimental isoimmunization to hemoantigens in man. J Immunol *87*:189, 1960.
62. Freda, V.J., Gorman, J.G., and Pollack, W.: Successful prevention of experimental Rh sensitization in man with an anti-Rh gamma 2-globulin antibody preparation. Transfusion *4*:26, 1963.
63. Clarke, C.A., Donohoe, W.T.A., McConnell, R.B., et al.: Further experimental studies in the prevention of Rh-haemolytic disease. Br Med J *1*:979, 1962.
64. Zipursky, A., and Israels, L.G.: The pathogenesis and prevention of Rh immunization. Can Med Assoc J *97*:1245, 1967.
65. Frigoletto, F.D., Jewett, J.F., and Konugres, A.A.: Rh Hemolytic Disease. Boston, G.K.M. Hall Medical Publishers, 1982.
66. Freda, V.J.: Karl Landsteiner Memorial Award Lecture, AABD 22nd Annual Meeting, Houston, Texas, 1969.
67. American College of Obstetricians and Gynecologists. Prevention of RHO(D) Isoimmunization. ACOG Technical Bulletin #79. Washington, D.C., August, 1984.
68. Pollack, W., Ascari, W.Q., Kochesky, R.J., et al.: Studies on Rh prophylaxis: Relationship between doses of anti-RH and size of antigenic stimulus. Transfusion *11*:333, 1971.
69. Pollack, W., Ascari, W.Q., Crispen, R.R., et al.: Studies on Rh prophylaxis: Rh immune prophylaxis after transfusion with Rh-positive blood. Transfusion *11*:340, 1971.
70. Bergstrom, H., Nilsson, L., and Ryttinger, L: Demonstration of Rh antigens in a 38-day-old fetal. Am J Obstet Gynecol *99*:130, 1967.
71. Steuart, F.H., Burnhill, M.S., and Bonorgi, N.: Reduced dose of Rh immunoglobulin following first trimester pregnancy termination. Obstet Gynecol *51*:318:1978.
72. Hensleigh, P.A., Leslie, W., Dixon, E., et al.: Reduced dose of Rho(D) immune globulin following induced first-trimester abortion. Am J Obstet Gynecol *129*:413, 1977.
73. Tabsh, K.M.A., Lebherz, T.B., and Crandall, B.F.: Risks of prophylactic anti-D immunoglobulin after second-trimester amniocenteses. Am J Obstet Gynecol *149*:225, 1984.
74. Lele, A.S., Carmedy, P.J., Hurd, M.E., et al.: Fetomaternal bleeding following diagnostic amniocentesis. Obstet Gynecol *60*:60, 1982.
75. Golbus, M.S., Stephens, J.C., Cann, H.M., et al.: Rh-isoimmunization following genetic amniocentesis. Prenat Diagn *2*:149, 1982.
76. Richman, L.K., and Chelles, J.M.: Enterically induced immunologic tolerance. J Immunol *121*:2429, 1978.
77. Biorne, S., and Blanc, M.: Oral treatment for severely immunized mothers. Lancet *1*:604, 1979.
78. Gold, W.R., Queenan, J.T., Woody, J., et al.: Oral desensitization in Rh disease. Am J Obstet Gynecol *146*:980, 1983.
79. Bowman, J.M.: Suppression of Rh isoimmunization. Obstet Gynecol *52*:385, 1978.

Chapter 8
LABORATORY EVALUATION OF HEMOSTASIS

Laurence Corash

NORMAL HEMOSTASIS AND PREGNANCY-ASSOCIATED EFFECTS ON HEMOSTASIS

Maintenance of normal hemostasis requires the complex interaction of both fluid phase plasma factors and blood cellular elements in a delicate balance of procoagulant and anticoagulant activities. The normal physiologic response to pregnancy superimposes additional complexity on these systems because of altered levels of multiple plasma factors. Recent years have seen a rapid expansion of information about both the cellular and the fluid phase of coagulation. Adequate utilization of laboratory tests to diagnose hemostatic disorders during pregnancy requires a thorough understanding of normal coagulation.

NORMAL HEMOSTASIS

Historical development of the elucidation of blood coagulation mechanisms has led to a division of the coagulation process into two basic pathways: the intrinsic and extrinsic (Fig. 8–1). While this dichotomy has proved useful, it is now clear that the two pathways are more interdependent than previously thought.

PLASMA FACTORS

The initial reactions of the intrinsic pathway are collectively thought of as the contact activation system and consist of Hageman factor (factor XII), prekallikrein (PK), high molecular weight kininogen (HMK), kallikrein (K), and factor XI.[1] The primary event in the activation of this pathway is the association and binding of Hageman factor to a negatively charged surface. This surface may be damaged endothelium basement membrane,[2] bacterial lipopolysaccharides,[3] or even pathologic crystals.[4] Upon binding to the charged surface, factor XII undergoes a conformational change and is cleaved by the plasma protein kallikrein. Kallikrein is produced by the cleavage of prekallikrein, thought to occur as a result of reciprocal activation by previously bound Hageman factor on the negatively charged surface.[5] Evidence now indicates that prekallikrein circulates as a complex with high molecular weight kininogen, which also binds to the negatively charged surface, bringing prekallikrein into proximity with Hageman factor. High molecular weight kininogen circulates in association with factor XI and serves as a cofactor in binding it to the negative surface proximate to activated Hageman factor, where it, in turn, will be cleaved and activated.[6]

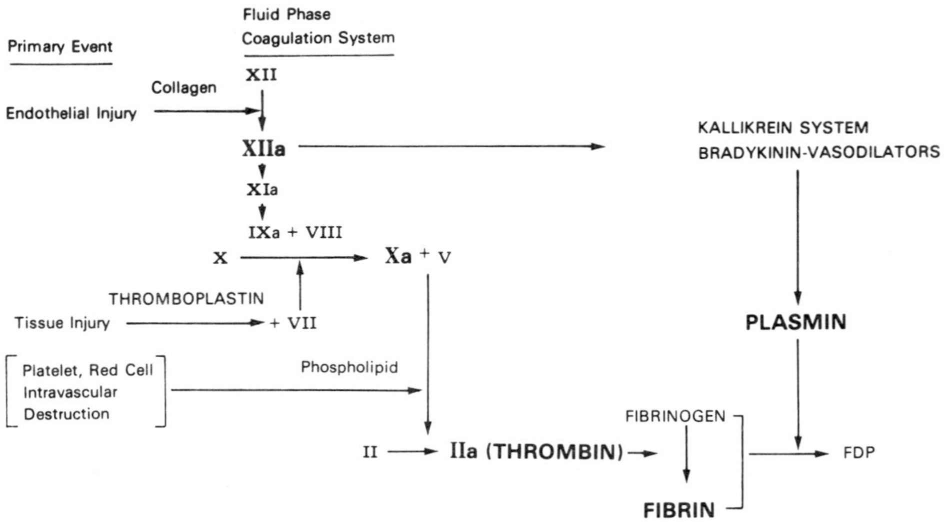

Figure 8–1. General schematic overview of the classic coagulation cascade. Factors indicated in bold type emphasize their central importance in the coagulation cascade.

This last reaction completes the process of contact activation and initiates the activation of the intrinsic pathway through activated factor XI (XIa).

Factor XIa, a serine protease, has as its principal substrate factor IX. The term serine protease connotes a serine residue at the active site and generally indicates sensitivity to the antithrombin III–heparin complex. This interaction of XIa and IX is calcium-dependent and may occur in solution with the production of factor IXa. Factor IXa is also a serine protease and, in the presence of factor VIII, calcium, and phospholipid, it converts factor X to its active form, factor Xa. At this juncture it is important to briefly clarify the biologic activities of the factor VIII complex.

Factor VIII possesses at least two distinct physiologic properties. The procoagulant activity is designated as VIII:C and is manifest by the cofactor activity with factor IXa in the activation of factor X. A second property of the factor VIII complex is attributable to the larger portion of the molecule, which supports platelet adhesion to subendothelial structures and is commonly called the von Willebrand factor (VWF). Various laboratory tests describe its activities: the ristocetin cofactor (VIIIR:RC) or factor VIII–related antigen (VIIIR:Ag). Full activity of the VIII:C moiety requires some degree of thrombin activation,[7] after which the activated species undergo rapid inactivation.

Activation of factor X in the presence of IXa, calcium, phospholipid, and factor VIII:C is a central part of the coagulation cascade. Activated factor X (Xa) subsequently participates with factor V, phospholipid, and calcium to convert prothrombin to thrombin. The phospholipid component has previously been designated as the ill-defined platelet factor 3. Current evidence now suggests that the production of prothrombinase, the Xa-V complex, may actually occur on the platelet surface.[8] Factor V is contained within platelet α-granules and binds to the cell surface after secretion. Platelet-bound factor V may actually serve as the factor Xa binding site, and the spatial orientation on the platelet surface forms the "prothrombinase complex," which converts prothrombin to thrombin. Thrombin is also a serine protease. It cleaves fibrinopeptide A from fibrinogen, resulting in the production of fibrin monomers. Fibrin monomers generated by the action of thrombin are cross-linked by the action of factor XIII, a transglutaminase that is directly activated by thrombin.[9] Production of thrombin and the subsequent proteolysis of fibrinogen culminate the coagulation process.

According to the classic concept of coagulation, the other major pathway is designated as the extrinsic system and is initiated by the action of tissue thromboplastin. Tissue thromboplastin is a cellular membrane lipoprotein whose separate protein and lipid moieties are devoid of procoagulant activity.[10] Factor VII, a plasma component, exists as a single chain proenzyme that is converted to an active two-chain form. Thrombin, factor Xa, or Hageman factor can serve as a stimulus for this conversion. However, the primary physiologic initiating stimulus to factor VII activation remains unclear, although it is known that even the single-chain form possesses some low level proteolytic activity.[11] In the presence of tissue thromboplastin liberated as a result of cell injury, two-chain factor VII activation of factor X is greatly accelerated. Activated factor Xa then enters the common pathway as described for the intrinsic system, with ultimate production of thrombin and consequent fibrinogen conversion to fibrin.

Historically the intrinsic and extrinsic pathways have been viewed as discrete, but recent data now support and confirm earlier observations that this separation may not be as complete as once thought. In the presence of tissue thromboplastin, activated factor XII is also capable of activating factor IX. This has been termed the "alternative extrinsic pathway." Its biologic significance may well be indicated by the observation that clotting factor deficiencies above factors IX, XI, and XII are mild because the "alternative extrinsic pathway" is left intact, whereas deficiencies of either factor VIII or IX seriously compromise factor X activation via this alternative pathway.[12]

Normal hemostasis also requires regulatory factors for the maintenance of antithrombotic conditions and control of the procoagulant properties described in the preceding section. Knowledge of these activities is rapidly growing and at present includes the plasminogen-plasmin system, antithrombin III, protein C, and the antiplasmin inhibitors α-2-antiplasmin and α-2-macroglobulin.

Maintenance of vascular integrity after a thrombotic event is facilitated by a system for the appropriate physiologic dissolution of fibrin clots. These processes are largely controlled by the plasminogen-plasmin system. Abnormalities among these factors may be associated with either prothrombotic disorders[13] or hemorrhagic disorders.[14] Congenital defects of these factors are rare, but partial defects due to acquired conditions may not be so infrequent and thus perhaps contribute to several pregnancy-related coagulation disorders. Plasminogen is synthesized in multiple tissues and is present in the plasma as an inactive form but is converted to its active form, plasmin, by activators. The major activators are present in the plasma or endothelial cells. Other minor activators may be derived from bacteria (e.g., streptokinase) or from the urinary tract (most notably urokinase). Thus far the tissue plasminogen activators derived from endothelial cells are poorly characterized but appear to be the most important for physiologic thrombus dissolution. Plasminogen activators have also been found in malignant tissues derived from the urinary tract, pancreatic tumors, and cultured carcinoma cells.[15] The activity of plasmin is in turn inhibited by the plasma protein α-2-plasmin inhibitor. Congenital deficiency of this protein results in a rare but severe hemorrhagic disorder.[14]

COAGULATION INHIBITORS

Two major inhibitors of the procoagulant pathway have been extensively characterized. Antithrombin III (ATIII) is a potent inhibitor of thrombin and the serine proteases in general,[16] and in the presence of heparin its activity is greatly enhanced. Absence of antithrombin III results in decreased heparin effectiveness, and both qualitative and quantitative abnormalities of ATIII can result in a severe congenital thrombotic disorder.[17, 18] ATIII appears to be a significant antithrombotic regulatory protein.

A second important inhibitor is protein C.[19] It inhibits activated factors V and VIII. This vitamin K–dependent protein also appears to have fibrinolytic properties through its ability to increase plasminogen activator levels.[20] Deficiency in protein C is associated with a thrombotic diathesis, and acquired protein C deficiency may be seen in the course of disseminated intravascular coagulation.[21, 22] Protein C is also regulated, and absence of the inhibitor-activated protein C may lead to the uncontrolled degradation of factors V and VIII with a resultant hemorrhagic diathesis.[23] Thus, protein C occupies a critical position in the modulation of coagulant activities but at a point different from that of ATIII.

PLATELET FUNCTION

Normal hemostasis is also dependent upon adequate platelet function. A reduction in the platelet count, usually to levels below 25×10^9 per L, or the presence of a qualitative platelet defect, may be associated with a severe hemorrhagic diathesis.[24, 25] Platelet function can be schematically divided into several different processes: adhesions, aggregation, secretion, and coagulant interactions. Platelets adhere to exposed subendothelial structures in the presence of the von Willebrand factor moiety of the factor VIII complex. Normal adhesion requires the presence of the platelet membrane glycoprotein GpIb and the large multimeric form of the von Willebrand factor.[26] Adhesion is the initial phase in the hemostatic process after endothelial disruption, and a defect in this function may be associated with a hemorrhagic diathesis. For example, homozygous von Willebrand's disease is characterized by defective platelet adhesion and clinically significant hemorrhage.[27] A second critical platelet function is that of aggregation with attendant secretion. Platelets secrete at least two classes of subcellular organelles, dense bodies and α-granules, which contain components involved in platelet function. These secreted products may act to recruit other platelets and may facilitate local platelet aggregation at the wound site.[28] Another major aspect of platelet function is participation in the fluid phase of coagulation. It now appears that the platelet surface is important for the generation of prothrombinase (as described earlier) and for the amplification of the coagulation cascade. Platelets also contain factor V, fibrinogen, and factor VIII–related antigen in α-granules, which may result in high local concentrations of these components after secretion. Localized secretion of high concentrations of factor VIII–related antigen may be required for effective platelet adhesion. Furthermore, the platelet surface constitutes the platelet factor 3 required for coagulation.[8] Impairment of platelet α-granule secretion or a deficiency of platelet factor V content is associated with a hemorrhagic diathesis.

CHANGES IN HEMOSTASIS ASSOCIATED WITH NORMAL PREGNANCY

PT AND aPTT

During normal pregnancy, a variety of changes occur that affect hemostasis. Interpretation of laboratory tests during pregnancy requires adjustment of the usual normal range values to reflect these special physiologic alterations. Nossel and co-workers[29] reported that both the kaolin-activated partial thromboplastin time (aPTT) and the one-stage prothrombin time (PT) were moderately shortened in pregnant women at delivery as compared with nonpregnant controls. No data were reported on the time-dependent relationship to the intervening gestational stage. These authors also observed elevated fibrinogen levels, factor VIII coagulant levels, and factors IX and X concentrations (Table 8–1). They found normal factor V and prothrombin levels with reduced factor XI activity. Factor XIII, as measured by monochloracetic acid solubility, was present in each subject. Pechet and Alexander have also reported that factors VII and X are elevated during pregnancy.[30] They observed no direct relationship between the degree of factor elevation and the gestational interval; however, most of the observations were made in the last trimester. Factor II was not elevated in the subjects in their study, findings similar to the Nossel data, and factors VII and X, while elevated, were found to return to normal range levels within two weeks of parturition.[30] Ganrot also measured the concentration of several hemostasis-associated proteins in pregnant women at the time of delivery. Plasminogen, α-2-macroglobulin, and fibrinogen levels were elevated, with the largest increase noted for fibrinogen.[31]

FACTOR XIII

Quantitation of factor XIII activity is difficult because of assay methodology limitations. The clot solubility tests are qualitative, and a very low level of activity—1 to 2%—is required for normal function.[32] Using a more quantitative assay, Duckert reported that at term maternal plasma contains a lower level of factor XIII activity than neonatal cord plasma: 67% versus 86%.[32] This observation has been confirmed by others, who found 50% levels at term.[33] Factor XIII deficiency is associated with chronic abortion, and there appears to be no transfer of fetal factor XIII to the maternal circulation. Factor XIII–deficient infants are delivered normally, and one case is reported in which a factor XIII–deficient female gave birth to an infant with normal factor XIII activity.[34] It is also known that placenta contains factor XIII activity of the α-subunit dimeric structure.[35]

ANTITHROMBINS

Antithrombin III is the major inhibitor of the serine protease coagulation factors II, IX, X, XI, and XII, except for factor VII,[36] which is not inhibited by ATIII. This protein is an important regulator of hemostasis in both the native physiologic state and during therapeutic anticoagulation. At least two studies have documented that antithrombin III levels do not change during pregnancy.[37,38] Women with familial antithrombin III deficiency are said to be at increased risk for thrombosis during pregnancy, but the data on actual ATIII concentrations are very limited.[39]

Alpha-2-Antiplasmin inhibitor (α2PI) is an important regulator of plasmin activity, but no data on α2PI concentrations in pregnancy are available. Alpha-2-Macroglobulin, a minor plasmin inhibitor, increases slightly during pregnancy. The case of α2PI

Table 8–1. Effect of Pregnancy on the Concentration of Plasma Coagulation Factors and Platelet α-Granule Proteins

Factor	Normal Values	First Trimester	Second Trimester	Third Trimester
Fibrinogen (I)	3.08 g/L[29]	3.48 ± 0.38 g/L[50]	3.59 ± 0.51 g/L[50]	378 ± 52 mg/dl[50] 5.32 g/L[29]
Prothrombin (II)	98%[31] 100%[29] 60–120%[30]			62–110%[30] 112%[31] 107%[29]
Factor V	100%[29]			108%[29]
Factor VIII:C	100%[44] 100%[29]			139–194%, x = 164%[44a] 156–208%, x = 180%[44b] 196%[29]
Factor VIIIR:Ag	1.09 U/ml[42] 100%[44]		1.23 ± 0.35 U/ml[42]	145–194%, x = 168%[44a] 180–231%, x −204%[44b]
Factor VIIIR:RC	100%[44]			142–199%, x = 168%[44a] 146–199%, x = 171%[44b]
Factor VII80	120%[30]		70–260%[31a]	70–260%, x = 162%[30]
Factor X	80–120%[30] 100%[29]			72–200%, x = 130%[30] 122%[29]
Factor IX	100%[29]			130%[29]
Factor XI	100%[29]			69%[29]
Factor XIII	100%[32]			67%[32]
AT III	Normal[29]	Normal[29]	Normal[38]	Normal[29]
Plasminogen	96.5% ± 15.1 SD[31]			128.7% ± 20.0 SD[31]
α-2-macroglobulin	99.2% ± 15.2 SD[31]			126.7% ± 25.4 SD[31]
Fibrin degradation products	6.5 ± 2.1 μg/dl[46]	6.6 ± 2.6 μg/dl[46]	8.2 ± 4.1 μg/dl[46]	14.0 ± 6.9 μg/dl[46]
F VIIIR:Ag/ VIII:C ratio		1.02 ± 0.24[50]	1.58 ± 0.54[50]	1.55 ± 0.44[50]
F VIII:CAg	0.97 U/ml[42]		1.17 ± 0.33 U/ml[42]	
β-thromboglobulin	20 ng/ml[51]	20 ng/ml[51]	27 ng/ml[51]	29 ng/ml[51]
Fibrinopeptide A	2–4 pmol/ml[48]			2 pmol/ml[48]

* Superscript numbers indicate reference source of data.
[a] Data from 28–34 weeks expressed as %.
[b] Data from 35–40 weeks expressed as %.

deficiency described by Aoki was in a male, and no mention was made of α2PI levels in pregnant female family members.[14] Elevated α2PI levels have been observed in a male patient with recurrent thrombosis, but there are no data that look at elevations of α2PI in pregnancy or its relationship to venous thrombosis. Protein C is an inhibitor of activated coagulation factors V and VIII.[21] Limited data are available about the absolute levels of protein C during normal pregnancy. Seligsohn and coworkers have described a large family in which two newborns, homozygous for protein C deficiency, died of massive venous thrombosis.[40] Fourteen heterozygotes who were partially deficient in protein C were also described in this kindred, and several have had normal pregnancies without venous thrombosis.[40] This is somewhat unusual, since in other kindreds the heterozygote state has been associated with thrombosis.[21] This study suggests that pregnancy does not increase the risk, but additional studies are required to fully evaluate the effect of pregnancy on normal and protein C–deficient patients.

FACTOR VIII COMPLEX

Of all the clotting factor activities, those of the factor VIII complex have been the most fully studied during normal and abnormal pregnancies. This emphasis is attributable in large part to the need to diagnose and to manage patients with suspected or documented von Willebrand's disease and hemophilia A during pregnancy. It is necessary to carefully define the different biologic activities that contribute to the factor VIII complex in order to clearly document their changes during pregnancy. Factor VIII coagulant activity (FVIII:C) is attributed to the smaller component of the complex, MW approximately 285,000 daltons.[41] The small procoagulant component is noncovalently bound to the larger portion, the von Willebrand factor protein, which has a molecular weight of more than 10^6 daltons.[41] This larger portion of the complex is defined by two biologic properties, factor VIII–related antigen (VIIIR:Ag) and the ristocetin-dependent platelet aggregation activity (VIIIR:RC).[41] Each of the activities is measured by an independent laboratory test, and each may fluctuate during pregnancy. Another factor VIII complex property that can now be measured independently is the procoagulant antigenic activity (VIII:CAg), which is immunologically distinct from the VIIIR:Ag molecule.[42] The VIII:CAg is stable compared with the VIII:C activity. The latter may be degraded while stored even at −80°C, and the VIII:CAg measurement improves the precision of hemophilia carrier detection.[43]

Fournie and coworkers[44] have reported that VIII:C activity increases during normal pregnancy. They observed at 28 to 34 weeks of gestation an average value of 164% (range 139% to 194%) compared with 100% for nonpregnant normal controls. The level of VIII:C increased further to an average value of 180% (range 156% to 208%) at term. Hoyer and colleagues[42] measured the VIII:CAg levels in pregnant normal controls during the 18th to 21st week of uncomplicated pregnancy and observed a mean value of 1.17 U*/ml ± 0.33 compared with a value of 0.97 U/ml for nonpregnant women. Fournie and associates[44] observed average VIIIR:Ag levels of 168% (range 145% to 194%) at 28 to 34 weeks, rising to an average of 204% (range 180% to 231%) at 35 to 40 weeks of pregnancy. Hoyer and coworkers[42] found an average factor VIIIR:Ag value of 1.23 ± .35 U/ml in normal pregnancy between the 18th and 21st week of pregnancy. The Fournie study also measured the functional ristocetin

* 1.0 U/ml = 100% activity level.

cofactor activity (VIIIR:RC), which was elevated at 28 to 34 weeks—average 168% (range 142% to 199%)—and remained similar up to 35 to 40 weeks at 171% (range 146% to 199%). Thus, all the properties associated with the factor VIII complex increase during pregnancy to approximately the same degree. The sole exception is the VIIIR:Ag, which exceeds the other activities at term, although as of this time there are no VIII:CAg data from normal women at term. The Fournie study[44] also measured the factor VIII complex activities on the second postpartum day and found little change from the levels at time of delivery.

Considerable interest has been devoted to coagulation changes associated with abnormal pregnancy states, especially the ratio of FVIIIR:Ag to FVIII:C activities. Among normal nonpregnant women this ratio is very close to 1.0.[42] Thornton and colleagues have observed that during normal pregnancy this ratio changes slightly—1.0 to 1.32 at 16 to 20 weeks and up to 1.45 at 36 weeks of pregnancy.[45] Thus, for the interpretation of any study that examines a change in this ratio as an index of abnormal pregnancy, a control group matched for gestational age is necessary for interpretation.

FIBRIN-FIBRINOGEN DEGRADATION PRODUCTS

Another index of coagulation activation during pregnancy that has been used is the presence of fibrin or fibrinogen degradation products. Woodfield and associates[46] reported that serum fibrin degradation products (FDP) rose during normal pregnancy from an average value of 6.6 ± 2.6 (SD) μg/dl during the first trimester to 14.0 ± 6.9 μg/dl in the third trimester. Their normal nonpregnant average value was 6.5 ± 2.1 μg/dl. Only values beyond 10.6 μg/dl, the 2SD level, would have achieved a level of significance. A second study[47] also demonstrated elevated FDP levels in the third trimester (5.3 μg/dl versus <4 μg/dl for normal), and the serial dilution protamine sulfate test (SDPS) was positive in up to one third of women with normal pregnancies. This last observation would indicate a low level of thrombin activation during normal pregnancy. However, conflict data have been reported by Borok and colleagues, who did not find an elevation beyond the normal nonpregnant range for FDP or for fibrinopeptide A, a sensitive index of thrombin activation, at time of delivery.[48]

PLATELETS

The platelet count does not change during normal pregnancy.[49] At least two investigators have reported that plasma levels of the platelet α-granule secretory protein β-thromboglobulin are increased during normal pregnancy.[50, 51] These increases occurred in the last two trimesters and may be indicative of low grade platelet activation in normal pregnancy.

USE OF LABORATORY TESTS IN THE DIAGNOSIS OF HEMOSTATIC DISORDERS DURING PREGNANCY

SCREENING TESTS

Congenital disorders of hemostasis, whether in the plasma or cellular phase, are rare disorders, and the routine laboratory screening of pregnant patients is of extremely low yield, as it is for other patient groups.[52] The most useful and cost-effective screening method to detect hemostatic disorders in pregnancy is a careful history with specific attention to spontaneous bleeding, thrombotic events, and previous surgical challenge.[53]

Since it is now recognized that certain coagulopathies are associated with spontaneous abortion, for example, factor XIII deficiency and the lupus inhibitor, specific inquiry for these events may also help to focus the subsequent choice of laboratory tests.[32, 54] If a history is obtained that indicates a hemostatic or a thrombotic disorder, then the first step would be to use a screening test. Frequently it is not possible to sort out a disorder of the fluid phase from a platelet-related disorder, and thus with a positive history the logical choices would be an activated partial thromboplastin time (aPTT), a quantitative platelet count, and a prothrombin time, in that order. If no abnormal results were detected at this level but the history was impressive, then a qualitative assessment of platelet function using a template bleeding time device would be a next logical choice. If the bleeding time is within normal limits but the history is significant, then a repeat bleeding time after aspirin challenge is a useful test, particularly when von Willebrand's disease is a suspected diagnosis.[55]

Once again, if these studies are negative but the history is clinically significant, then several additional tests may be selected, depending upon the history. If a pattern of delayed bleeding after surgical challenge or deep tissue hemorrhage is elicited, a clot solubility test to screen for factor XIII activity is warranted. Other possible options are to measure the fibrinogen level by a functional assay and to perform a thrombin time with a dilute thrombin solution to detect abnormal fibrinogens. If these tests are negative and a hemorrhagic diathesis is strongly suspected, then consideration may be given to measuring α-2-antiplasmin. However, deficiency of this protein is so unusual that use of this test should only be reserved for highly selected patients with a significant positive bleeding history.

Screening for prothrombotic disorders is an even more difficult task. These diseases are rare, and consideration to test for them should be guided by the patient history. The combination of a positive history of documented thrombosis tendency and a shortened aPTT is suggestive, but the aPTT is a nonspecific test and of little diagnostic use.[56] In a patient with a strong familial history, consideration should be given to measuring antithrombin III (ATIII) concentration.[39] It is possible that the antigenic level of ATIII could be normal, but a qualitative abnormality must be sought with a functional assay or crossed immunoelectrophoresis in the presence of the heparin cofactor.[57] If the ATIII levels are normal and there is a history of congenital disorders, then the presence of an abnormal fibrinogen function should also be considered.[58] This can be detected by use of the thrombin time at a low thrombin concentration (1.5 U/ml), a reptilase time, and the use of simultaneous functional and immunologic fibrinogen determinations.[59] Other possible tests to detect abnormal fibrinogens are crossed immunoelectrophoresis and prolonged englobulin clot lysis.[59, 60] Abnormal fibrinogens may clot readily but will resist plasmin digestion.[60] Protein C is a rare cause of recurrent thrombosis, and it can be directly assayed by an immunologic method.[21] An abnormal plasminogen-plasma system can also cause thrombosis and would be detected by either functional or immunologic assays.[13] In both of these disorders the routine screening tests are normal, and the physician should feel compelled to select these specific tests only in the face of a strong history.

SPECIFIC DIAGNOSTIC TESTS, FACTOR DEFICIENCIES

Fortunately many patients with a significant bleeding history will have positive findings on a screening test, which directs further diagnostic evaluation. If only the aPTT is prolonged, then consideration must be given to a differential diagnosis of acquired versus congenital disorders of the intrinsic pathway. The congenital disorders are rare, and if they are suspected the appropriate diagnostic test would be the specific factor assay, usually done in order for factors VIII, IX, XI, and XII. A deficiency of the last is not associated with a hemorrhagic diathesis and would only be resorted to as a last choice to explain a prolonged aPTT.[61] If family history points to a previously recognized selected factor deficiency, then the choice is obvious. If only the PT or both the aPTT and PT are prolonged, then consideration must be given to an extrinsic pathway defect or to a common pathway defect. Vitamin K deficiency is the most common cause of these defects, and its complications will be discussed. All the common pathway and extrinsic factor deficiency disorders are extremely rare and selected assay for factors X, V, and prothrombins would be reasonable if both the PT and aPTT are prolonged and for factor VII if only the PT is prolonged. Hypofibrinogenemia or dysfibrinogenemia may be associated with a hemorrhagic diathesis and rarely cause a prolonged PT or aPTT, and other more sensitive tests described earlier would be more appropriate.

Frequently the historical distinction between an acquired and a congenital disorder is not clear, and rather than systematically assay all the intrinsic factors, a mixing study to differentiate a deficiency from an acquired inhibitor is useful. This can be easily accomplished in most laboratories by mixing citrated patient plasma 1:1 with a citrated normal plasma and performing an aPTT on the mixture immediately and after 60 minutes of incubation at 37°C. A factor deficiency should exhibit complete correction (Table 8–2), whereas an acquired inhibitor will not be corrected, and depending on the type of inhibitor, a distinctive pattern of prolongation may occur (Tables 8–3 and 8–4).

It should be remembered that the most common acquired inhibitor detected in a clinical laboratory is heparin contamination, and perhaps the second most common is fibrin degradation products (FDP) caused by disseminated intravascular coagulation (DIC). The first can be evaluated by the performance of a thrombin time (TT) that will be prolonged due to heparin but will correct with the addition of toluidine blue. FDP can be identified most easily with a latex agglutination test.[62]

The remaining significant acquired inhibitors may be directed against a specific clotting factor[63] or will appear to be nonspecific if due to the lupus type anticoagulant.[64] The factor-specific inhibitors usually do not show immediate inhibition but require time for potentiation (see Table 8–3). In contrast, the lupus anticoagulant almost always reacts immediately, with little time-dependent potentiation (see Table 8–4).[65]

Table 8–2. Factor VIII–Deficient Plasma, Inhibitor Screen Mixing Study; Noninhibitory Plasma with Complete Correction*

	0 Min	**60 Min**
Patient	127.5 s	120.6 s
Control	33.6 s	34.6 s
Patient:Control	35.1 s	35.2 s
Deficient Control:Control	34.6 s	37.1 s

* Plasma or equal part mixtures of plasmas were tested using the aPTT as the assay system. The deficient control:control mixture represents a mixture of a known factor VIII–deficient plasma without any inhibitory activity and a normal control plasma. The assay is performed immediately upon mixing the plasmas (0 min) and after incubation at 37°C (60 min). Test results are expressed in seconds. Laboratory normal aPTT range is 24–38 s, which encompasses 2 SD around the normal mean aPTT. A result is interpreted as abnormal when it exceeds this range.

Table 8–3. Factor VIII–Deficient Plasma, Inhibitor Screen Mixing Study; Inhibitory Plasma without Complete Correction*

	0 Min	60 Min
Patient	90.5 s	89.8 s
Control	32.3 s	32.6 s
Patient:Control	39.0 s	44.6 s
Deficient Control:Control	35.9 s	36.9 s

* Same assay conditions as in Table 8–2. Results demonstrate poor initial correction and time-dependent potentiation at 60 min, at which point the patient plasma has further prolonged control plasma. The deficient control demonstrates appropriate correction and no inhibitory activity. This result is consistent with an acquired factor VIII inhibitor subsequently confirmed by a specific antifactor VIII assay.

When a factor-specific inhibitor is suspected, a substrate deficient assay system is used. Eventually the strength of the inhibitor can be determined in a specific, mixing assay that measures how much normal factor can be inactivated by the specific factor inhibitor.[66]

If the preliminary mixing study is more consistent with the lupus type anticoagulant or if other indicators such as a false-positive serologic test for syphilis or multiple abnormal specific factor assays are found, then a more specific test for the lupus anticoagulant may be carried out. The presence of multiple abnormal factor assays is caused by the fact that all these assays are performed using a modified single stage aPTT; thus each assay will be inhibited as would the standard aPTT. Generally the aPTT is prolonged in the presence of the lupus anticoagulant and is a more sensitive screening test than the PT. When the PT is prolonged, the occurrence of acquired hypoprothrombinemia must also be considered, especially when the ratio of the patient PT to the upper limit of the normal range PT is greater than 1.5.[64] In the past, several specific tests for the lupus anticoagulant have been recommended based on either the dilute thromboplastin time or a whole blood thromboplastin inhibition test.[67] Currently the most specific assay appears to be the dilute Russell's viper venom test, which Shapiro and Thiagarajan found to be a highly sensitive and specific test.[64] This test uses Russell's viper venom to directly activate factor X in the presence of dilute phospholipid. Since the lupus anticoagulant is primarily directed against phospholipid, this test is very selective for the detection of this inhibitor. A test based on the kaolin-activated clotting time has also been successful.[68] Typical data for a mixing study and the diluted Russell's viper venom test are presented for a factor VIII specific inhibitor and the lupus anticoagulant in Table 8–5. Clinically the lupus anticoagulant is not associated with a bleeding diathesis but more commonly with an increased incidence of venous thrombosis[69] and spontaneous abortion.[54] Thus accurate diagnosis of the

Table 8–4. Lupus-Type Anticoagulant, Inhibitor Screen Mixing Study with Inhibition*

	0 Min	60 Min
Patient	73.4 s	79.2 s
Control	32.9 s	33.2 s
Patient:Control	45.2 s	45.4 s
Deficient Control:Control	35.7 s	35.2 s

* Same conditions as for Table 8–3. Results demonstrate an immediate acting inhibitor that does not show time- or temperature-dependent potentiation.

Table 8–5. Russell's Viper Venom Test (RVVT) to Evaluate the Presence of the Lupus Anti-coagulant*

Patient MC	
aPTT	67.0 s
RVVT—Patient	72.9 s
Patient:Control plasmas RVV	48.0 s
RVVT—Control	31.0 s
aPPT (ionophore-treated platelets)	40.6 s
Patient AW	
aPTT	48.0 s
RVVT—Patient	55.8 s
Patient:Control plasma RVV	31.5 s
RVVT—Control	217.0 s

* Patient MC has prolonged RVVT that does not correct after mixing with normal plasma. Patient AW has a prolonged RVVT that completely corrects after mixing with normal plasma. Patient AW was found to be deficient in factor X. A prolonged RVVT caused by the lupus anticoagulant should not correct upon mixing.

disorder will frequently alter the therapeutic approach. Documentation of acquired prothrombin deficiency associated with the lupus anticoagulant syndrome can be demonstrated using both functional and immunologic factor II assay.[70]

Under very unusual circumstances inhibitors with heparin-like activity may occur, but none have been reported during pregnancy. These inhibitors are usually proteoglycans and have the generic label of "heparinoids" because of their heparin-like antithrombin activity. Classically they are associated with a dramatically prolonged thrombin time[71] and normal reptilase time and can be neutralized by adding exogenous platelet factor 4 (PF4).

DISSEMINATED INTRAVASCULAR COAGULATION

Disseminated intravascular coagulation (DIC) is the most common cause of an acquired hemorrhagic diathesis during pregnancy. The disorder is usually associated with a variety of abnormal screening tests that suggest the diagnosis: prolonged aPTT, hypofibrinogenemia, and thrombocytopenia. The presence of FDP can be confirmed with the latex agglutination test, which is rapid and simple.[62] False-positive results can occur with this test because of rheumatoid factor, but this can be eliminated by repeating the test in the presence of a reducing substance such as 2-mercaptoethanol.[72] Additional tests to confirm the presence of DIC may detect the presence of fibrin monomers via the protamine sulfate paracoagulation test[73] or the radioimmunoassay for fibrinopeptide- A (FPA).[74] The former is only 50% sensitive and the latter, while extremely sensitive, is too costly for the routine laboratory. FDP can also be produced as a result of another rare syndrome, primary fibrinogenolysis. This disorder can be seen with excessive release of tissue plasminogen activator (TPA) caused by genitourinary tract tumors.[15] Placental tissue is also rich in TPA and could theoretically produce excessive fibrinogenolysis. Plasmin activity does not cause thrombocytopenia or the production of fibrin monomers. It does cause the production of a specific fibrinopeptide derived from the fibrinogen β chain, B β-1–42 fragment.[48] Unfortunately, this very sensitive and specific test is not readily available.

VON WILLEBRAND'S DISEASE

The diagnosis of von Willebrand's disease is complicated by the changes in the various factor VIII complex activities during pregnancy superimposed upon the molecular and clinical heterogeneity of the disease.[75] In addition, there is biologic variation in the expression of the factor VIII complex activities within a given individual patient over time that is beyond the intrinsic variability of the assay itself.[76] This latter feature makes it necessary to retest a suspected von Willebrand's disease patient a number of times in order to ensure the correct diagnosis. The following laboratory tests are commonly utilized in the evaluation of this disorder: bleeding time (BT), factor VIII coagulant activity (FVIII:C), factor VIII–related antigen (FVIIIR:Ag), factor VIII ristocetin cofactor (FVIIIR:RC), factor VIII–related antigen by crossed immunoelectrophoresis,[77] and factor VIII–related antigen multimeric structure.[78] The older tests of glass bead platelet retention and direct platelet aggregation by ristocetin using platelet-rich plasma have largely been replaced by the newer tests.

Phenotypic von Willebrand's disease is generally defined by the activities which are tested for. Classic von Willebrand's disease (type I) is characterized by a decrease, usually of equal proportions, in all the factor VIII complex activities and with a prolonged bleeding time. Measurement of the qualitative properties of the factor VIII–related antigen by either crossed immunoelectrophoresis or multimer composition demonstrates a normal pattern with reduced quantity. The second major group of von Willebrand patients are classified as variant (type II) because of a number of atypical features. Generally the level of FVIII:C is within the normal range and FVIIIR:Ag is also normal or at most moderately reduced, but the FVIII:RC is markedly decreased, the BT is prolonged, and crossed immunoelectrophoresis demonstrates an anodal shift[79] (Fig. 8–2). Multimeric analysis reveals the complete absence of large and intermediate molecular weight forms. After the initial characterization of the type II variant, a second variant von Willebrand phenotype was described in

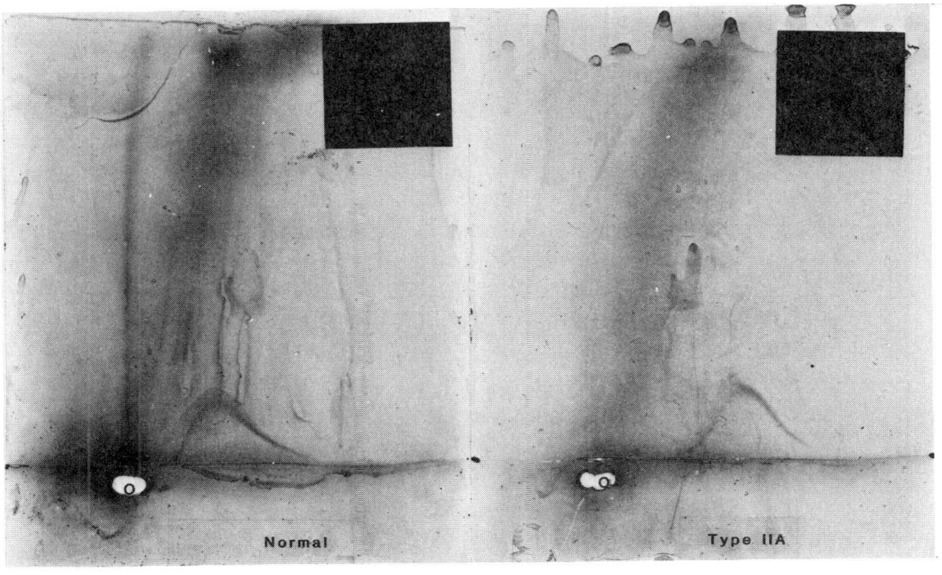

Figure 8–2. Crossed immunoelectrophoresis of factor VIII–related antigen from a normal patient (N) and a patient with variant von Willebrand's disease type IIA. The origin is indicated by 0 and the anodal direction of migration is away from the origin in the first direction and from bottom to top in the second direction. Note that the IIA pattern is more anodal and is missing the larger, slower migrating VWF molecules.

which the FVIII:C ranged from normal to moderately reduced, FVIII:Ag was normal or moderately reduced, FVIIIR:RC was normal or moderately reduced, and the bleeding time was variable from prolonged to normal.[79] Further study using direct ristocetin-induced platelet aggregation (RIPA) showed this patient group to have enhanced platelet aggregation at low ristocetin concentrations (1.2 g/L).[61] Crossed immunoelectrophoresis of the factor VIIIR:Ag of these patients also demonstrated an anodal shift, and multimeric analysis confirmed the absence of the larger forms, although intermediate size multimers were observed. On the basis of the increased RIPA, the variant type II classification was split into IIA and IIB subtypes, IIB now designating the patients with increased RIPA.[79] A third variant labeled type IIC has also recently been described in which the larger multimers are absent but the remaining multimer subunit pattern appears abnormal.[80] A third variant, now called pseudo-von Willebrand's disease, has also been reported.[81] These patients have a bleeding diathesis but the BT is within the normal range. Factor VIII:C is normal or moderately reduced and plasma FVIIIR:Ag by standard electroimmunoassay is within the normal range, although upon re-examination by immunoradiometric assay two subjects had a decreased level. Ristocetin cofactor activity (FVIIIR:RC) is normal or reduced. Crossed immunoelectrophoresis of the plasma FVIIIR:Ag demonstrated increased anodal mobility, but the platelet FVIIIR:Ag exhibited normal mobility in spite of a slight reduction in absolute FVIII:Ag.[81] The platelets from these patients adsorbed increased amounts of high molecular weight FVIII:VWF multimer and were aggregated spontaneously by purified FVIII:VWF in the absence of ristocetin.[81] Both of these properties are not seen with normal platelets or platelets from patients with type I, type IIA, type IIB, or type IIC von Willebrand's disease. Another unique characteristic of this phenotype is the occurrence of intermittent thrombocytopenia. A second group of patients with similar laboratory characteristics has also been described, with the additional observation of increased mean platelet volumes (MPV).[82] Measurement of MPV is now available in many laboratories and may be of diagnostic use in this syndrome. A rare, third type of von Willebrand's disease (type III) has been reported in which no ristocetin cofactor activity or factor VIII–related antigen is present. This is a very severe hemorrhagic disorder.[83] Other variants that do not readily fit into the described classification scheme for von Willebrand's disease have also been reported, and undoubtedly new variants will continue to be reported as the molecular basis of this complex disorder is elucidated.[84] The laboratory tests described will continue to define these phenotypic variants, and new tests such as the recent FVIII:VWF binding studies will evolve.

The diagnosis of classic severe von Willebrand's disease during pregnancy is complicated because of the potential normalization of the various laboratory tests. Patients have been reported with severe, classic von Willebrand's disease in which factors VIII:C, VIIIR:Ag, and VIIIR:RC all rose from abnormal values well into the normal range at time of delivery, although the BT did remain prolonged.[85] Obviously such normalization during the physiologic response to pregnancy will make diagnosis during this time extremely difficult.

The data on the changes in the various components of the factor VIII complex for variant von Willebrand's disease are limited. Hanna and colleagues have described a case of type IIA von Willebrand's disease.[86] The factor VIII:C and VIIIR:Ag levels gradually increased during pregnancy, although not as much as those of two normal pregnant controls. Near term the factor VIIIR:RC activity became "normal" but was still subnormal considering the gestational age, and the bleeding time was transiently reduced but never entirely normal at term. In spite of the normalization of the ristocetin cofactor activity, the multimeric composition remained abnormal throughout pregnancy and during the postpartum period.[86] The authors concluded that the multimeric structure and the ristocetin cofactor activity were dissociated. Also of interest was the observation that the factor VIIIR:RC activity declined precipitously after delivery compared with that of the normal pregnant controls. This effect had not been observed for the two classic von Willebrand's patients previously described, in whom factor VIIIR:RC activity stayed elevated in the immediate postpartum period.[85] This observation is of special note because generally it is the assay of factor VIIIR:RC that tends to correlate best with the bleeding time and clinical bleeding; thus its rapid decline may predict an increased risk of postpartum hemorrhage.[87]

Diagnosis of von Willebrand's disease during pregnancy requires measurement of each of the factor VIII complex associated activities. The results must be interpreted in light of the changes known to occur for the factor VIII complex in pregnancy. Yet with the extreme variability of this disease, diagnosis remains difficult. These changes are best characterized for the VIII:C and VIIIR:Ag activities. Unfortunately there are only limited data for the VIIIR:RC and very little data exist on normal crossed immunoelectrophoresis FVIIIR:Ag or multimer patterns during pregnancy. Additionally, the normal ranges for these assays in pregnancy are quite broad, and thus the statistical certainty with which von Willebrand's disease can be diagnosed or excluded may be tenuous. Management of patients with previously diagnosed von Willebrand's disease requires assay of each factor VIII complex activity that can be quantitated. The single test that seems to correlate best with clinical bleeding appears to be the factor VIIIR:RC level.[85, 88] Repetition of the bleeding time for therapeutic management is not very useful because frequently correction is transient or only partial and does not appear to correlate highly with clinical bleeding.[85] Repeat assay of the factor VIII procoagulant activity is frequently performed because it is readily available, but the levels do not correlate well with bleeding tendency and frequently will be in the normal range during pregnancy.[88] The overshoot in coagulant activity after cryoprecipitate infusion that is typically seen with von Willebrand's disease may be of some diagnostic value on rare occasions and has been described in pregnancy. Monitoring the presence of the larger multimers during pregnancy is too difficult for routine care of these patients.

DIAGNOSIS OF THE HEMOPHILIA CARRIER STATE DURING PREGNANCY

Detection of the hemophilia carrier state is frequently required during pregnancy, since this is the time when many individuals who are at risk may present for testing.[89] Previous diagnostic techniques relied upon the discordance between the factor VIII:C activity and the factor VIIIR:Ag level as a means to detect carriers. Because VIII:C is controlled by the X chromosome gene while VIIIR:Ag is autosomal, there is a reduction in one but not the other. Earlier techniques have used the ratio between the factor VIII:C procoagulant activity and the factor VIII:RAg level or a discriminant analysis technique using these two activities to classify hemophilia A carriers.[90, 91] More recently Hoyer and coworkers have demonstrated that the use of an assay to measure antigenic procoagulant VIII concentration (VIII:CAg) is more reliable than the functional VIII:C coagulant assay.[92] The latter is less reliable because of activity changes caused by sample degradation during transportation and storage. Using an immunoradiometric assay to detect antigenic VIII:C (VIII:CAg) and a similar assay to detect VIIIR:Ag in frozen samples, the classification accuracy of 96% was similar to that using freshly drawn blood from nonpregnant subjects. Thus, the ability to use frozen samples permits a much more uniform assay method in a limited number of reference laboratories. This now makes available a highly reliable method to diagnose the hemophilia carrier state during pregnancy.

LIVER DISEASE AND DEFICIENCY OF VITAMIN K–DEPENDENT COAGULATION FACTORS

Factors II, V, VII, IX, X, XI, XII, XIII, fibrinogen, prekallikrein, HMK, and antithrombin III are synthesized in the liver.[93] In addition, the liver functions as a site for clearance of activated coagulation factors. Coagulation factors II, VII, IX, and X require vitamin K for posttranslational modification in the liver to become functional.[93] Defects in the vitamin K–dependent step appear to be more sensitive to hepatic dysfunction than failure of protein synthesis. A severe reduction in factor II, VII, or X will result in a prolonged prothrombin time, which can be corrected by mixing with normal plasma. Factor VII is most sensitive to hepatic dysfunction because it exhibits the shortest plasma turnover rate and thus the PT is most sensitive to its concentration. A deficiency of factor IX caused by vitamin K or liver disease will cause prolongation of the partial thromboplastin time (aPTT), but because of its relatively long half-life, the deficiency develops slowly and the aPTT is not a very sensitive test. Acquired factor X deficiency is associated with both a long PT and aPTT because of its position in the common pathway. In each case direct assay for the suspected absent factor will substantiate the diagnosis. If vitamin K deficiency is suspected clinically, a repeat measurement of the PT after vitamin K replacement will be useful, or it can be demonstrated that the vitamin K–dependent factors are immunologically present but functionally inactive. Using direct Russell's viper venom activation of factor X, the Stypven time can be used to discriminate factor VII deficiency from factor X deficiency by its differential site of action.

Discrimination of liver disease from DIC as the sole cause of a coagulopathy may be difficult. In both disorders there may be low levels of FDP. In liver disease this is postulated to be produced by defective hepatic clearance of activated factors, and hepatic necrosis may also serve to initiate DIC.[94] Earlier it was felt that factor VIII:C levels could be used to separate liver disease from DIC, but since factor VII:C is elevated in pregnancy and may not necessarily decrease in DIC, it is not a reliable test. The implication of intrinsic hepatic dysfunction as a cause of coagulopathy is best supported by the demonstration of multiple hepatic–dependent clotting factor deficiencies in spite of adequate vitamin K repletion. Ancillary laboratory evidence of other hepatic dysfunction will also assist in establishing the diagnosis. In general, the absence or presence of FDP will not be very helpful in identifying hepatic disease as the primary cause of a coagulopathy.

DIAGNOSIS OF PLATELET DISORDERS IN PREGNANCY

Both qualitative and quantitative platelet disorders may occur during pregnancy. The congenital qualitative platelet disorders are rare, whereas acquired qualitative and quantitative platelet disorders are much more common and warrant a more extensive discussion. The leading cause of qualitative platelet dysfunction after iatrogenic pharmacologic causes is probably immune-mediated platelet dysfunction, and this is probably the leading cause of quantitative platelet disorders as well. Immune-mediated thrombocytopenia can occur as a result of a variety of etiologies, but the most common are autoimmune thrombocytopenia, drug-induced thrombocytopenia, and immune thrombocytopenia secondary to a variety of autoimmune disorders, including systemic lupus erythematosus, rheumatoid arthritis, and Hashimoto's thyroiditis. In addition, fetal-maternal genetic differences can give rise to alloimmune platelet disorders. The commonest case finding laboratory index for these disorders is a reduced platelet count, although these patients may present with a normal platelet count and only a qualitative disorder, as evidenced by easy bruising and a prolonged bleeding time.[95] Until recently the laboratory documentation of platelet immune disorders has lacked adequate sensitivity, and although questions about the specificity of platelet antibodies have been raised, the current consensus indicates that the increased platelet-associated immunoglobulin (PAIg) is highly correlated with platelet destruction.[96, 97]

Two basic forms of immune-mediated thrombocytopenia occur during pregnancy: autoimmune and alloimmune. In the first, both mother and fetus may be affected and the diagnosis of the etiology of the thrombocytopenia may affect management.[98] The second disorder only affects the fetus, and accurate diagnosis may dramatically affect choice of therapy.

Traditionally the diagnosis of autoimmune thrombocytopenia depended upon the clinical setting and the demonstration of increased megakaryocytes in bone marrow. A variety of assays to detect serum antibodies had been developed but lacked adequate sensitivity. Newer assays that directly measure platelet-associated hemoglobulin (PAIg) are more sensitive for the detection of immune-mediated platelet destruction.[97] The absolute amount of immunoglobulin deposited on the platelet surface in these disorders does not appear to correlate well with the degree of thrombocytopenia, but the assay is specific in that platelets from patients with nonimmune thrombocytopenia contained normal amounts of PAIg.[97] Questions about the specificity of these assays have been raised, and the issue is further complicated by the multiplicity of assays described in the literature.[96] Assessment of the validity of an available assay is therefore important, and one significant criterion is that the assay specificity be demonstrated. It appears that assays that use monoclonal reagents or exhibit low nonspecific binding provide reliable data. Using these assays, pregnant patients with immune thrombocytopenia can be identified.

Once these patients are detected a second problem is to determine whether the fetus will be affected. Controversy exists as to the best test with which to predict whether fetal thrombocytopenia is present without actual fetal blood sampling. A direct fetal platelet count can be obtained at the time of labor, but it requires an invasive procedure and is only available once the cervix has dilated enough to permit sampling.[99] If the fetal platelet count is above $50 \times 10^9/L$, vaginal delivery appears to be a safe procedure.[99] Several laboratories have used either direct platelet-associated immunoglobulin or the serum antiplatelet antibody concentration as measured by an indirect test to predict the effect on fetal platelet count. Kelton and associates reported that the maternal platelet–associated IgG level correlated poorly with the fetal platelet count.[100] The poor correlation between maternal and fetal platelet count has been generally observed. Cines and coworkers observed that maternal PAIgG was not a good predictor of fetal platelet count but instead that the maternal serum antiplatelet antibody concentration, as measured by their indirect radioactive Coombs' type test, was a good indicator of the fetal platelet status.[101] Using a different assay, other workers have found a trend between the maternal indirect test and fetal platelet count but have felt that the correlation was too imprecise to be used as a clinical tool.[102]

As of this time it appears that measurement of maternal PAIgG is useful to establish the diagnosis of immune-mediated thrombocytopenia. The assay to be selected should utilize reagents that give a very low false-positive rate. If accurate platelet sizing is also available, the combined use of the PAIgG and mean platelet volume should be adequate to establish the diagnosis without the need for a bone marrow aspirate. There is adequate evidence to substantiate that increased mean platelet volume correlates with disorders of increased platelet destruction, with the rare exception of myeloproliferative syndromes and severe megaloblastic anemia.[103] It appears to be more difficult to predict fetal risk for thrombocytopenia. The weight of evidence shows that maternal platelet count and probably the concentration of maternal PAIgG (direct test) are not predictive. The serum concentration of platelet antibody may be useful to determine fetal risk, but the value of this test is unsettled. In the face of these limitations, direct sampling of fetal platelet count remains the most precise predictor of fetal risk. Obviously if other autoimmune disorders such as systemic lupus erythematosus are suspected, additional tests should be done to establish these diagnoses.

The demonstration of alloimmune fetal thrombocytopenia is more difficult. Before delivery of a thrombocytopenic infant, the disease may not be suspected.[104] Establishing the correct diagnosis is important, since the management is different from that of maternal autoimmune thrombocytopenia. Measurement of fetal platelet-associated IgG should establish an immune basis for this disorder. Maternal PAIgG level should be normal, but an indirect assay using maternal serum against paternal platelets should be positive.[98] Measurement of fetal mean platelet volume should also help to establish that increased fetal platelet volume is within the normal adult ranges.[105] Platelet antigen systems are complex, and very few laboratories have the ability to specifically identify the immunogen in neonatal alloimmunization. Thus the use of paternal platelets in the test system simplifies the diagnosis. If transfusion support is required the most appropriate form of therapy would be washed maternal platelets.[98]

Maternal autoimmune thrombocytopenia with passive fetal transfer caused by drug-induced sensitization has also been described.[106] There are assays similar to those described for the diagnosis of the above disorders that can demonstrate drug-mediated platelet destruction.[107]

THROMBOTIC THROMBOCYTOPENIA PURPURA AND PRE-ECLAMPSIA-ECLAMPSIA SYNDROMES

Thrombotic thrombocytopenia purpura (TTP) is a rare disorder characterized by the clinical pentad of thrombocytopenia, hemolytic anemia, fever, fluctuating neurologic deficits, and renal disease. There is no single laboratory test that is diagnostic in all cases. Generally only a low level of fibrin degradation products is seen, adequate bone marrow megakaryocytes are observed, and a normal PAIgG level is found.[108] Gingival biopsy or biopsy of other tissue may demonstrate hyalin thrombi in small arterioles in 50% of cases.[109] More recently Moake and coworkers have reported that abnormally large factor VIII:VWF multimers are present during remission in patients with chronic relapsing TTP.[110] Exacerbation of disease may be associated with pregnancy; thus the factor VIII:VWF multimer pattern could be of potential diagnostic value.[110, 111]

Changes in hemostasis occur in patients with pre-eclampsia-eclampsia syndromes. Some reports have emphasized evidence for low grade DIC, but the most consistent observation appears to be an effect on platelets. No specific changes are known, but there is evidence of platelet consumption and platelet activation with secretion of platelet α-granule proteins.[112] Several groups of workers have also reported elevated PAIgG levels in patients with eclampsia as evidence of an autoimmune etiology.[112] β-Thromboglobulin has been the most commonly measured α-granule protein, and commercial reagents to perform the assay are available, although meticulous care in sample collection is required to avoid false positive results caused by spurious platelet secretion.[48, 113] Studies of coagulation changes in eclampsia have also suggested that thrombin activation is important in the pathogenesis of this syndrome. This was manifest by activation of factor VIII coagulant activity, which caused the FVIII:C to FVIIIR:Ag ratio to fall as the result of procoagulant activity.[114] More recent studies, however, indicate that plasmin activation is more important, and platelet activation may be due to mechanisms other than thrombin.[48] Determination of plasmin activation is difficult because sensitive, precise tests are not routinely available in most clinical laboratories. The most sensitive specific test is the measurement of thrombin increasable fibrinopeptide B, but its availability is severely limited. Thus, specific laboratory documentation of the eclampsia syndromes is not possible, although a variety of indirect tests such as platelet BTG or PAIgG may be useful.

RARE QUALITATIVE DISORDERS OF PLATELET DYSFUNCTION

It is well established that a defect in certain specific platelet membrane glycoproteins is associated with platelet dysfunction.[115] The Bernard-Soulier syndrome (BSS) is a hereditary platelet disorder characterized by fluctuating thrombocytopenia, large platelets, and defective platelet adhesion. BSS platelets are lacking in glycoprotein Ib and exhibit defective platelet aggregation of platelet-rich plasma in response to ristocetin.[116] Glanzmann's thrombasthenia is a severe hemostatic disorder caused by a defect in glycoprotein IIb–IIIa. Glanzmann thrombasthenic platelets do not aggregate in response to the common platelet agonists—epinephrine, ADP, or collagen.[117] Both Glanzmann's thrombasthenia and the Bernard-Soulier syndrome can be diagnosed by gel electrophoresis of platelet membranes, but platelet aggregation using PRP is a simpler and more available method.

A deficiency in at least two classes of platelet subcellular granules is associated with defective platelet function.[118] A decrease in dense bodies is associated with mild, spontaneous bleeding that can be severe after surgical challenge. There may be moderate defects in platelet aggregation to standard agonists, but the diagnosis is best established by demonstrating a reduced number of dense bodies by electron microscopy or a decrease in dense body composition such as serotonin or adenine nucleotides.[119] A reduced number of alpha granules is associated with a mild bleeding diathesis, and the platelets may have a monochromatic appearance in routine Wright-Giemsa smears because of the absence of azurophilic granules, giving rise to the term gray platelet syndrome.[120] These platelets demonstrate aggregation defects, but the lack of α-granules is best diagnosed by showing a reduced content of platelet α-granule proteins either β-thromboglobulin or platelet factor 4.[120] As mentioned previously, these disorders are rare and there is little information about the effect of pregnancy upon their severity. However, the diagnostic approach would remain the same as for nonpregnant subjects.

THROMBOTIC DISEASE CAUSED BY HYPER-REACTIVE PLATELETS

Numerous reports have emphasized that platelet hyperaggregability is important to the pathogenesis of arterial thromboembolism.[121] The sensitivity and specificity of platelet aggregation to detect and to correlate with the clinical stages of these disorders is questionable.[122] The detection of circulating platelet aggregates, as described by the method of Wu and Hoak,[121] has been reported to correlate with clinically significant arterial disease and may be a useful test to evaluate pregnant patients with suspected platelet-induced occlusive vascular disease. However, a more recent study suggests that the presence of "circulating platelet aggregates" may be due to an artifact of collection and that circulating aggregates may not be an in vivo physiologic mechanism of vascular disease.[123]

LABORATORY TESTS TO MONITOR ANTICOAGULATION DURING PREGNANCY

Since the 4-hydroxycoumarin derivatives that constitute the oral anticoagulants cross the placental-fetal barrier, they are not used during pregnancy. Heparin is the anticoagulant of choice for treating thrombotic disease during pregnancy. Heparin may be used in a variety of dosage regimens to treat and to provide prophylaxis against thrombosis, and the therapeutic goal selected will, to a large extent, determine which laboratory test is selected to monitor the therapeutic effect.

FULL DOSE HEPARIN ANTICOAGULATION

Active venous thrombosis generally requires a full heparin dose, which means in the range of 1000 U per hour by continuous infusion intravenously. The level of anticoagulation effect is most commonly regulated by following the effect upon the activated partial thromboplastin time.[124] Prior to the initiation of heparin therapy, it is necessary to ascertain that there is no pre-existing bleeding diathesis. This is best accomplished by a careful history and a quantitative platelet count, PT, and aPTT. The baseline aPTT is necessary because it will be used to regulate heparin dosage. With a sensitive thromboplastin reagent the normal range aPTT should be 25 to 35 sec; this may be slightly shorter in pregnant patients, as previously noted.[2] When heparin is given by continuous intravenous infusion, the goal is to maintain the aPTT at 1½ to 2 times the patient's baseline aPTT.[125, 126] The metabolism of heparin can vary, depending upon the presence of hepatic or renal disease and the extent of thrombosis. Guidelines for the frequency with which the aPTT is followed are difficult to find. In general, the level should be checked one to two hours after initiation of therapy, then every 12 hours for the first 24 hours, and then daily. Resistance to heparin infusion may suggest the presence of acquired antithrombin III deficiency, since adequate levels are required for a full heparin therapeutic effect.[127] If heparin is used by the intermittent route, the aPTT should be checked three hours after an intravenous injection or six hours after a subcutaneous injection.

Hemorrhage is a major complication of heparin administration, although there are no data to show that the degree of aPTT prolongation correlates with the risk of hemorrhage; however, there is general agreement that there is reduced hemorrhage with reduction in the total heparin dosage given.[127] Regular monitoring of the hemoglobin or hematocrit value should be carried out to detect clinically occult blood loss. In addition, since heparin-associated thrombocytopenia is now a recognized complication of heparin therapy, the platelet count should be followed at least every third day during therapy.[128, 129] Testing of stool and urine for occult blood loss is also useful, since it may herald the later onset of severe hemorrhage.

LOW DOSE HEPARIN PROPHYLAXIS

Heparin is also used for prophylaxis against venous thromboembolism in a wide variety of disorders, many of which may arise coincidentally during pregnancy.[127] When heparin is used in this manner, its effect upon the coagulation system is usually not followed. Recently newer data looking at adjusted low dose heparin therapy in the long-term management of venous thrombotic disease have been presented.[130] This approach is important in pregnancy and the postpartum period because it avoids the need for 4-hydroxycoumarin derivatives and appears to provide adequate protection against recurrent venous thrombosis.[130] The dose of subcutaneous heparin is adjusted so that at midinterval after the injection (six hours), the aPTT is 1½ times the baseline level.[130] In this study, the dosage adjustment took place over the first three days, and thereafter the heparin was used at a fixed dose. The mean dose required was 10,000 ± 1000 units (SD) given on a 12 hourly schedule. The peak anticoagulant effect occurred at four hours after the subcutaneous injection.[127] Using this regimen in nonpregnant patients, both the rate of recurrent disease and the bleeding complication rate were low and superior to those of other regimens tested.[130] As the authors point out, this study is especially useful in pregnancy because various high dose subcutaneous regimens have been used in pregnant patients without adequate documentation of therapeutic effect.[130]

There may be occasions when a patient with the lupus anticoagulant will require heparin administration with dose adjustment. This complicates the laboratory management, because the aPTT is already prolonged as a result of the inhibitor; yet it is quite clear that this prolongation is not a biologic anticoagulant effect but merely a laboratory artifact.[64] In these patients the prolonged aPTT can be corrected by using ionophore-treated platelets as the phospholipid source.[64] This then normalizes the aPTT and permits using the test to adjust heparin dosage provided that the ionophore-treated platelet reagent is used for all assays.

ACKNOWLEDGEMENTS

The author wishes to acknowledge the efforts of Ms. Jeanne Elliott in typing and editing the manuscript. I am indebted to Ms. Fay Weimer for the supervision and performance of the specialized coagulation tests used to illustrate the text.

REFERENCES

1. Cochrane, C.G., and Griffin, J.H.: Molecular assembly in the contact phase of the Hageman factor system. Am J Med *67*:657, 1979.
2. Cochrane, C.G., and Wuepper, K.D.: The kinin forming system: Delineation and activation in immunopathology. *In* Immunopathology, Vol. VI. Edited by P. Miescher. Basel, Switzerland, Schwab & Co 1972, p 220.
3. Manson, D.C., and Cochrane, C.G.: Direct evidence for Hageman (factor XII) activation by bacterial lipopolysaccharides. J Exp Med *140*:797, 1974.
4. Kellermeyer, R.W., and Breckenridge, R.T.: The inflammatory process in acute gouty arthritis I. Activation of Hageman factor by sodium urate crystals. J Lab Clin Med *65*:307, 1965.
5. Griffin, J.H.: The role of surface in the surface dependent activation of Hageman factor (factor XII). Proc Natl Acad Sci USA *75*:1998, 1978.
6. Griffin, J.H., and Cochrane, C.G.: Mechanisms for involvement of high molecular weight kininogen in surface dependent reactions of Hageman factor (coagulation factor XII). Proc Natl Acad Sci USA *73*:2554, 1976.

7. Hultin, M.B., and Nemerson, Y.: Activation of factor X by factors IXa and VIII: A specific assay for factor IXa in the presence of thrombin activated factor VIII. Blood *52*:928, 1978.
8. Miletich, J.P., Majerus, D.W., and Majerus, P.W.: Patients with congenital factor V deficiency have decreased factor Xa binding sites on their platelets. J Clin Invest *62*:824, 1978.
9. Falk, J.E., and Chung, S.I.: Molecular and catalytic properties of transglutaminases. Adv Enzymol *38*:109, 1973.
10. Nemerson, Y.: Characteristics and lipid requirements of coagulant proteins extracted from brain and lung: The specificity of the protein component of tissue factor. J Clin Invest *48*:322, 1969.
11. Radcliffe, R., and Nemerson, Y.: Activation and control of factor and thrombin. Isolation and characterization of a single chain form of factor VII. J Biol Chem *250*:388, 1974.
12. Marlar, R.A., Kleiss, A.J., and Griffin, J.H.: An alternative extrinsic pathway of human blood coagulation. Blood *60*:1353, 1982.
13. Aoki, N., Massi, M., Sakata, Y., et al.: Abnormal plasminogen. A hereditary molecular abnormality found in a patient with recurrent thrombosis. J Clin Invest *61*:1186, 1978.
14. Aoki, N., Saito, H., Kanuya, T., et al.: Congenital deficiency of α_2-plasmin inhibitor associated with severe hemorrhagic tendency. J Clin Invest *63*:877, 1979.
15. Rifkin, D.B., Loeb, J.N., Mosse, G., et al.: Properties of plasminogen activators formed by neoplastic human cell cultures. J Exp Med *139*:1317, 1974.
16. Abildgaard, U.: Purification of two progressive antithrombins of human plasma. J Clin Lab Invest *19*:190, 1967.
17. Marciniak, E., Farley, C.H., and DeSimone, P.A.: Familial thrombosis due to antithrombin III deficiency. Blood *43*:219, 1974.
18. Sas, G., Pepper, D.S., and Cash, J.C.: Plasma and serum antithrombin III: Differentiation by crossed immunoelectrophoresis. Thromb Res *6*:87, 1975.
19. Marlar, R.A., Kleiss, A.J., and Griffin, J.H.: Anticoagulant action of human protein C. Protides Biol Fluids Proc Colloq *28*:341, 1980.
20. Comp, P.C., and Esmon, C.T.: Generation of fibrinolytic activity by infusion of activated protein C into dogs. J Clin Invest *68*:1221, 1981.
21. Griffin, J.H., Evatt, B., Zimmerman, T.S., Kleiss, A.J., and Wideman, C.: Deficiency of protein C in congenital thrombotic disease. J Clin Invest *68*:1370, 1981.
22. Griffin, J.H., Mosher, D.F., Zimmerman, T.S., et al.: Protein C, an antithrombotic protein, is reduced in hospitalized patients with intravascular coagulation. Blood *60*:261, 1982.
23. Marlar, R.A., and Griffin, J.H.: Deficiency of protein C inhibitor in combined factor V/VIII deficiency disease. J Clin Invest *68*:1221, 1980.
24. Weiss, H.J.: Biological properties of platelets. *In* Platelets: Pathophysiology and Antiplatelet Drug Therapy. Edited by H.J. Weiss. New York, Alan R Liss, 1982, pp 29–43.
25. Malpass, T.W., and Harker, L.A.: Acquired disorders of platelet function. Sem Hematol *17*:242, 1980.
26. Hagen, I., Nurden, A., Berrjun, O.J., et al.: Immunochemical evidence for protein abnormalities in platelets from patients with Glanzmann's thrombasthenia and Bernard-Soulier syndrome. J Clin Invest *65*:722, 1980.
27. Bloom, A.L.: The von Willebrand syndrome. Sem Hematol *17*:215, 1980.
28. Weiss, H.J.: Inherited disorders of platelet secretion. *In* Hemostasis and Thrombosis. Edited by R.W. Colman, J. Hirsh, V.J. Marder, and E.W. Salzman. Philadelphia, JB Lippincott Company, 1982, p 507.
29. Nossel, H.L., Langkowsky, P., Levy, S., Mibashan, R.S., and Hansen, J.D.L.: A study of coagulation factor levels in women during labor and their newborn infants. Thromb Diathes Hemorrhag *16*:185, 1966.
30. Pechet, L., and Alexander, B.: Increased clotting factors in pregnancy. N Engl J Med *265*:1093, 1961.
31. Ganrot, P.D.: Variation in the concentration of some plasma proteins in normal adults, in pregnant women, and in newborns. Scand J Clin Lab Invest *29*:Suppl *124*:83, 1972.
32. Duckert, F.: Documentation of the plasma factor XIII deficiency in man. Ann NY Acad Sci *202*:190, 1972.
33. Coopland, A., Alkjoersig, N., and Fletcher, A.P.: Reduction in plasma XIII (fibrin stabilizing factor) concentration during pregnancy. J Lab Clin Med *73*:144, 1969.
34. Fisher, S.M., Rikover, M., and Naor, S.: Factor XIII deficiency with severe hemorrhagic diathesis. Blood *28*:34, 1966.
35. Bohn, H.: Comparative studies of the fibrin-stabilizing factors from human plasma, platelets and placentas. Ann NY Acad Sci *202*:256, 1972.
36. Rosenberg, R.D.: Heparin-antithrombin system. *In* Hemostasis and Thrombosis. Edited by R.W. Colman, J. Hirsh, V.J. Marder, and E.W. Salzman. Philadelphia, J.B Lippincott Co, 1982, p 965.
37. Weiner, C.P., and Brandt, J.: Plasma antithrombin III activity in normal pregnancy. Obstet Gynecol *56*:601, 1980.
38. Weenink, G.H., Treffers, P.E., et al.: Antithrombin III in normal pregnancy. Thomb Res *26*:281, 1982.

39. Cosgriff, T.M., Bishop, D.T., Hershgold, E.J., et al.: Familial antithrombin III deficiency: Its natural history, genetics, diagnosis and treatment. Medicine *62*:209, 1983.
40. Seligsohn, U., Berger, A., Abend, M., et al.: Homozygous protein C deficiency manifested by massive venous thrombosis in the newborn. N Engl J Med *310*:559, 1984.
41. Hoyer, L.W.: The factor VIII complex: Structure and function. Blood *58*:1, 1981.
42. Hoyer, L.W., Carta, C.A., and Mahoney, M.J.: Detection of hemophilia carriers during pregnancy. Blood *60*:407, 1982.
43. Peake, I.R., Newcombe, R.G., Davies, B.L., et al.: Carrier detection in haemophilia A by immunological measurement of factor VIII related antigen (VIIIRAg) and factor VIII clotting antigen (VIIICAg). Br J Haematol *48*:651, 1981.
44. Fournie, A., Monrozies, M., Pontonnier, G., et al.: Factor VIII complex in normal pregnancy, pre-eclampsia, and fetal growth retardation. Br J Obstet Gynaecol *88*:250, 1981.
45. Thornton, C.A., and Bonnar, J.: Factor VIII related antigen and factor VIII coagulant activity in normal pregnancy, pre-eclampsia and abruptio placentae. *In* Pregnancy Hypertension. Edited by J. Bonnar, I. MacGillivray, and M. Symonds. Baltimore, University Park Press, 1980, pp 419–425.
46. Woodfield, D.G., Cole, S.K., Allan, A.G.E., et al.: Serum fibrin degradation products throughout normal pregnancy. Br Med J *4*:665, 1968.
47. Hyde, E., Joyce, D., Gurewich, V., et al.: Intravascular coagulation during pregnancy and the puerperium. J Obstet Gynaecol Br Commonw *80*:1059, 1973.
48. Borok, Z., Weitz, J., Owen, J., et al.: Fibrinogen proteolysis and platelet α-granule release in pre-eclampsia/eclampsia. Blood *63*:525, 1984.
49. Fenton, V., Saunders K., and Cavill, I.: The platelet count in pregnancy. J Clin Pathol *30*:68, 1977.
50. Ingles, J.C.M., Stuart J., George, A.J., et al.: Haemostatic and rheological changes in normal pregnancy and pre-eclampsia. Br J Haematol *50*:461, 1981.
51. Douglas, J.T., Shah, M., Lowe, G.D.O., et al.: Plasma fibrinopeptide A and beta thromboglobulin in pre-eclampsia and pregnancy hypertension. Thromb Haemost *47*:54, 1982.
52. Robbins, J.A., and Rose, S.D.: Partial thromboplastic time as a screening test. Ann Intern Med *90*:796, 1979.
53. Rapaport, S.I.: Preoperative hemostatic evaluation: Which tests, if any? Blood *61*:229, 1983.
54. Lubbe, W.F., Palmer, S.J., Butler, W.S., et al.: Fetal survival after prednisone suppression of maternal lupus-anticoagulant. Lancet *ii*:1361, 1983.
55. Stuart, M.J., Miller, M.L., Davey, F.R., et al.: The post aspirin bleeding time: A screening test for evaluating hemostatic disorders. Br J Haematol *43*:649, 1979.
56. McKenna, R., Bachman, F., and Miro-Quesada, M.: Thromboembolism in patients with abnormally short activated partial thromboplastin time. Thromb Haemost *38*:893, 1977.
57. Sas, G., Pepper, D.S., and Cash, J.D.: Investigation on antithrombin III in normal plasma and serum. Br J Haematol *30*:265, 1975.
58. Beck, E.A., Shainoff, J.R., Vogel, A., et al.: Functional evaluation of an inherited abnormal fibrinogen: Fibrinogen "Baltimore." J Clin Invest *50*:1874, 1971.
59. Gralnick, H.R., Coller, B.S., Fratantoni, J., et al.: Fibrinogen Bethesda III: A hypodysfibrinogenemia. Blood *58*:28, 1979.
60. Carrell, N., Gabriel, D.A., Blatt, P.M., et al.: Hereditary dysfibrinogenemia in a patient with thrombotic disease. Blood *62*:439, 1983.
61. Ratnoff, O.D., and Colopy, J.E.: A familial hemorrhagic trait associated with a deficiency of a clot promoting fraction of plasma. J Clin Invest *34*:602, 1955.
62. Wilson, J.E., III, and Thornton, R.D.: Comparison of a direct latex-agglutination technique with the tanned red cell hemagglutination inhibition immunoassay (TRHII) for semiquantitation of fibrinogen/fibrin degradation products. Am J Clin Pathol *65*:528, 1976.
63. Shapiro, S.S., and Hultin, M.: Acquired inhibitors to the blood coagulation factors. Sem Thromb Hemost *1*:336, 1975.
64. Shapiro, S.S., and Thiagarajan, P.: Lupus anticoagulants. Prof Hemost Thromb *6*:263, 1982.
65. Feinstein, D.I., and Rapaport, S.I.: Acquired inhibitors of blood coagulation. Prog Hemost Thromb *1*:75, 1972.
66. Kasper, C.K., Aledert, L.M., Counts, R.B., et al.: A more uniform measurement of factor VIII inhibitors. Thromb Diathes Haemost *34*:869, 1975.
67. Schleider, M.A., Nachman, R.L., Jaffe, E.A., et al.: A clinical study of the lupus anticoagulant. Blood *48*:499, 1976.
68. Exner, T., Richard, A., and Kronenberg, H.: A sensitive test demonstrating lupus anticoagulant and its behavioral patterns. Br J Haematol *40*:143, 1978.
69. Mueh, J.R., Herbst, K.D., and Rapaport, S.I.: Thrombosis in patients with the lupus anticoagulant. Ann Intern Med *92*:156, 1980.
70. Bajaj, S.P., Rapaport, S.I., Fierer, D.S., et al.: A mechanism for the hypoprothrombinemia of the acquired hypoprothrombinemia-lupus anticoagulant syndrome. Blood *61*:684, 1983.

71. Khoory, M.S., Nesheim, M.E., Bowie, E.J.W., et al.: Circulating heparin sulfate proteoglycan anticoagulant from a patient with a plasma cell disorder. J Clin Invest *65*:666, 1980.
72. Rutstein, J.E., Holahan, J.R., Lyons, R.M., et al.: Rheumatoid factor interference with the latex agglutination test for fibrin degradation products. J Lab Clin Med *92*:529, 1978.
73. Seaman, A.J.: The recognition of intravascular clotting, the plasma protamine paracoagulation test. Arch Intern Med *125*:1016, 1970.
74. Nossel, H.L., Yudelman, I., Canfield, R.E., et al.: Measurement of fibrinopeptide A in human blood. J Clin Invest *54*:43, 1974.
75. Nilsson, I.M., and Holmberg, L.: Von Willebrand's disease today. Clin Haematol *8*::147, 1979.
76. Abildgaard, C.F., Suzuki, Z., Hairrison, J., et al.: Serial studies in von Willebrand's disease: Variability versus "variants." Blood *56*:712, 1980.
77. Sultan, Y., Simeon, J., and Caen, J.P.: Electrophoretic heterogeneity of normal factor VIII/von Willebrand protein, and abnormal electrophoretic mobility in patients with von Willebrand's disease. J Lab Clin Med *87*:185, 1976.
78. Ruggieri, Z.M., and Zimmerman, T.S.: Variant von Willebrand's disease. Characterization of two subtypes by analysis of multimeric composition of factor VIII/von Willebrand factor in plasma and platelets. J Clin Invest *65*:1318, 1980.
79. Ruggieri, Z.M., Pareti, F.I., Mannucci, P.M., et al.: Heightened interaction between platelets and factor VIII/von Willebrand factor in a new subtype of von Willebrand's disease. N Engl J Med *302*:1047, 1980.
80. Ruggieri, Z.M., Nilsson, I.M., Lombardi, R., et al.: Aberrant multimeric structure of von Willebrand factor in a new variant of von Willebrand's disease (type IIC). J Clin Invest *70*:1124, 1982.
81. Weiss, H.J., Meyer, D., Rabinowitz, R., et al.: Pseudo-von Willebrand's disease. N Engl J Med *306*:326, 1982.
82. Gralnick, H.R., Williams, S.B., Shafer, B.C., et al.: Factor VIII/von Willebrand factor binding to von Willebrand's disease platelets. Blood *60*:328, 1982.
83. Italian Working Group: Spectrum of von Willebrand's disease: A study of 100 cases. Br J Haematol *35*:101, 1977.
84. Howard, M.A., Salem, H.H., Thomas K.B., et al.: Variant von Willebrand's disease type B—revisited. Blood *60*:1420, 1982.
85. Lipton, R.A., Ayromlooi, J., and Coller, B.S.: Severe von Willebrand's disease during labor and delivery. JAMA *248*:1355, 1982.
86. Hanna, W., McCarroll, D., McDonald, T., et al.: Variant von Willebrand's disease and pregnancy. Blood *58*:873, 1981.
87. Weiss, H.J.: Relation of von Willebrand factor to bleeding time. N Engl J Med *291*:420, 1974.
88. Green, D., and Potter, E.V.: Failure of AHF concentrate to control bleeding in von Willebrand's disease. Am J Med *60*:357, 1976.
89. Barrow, E.S., Miller, C.H., Reisner, H.M., et al.: Genetic counseling in hemophilia by discriminant analysis. J Med Genet *19*:26, 1982.
90. Bouma, B.N., van der Kloauw, M.N., Veltkamp, J.J., et al.: Evaluation of the detection rate of hemophilia carriers. Thromb Res *7*:339, 1975.
91. Klein, H.G., Aledort, L.M., Bouma, B.N., et al.: A cooperative study for the detection of the carrier state of classic hemophilia. N Engl J Med *296*:959, 1977.
92. Hoyer, L.W., Carta, C.A., and Mahoney, M.J.: Detection of hemophilia carriers during pregnancy. Blood *60*:1407, 1982.
93. Mannucci, P.M., and Farman, S.P.: Hemostasis and liver disease. In Hemostasis and Thrombosis. Edited by R.W. Colman, J. Hirsh, V.J. Marder, and E.W. Salzman. Philadelphia, JB Lippincott Company, 1982, p 595.
94. Verstraete, M., Vermylen, J., and Collen, D.: Intravascular coagulation in liver disease. Ann Rev Med *25*:447, 1974.
95. Lackner, H., and Karpatkin, S.: On the "easy bruising" syndrome with normal platelet count. Ann Intern Med *83*:190, 1975.
96. Kelton, J.G., Powers, P.G., and Carter, C.J.: A prospective study of the usefulness of the measurement of platelet associated IgG for the diagnosis of idiopathic thrombocytopenic purpura. Blood *60*:1050, 1982.
97. LoBuglio, A.F., Court, W.S., Vinocur, L., et al.: Immune thrombocytopenia purpura. Use of a ^{125}I-labeled antihuman IgG monoclonal antibody to quantify platelet bound IgG. N Engl J Med *309*:459, 1983.
98. Kelton, J.G., Blanchette, V.S., Wilson, W.E., et al.: Neonatal thrombocytopenia due to passive immunization. N Engl J Med *302*:1401, 1980.
99. Scott, J.R., Cruikshank, D.P., Kochenoar, N.K., et al.: Fetal platelet counts in the obstetric management of immunologic thrombocytopenic purpura. Am J Obstet Gynecol *136*:495, 1980.
100. Kelton, J.B., Inwood, M.J., Barr, R.M., et al.: The prenatal prediction of thrombocytopenia in infants of mothers with clinically diagnosed immune thrombocytopenia. Am J Obstet Gynecol *144*:449, 1982.

101. Cines, D.B., Dusak, B., Tomaski, A., et al.: Immune thrombocytopenic purpura and pregnancy. N Engl J Med *306*:826, 1982.
102. Scott, J.R., Rote, N.S., and Cruikshank, D.P.: Antiplatelet antibodies and platelet counts in pregnancies complicated by autoimmune thrombocytopenia purpura. Am J Obstet Gynecol *145*:932, 1983.
103. Corash, L.: Platelet sizing techniques, biologic significance and clinical applications. Curr Top Hematol *4*:99, 1983.
104. Perason, H.A., Shulman, N.R., Marder, V.J., et al.: Isoimmune neonatal thrombocytopenic purpura: Clinical and therapeutic considerations. Blood *23*:154, 1964.
105. Holmberg, L., Gustavii, B., and Jonsson, A.: A prenatal study of fetal platelet count and size with application to fetus at risk for Wiskott-Aldrich syndrome. J Pediatr *102*:773, 1983.
106. Gynn, T.N., Messmore, H.L., and Friedman, I.A.: Drug-induced thrombocytopenia. Med Clin North Am *56*:65, 1972.
107. Faig, D., and Karpatkin, S.: Cumulative experience with a simplified solid phase radioimmunoassay for the detection of bound antiplatelet IgG, serum auto-, allo-, and drug-dependent antibodies. Blood *60*:807, 1982.
108. Jaffe, E.A., Nachman, R.L., and Mersky, C.: Thrombotic thrombocytopenic purpura—coagulation parameters in twelve patients. Blood *42*:499, 1973.
109. Myers, T.H., Waken, C.T., Ball, E.D., et al.: Thrombotic thrombocytopenia purpura: Combined treatment with plasmapheresis and antiplatelet agents. Ann Intern Med *92*:149, 1980.
110. Moake, J.L., Rudy, C.K., Troll, J.H., et al.: Unusually large plasma factor VIII: Von Willebrand factor multimers in chronic relapsing thrombotic thrombocytopenic purpura. N Engl J Med *307*:1432, 1982.
111. Thiagarajan, S., Harbert, G.M., Caudle, M.R., et al.: Thrombotic thrombocytopenic purpura in pregnancy: A reappraisal. Am J Obstet Gynecol *141*:20, 1981.
112. Gibson, B., Hunter, D., Neane, P.B., et al.: Thrombocytopenia in pre-eclampsia and eclampsia. Sem Thromb Hemost *8*:234, 1982.
113. Douglas, J.T., Shah, M., Lowe, G.D.O., et al.: Plasma fibrinopeptide A and beta thromboglobulin in pre-eclampsia and pregnancy hypertension. Thromb Haemost *47*:54, 1982.
114. Thornton, C.A., and Bonnar, J.: Factor VIII-related antigen and factor III coagulant activity in normal pregnancy, pre-eclampsia and abruptio placentae. *In* Pregnancy Hypertension. Edited by J. Bonnar, I. MacGillivray, and M. Symmonds. Baltimore, University Park Press, 1980, pp 419–425.
115. Brendt, M.C., and Phillips, D.R.: Platelet membrane proteins composition and receptor function. *In* Platelets in Biology and Pathology 2. Edited by J.L. Gordon. Amsterdam, Elsevier, 1981, p 43.
116. Nurden, A.T., and Caen, J.P.: Specific roles for platelet surface glycoproteins. J Clin Invest *60*:535, 1977.
117. Phillips, D.R., and Agin, P.P.: Platelet membrane defects in Glanzmann's thrombasthenia: Evidence for decreased amounts of two major glycoproteins. J Clin Invest *60*:535, 1977.
118. Weiss, H.J.: Biological properties of platelets. *In* Platelets: Pathophysiology and Antiplatelet Drug Therapy. Edited by H.J. Weiss. New York, Alan R. Liss, 1982, pp 29–43.
119. Weiss, H.J., Witte, L.D., Kaplan, K.L., et al.: Heterogeneity in storage pool deficiency: Studies on granule bound substances in 18 patients including variants deficient in α-granules, platelet factor 4, Δ-thromboglobulin and platelet derived growth factor. Blood *54*:1296, 1979.
120. Nurden, A.T., Kunicki, T.J., Dupius, D., et al.: Specific protein and glycoprotein deficiencies in platelets isolated from two patients with the gray platelet syndrome. Blood *59*:709, 1982.
121. Wu, K.K., and Hoak, J.C.: A new method for the quantitative detection of platelet aggregates in patients with arterial insufficiency. Lancet *ii*:924, 1974.
122. Corash, L., Andersen, J., Poindexter, B., et al.: Platelet function and survival in patients with severe hypercholesterolemia. Arteriosclerosis *1*:443, 1981.
123. Kohanna, F.H., Smith, M.H., and Salzman, E.W.: Do patients with thromboemobolic disease have circulating platelet aggregates? Blood *64*:204, 1984.
124. Salzman, E.W., Deykin, D., Shapiro, R.M., et al.: Management of heparin therapy. N Engl J Med *292*:1046, 1975.
125. Basu, D., Gallus, A. and Hirsh, J.: A prospective study of the value of monitoring heparin treatment with the activated partial thromboplastin time. N Engl J Med *287*:324, 1972.
126. Zucker, S., and Cathey, M.H.: Control of heparin therapy: Sensitivity of the activated partial thromboplastin time for monitoring the antithrombotic effects of heparin. J Lab Clin Med *73*:320, 1969.
127. Thomas, D.P.: Heparin in the prophylaxis and treatment of venous thromboembolism. Sem Hematol *15*:1, 1978.
128. Bell, W.R.: Thrombocytopenia occurring during heparin therapy. N Engl J Med *295*:276, 1976.
129. Bell, W.R., Tomasulo, P.A., and Alving, B.M.: Thrombocytopenia occurring during the administration of heparin. A prospective study in 52 patients. Ann Intern Med *85*:155, 1976.
130. Hull, R.B., Delmore, T., Carter, C., et al.: Adjusted subcutaneous heparin versus warfarin sodium in the long term treatment of venous thrombosis. N Engl J Med *306*:189, 1982.

Chapter 9

CONGENITAL DISORDERS OF HEMOSTASIS

Charles A. Linker

Although congenital disturbances of hemostasis are uncommon, it is important that they be recognized because the morbidity and mortality they can cause is essentially completely preventable by correct diagnosis and treatment. Severe congenital disturbances of hemostasis are almost always clinically apparent early in life and hence will have been diagnosed by the time an obstetrician or gynecologist deals with the patient. The physician will then need to confirm the diagnosis and apply therapeutic or prophylactic agents, as described later in this chapter. Milder forms of congenital hemostatic disorders are more of a diagnostic challenge and often go unrecognized until problems arise in adult life. Most of these disorders do not result in spontaneous bleeding or bleeding following the mild trauma encountered in everyday life. Often these patients are able to engage in a full range of activities, including athletics. However, they may still experience significant morbidity from bleeding complications of surgery, since surgery imposes a challenge on the hemostatic mechanism that far exceeds anything encountered in everyday life. It is by no means uncommon for adult patients to have significant bleeding following surgery because of congenital disorders that have previously been unrecognized. Before embarking on surgery, invasive procedures, or even vaginal delivery, the physician should look for clues to a previously unrecognized disorder.

Since mild bleeding disorders may be clinically silent, the patient should be questioned about prior hemostatic challenges such as surgery, major trauma, or dental extractions. A patient's prior experience with dental extractions is especially useful in assessing the probability of a hemostatic disorder because such dental work is commonly performed. If a patient has bled for more than three days following an extraction or has bled to the point of requiring a red blood cell transfusion, a higher degree of suspicion is justified. Conversely, if the patient has experienced prior surgery or several prior dental extractions with no bleeding difficulties, the chance of a bleeding disorder is minimal. The patient should be asked for a family history of bleeding disorders, although the absence of a known familial problem is by no means conclusive. The patient should be further questioned about her experience with aspirin and nonsteroidal anti-inflammatory drugs, since the platelet dysfunction these drugs can produce will frequently unmask clinically silent disorders. Last, the patient should be questioned about the history of menstrual bleeding, since menorrhagia is one of the most common clinical manifestations of congenital bleeding disorders. It should be noted that a history of previous uneventful vaginal deliveries does not exclude the possibility of a factor VIII-related bleeding disorder, since (as will be discussed further on) factor VIII disorders frequently improve or normalize late in pregnancy. Patients who have uneventful deliveries while transiently corrected may still have significant bleeding early in pregnancy or when not pregnant.

The coagulation and platelet arms of the hemostatic mechanism will be considered separately because the type of bleeding encountered clinically differs in these different types of disorders. Patients with defective platelet function or number primarily have mucosal bleeding, with epistaxis, gingival bleeding, menorrhagia, and gastrointestinal bleeding being frequent manifestations. Bleeding tends to occur immediately after trauma or surgery, and aspirin will commonly provoke overt bleeding. Patients with defective platelet function may not have surgical bleeding provided that primary hemostasis can be achieved with suturing. In contrast, bleeding caused by coagulation disturbances may be either immediate or delayed. Deep muscle hematomas and hemarthroses are seen almost exclusively in coagulation disturbances. Bleeding following dental extractions is not specific for coagulation disturbances and may occur either in these disorders or in platelet disorders. Disorders of fibrinolysis are much harder to detect, since results of screening laboratory tests such as the prothrombin time and partial thromboplastin time are normal. Disorders of fibrinolysis should be suspected in cases of delayed bleeding, especially when this is accompanied by poor wound healing.

Because the laboratory evaluation of patients with suspected bleeding disorders is time-consuming and expensive, the clinician should rely heavily on the history in deciding how far to pursue a laboratory evaluation.[1] Patients who have had repeated hemostatic challenges and have not exhibited excessive bleeding require no laboratory evaluation prior to routine procedures. In contrast, a patient with a history strongly suggestive of abnormal bleeding should have a diagnosis vigorously pursued in consultation with a hematologist, even when initial laboratory tests are entirely normal. Patients with a history suggestive of a bleeding disorder should be screened initially with a prothrombin time, partial thromboplastin time, platelet count, and template bleeding time. Depending on the results of these tests and the level of clinical suspicion, further specific laboratory tests may be necessary, as described later on.

The most common congenital coagulation disorders are von Willebrand's disease, factor VIII deficiency (hemophilia A), and factor IX deficiency (hemophilia B). Less common coagulation disorders are factor XI deficiency and deficiency or abnormalities in fibrinogen. Other factor deficiencies are extremely rare. The most common disorder of fibrinolysis is factor XIII deficiency, but other rare disorders have been described. The most common disorders of platelet function are von Willebrand's disease and storage pool disease.

VON WILLEBRAND'S DISEASE

Von Willebrand's disease is the most common congenital coagulation disorder, with an incidence of overt disease of more than one per 10,000 population.[2] The incidence of overt disease is equivalent to that of hemophilia A, but since subclinical von Willebrand's disease is common, the total incidence of von Willebrand's disease is greater than that of hemophilia. Since von Willebrand's disease, in contrast to the hemophilias, is an autosomal disorder, it is by far the most significant congenital coagulation problem seen in women. Von Willebrand's disease is best defined as a group of hereditary bleeding disorders characterized by a deficiency or defect in a plasma factor necessary to support platelet adhesion.[3,4] In addition to being a platelet disorder, von Willebrand's disease may also cause a secondary decrease in the factor VIII coagulant factor and the clinical manifestations of a coagulation disorder. It is almost always an autosomal dominant disorder, although one rare subtype of autosomal recessive disease has been described in which homozygotes are severely affected.

Clinically, the disorder is variable in expression. Many cases are clinically silent or result in only trivial bleeding, but severe and even fatal bleeding can be seen. Most commonly, the disorder is mild, and most morbidity occurs in the setting of surgery. In addition to being variable among patients, the disorder is notoriously variable for a given patient at different points in time. The most common type of bleeding encountered clinically is that associated with platelet dysfunction, namely, epistaxis, gingival bleeding, menorrhagia, and gastrointestinal bleeding. Gastrointestinal bleeding may rarely be due to the coexistence of the hemostatic disorder and angiodysplasia, a syndrome of a more general disorder of endothelial cells in some kindreds.[5] Patients with von Willebrand's disease commonly bleed following challenges with surgery, dental extractions, and delivery and following administration of aspirin. Two cases of spontaneous ovarian hemorrhage, analogous to that seen during anticoagulation with warfarin, have been reported.[6,7]

PATHOPHYSIOLOGY

The defect of von Willebrand's disease lies in von Willebrand's factor, which is one of two major components of the human factor VIII complex. Von Willebrand factor and factor VIII coagulant activity have been conclusively identified as two separate proteins that are the products of two separate genes.[8] Von Willebrand factor is encoded by a gene on an autosomal chromosome and is synthesized in endothelial cells and megakaryocytes.[9–11] It is composed of a subunit of a molecular weight of 230,000 daltons but circulates in multimers ranging in size from 800,000 daltons to more than 10,000,000 daltons. Von Willebrand factor constitutes approximately 99% of the mass of factor VIII complex in humans and circulates in plasma in a concentration of 5 to 10 μg/ml. When one measures the factor VIII complex by immunologic means (factor VIII antigen), it is almost exclusively von Willebrand factor.

In contrast, factor VIII coagulant activity is a smaller protein that constitutes approximately 1% of the weight of the factor VIII complex and circulates in a concentration of approximately 50 ng/ml. This protein is encoded by a gene on the long arm of the X chromosome, and the site of synthesis is still not determined. The protein has a molecular weight of 280,000 daltons and circulates in plasma closely associated with von Willebrand factor. Von Willebrand factor appears to stabilize the smaller coagulant protein or perhaps protect it from proteolytic digestion, and reduced levels of von Willebrand factor usually lead to a comparable decrease in the level of circulating factor VIII coagulant activity.[12] This reduction in factor VIII coagulant activity may also be related to a relationship in the synthetic rate of these two proteins.

Von Willebrand factor is the major protein in plasma that mediates platelet adhesion. Platelet adhesion is the initial step in hemostasis, in which disruption of the non-thrombogenic endothelial cell surface of a blood vessel leads to adhesion of platelets to collagen. Von Willebrand factor forms a bridge between the subendothelial collagen and a specific receptor on the platelet membrane that is composed largely of glycoprotein Ib. The large multimeric forms of von Willebrand factor appear to have the greatest physiologic ability to mediate this adhesion. Platelet adhesion is distinct from aggregation. Platelets adhere to a foreign surface but aggregate with each other. Platelet aggregation occurs when activated platelets express specific receptors for fibrinogen. These fibrinogen receptors are composed of glycoproteins IIb and IIIa of the platelet membrane. Standard in vitro tests of platelet aggregation using collagen, ADP, or thrombin as platelet agonists will be entirely normal in von Willebrand's disease, since an entirely different mechanism and platelet receptor are involved. Platelet aggregation can be studied in vitro using the antibiotic ristocetin. However, the process involved here should more accurately be termed platelet agglutination, since unlike true aggregation, no metabolic activity is required and the assay can be equally well performed with formalin-fixed platelet membranes. The tests employing ristocetin take advantage of the fact that it will agglutinate platelets by a mechanism involving von Willebrand factor and its receptor composed of glycoprotein Ib of the platelet membrane.

MEASUREMENT OF VON WILLEBRAND FACTOR AND FACTOR VIII

Factor VIII coagulant activity (factor VIII:C), commonly called factor VIII activity, is measured by a functional coagulation assay. Reductions in factor VIII:C are the primary defect in hemophilia A but are seen as a secondary manifestation in von Willebrand's disease. Factor VIII:C levels are normal in at least one third of cases of von Willebrand's disease and hence are neither very sensitive nor very specific.

Factor VIII antigen (FVIIIR:Ag) is commonly measured using a polyspecific, rabbit antibody against human factor VIII. Since human factor VIII is composed of at least 99% von Willebrand factor, the factor VIII antigen assay primarily measures the immunologic presence of von Willebrand factor. Since von Willebrand factor levels and consequently factor VIII antigen levels are entirely normal in patients with factor VIII hemophilia (hemophilia A), the coexistence of reduced factor VIII:C levels and normal factor VIII antigen levels confirms the diagnosis of hemophilia and differentiates hemophilia from von Willebrand's disease. Factor VIII antigen levels are normal in approximately 20% of patients with von Willebrand's disease and hence are not extremely sensitive for detection of this disorder.

The most sensitive test for detection of von Willebrand's disease is the ristocetin cofactor assay (FVIIIR:RC), a functional assay for von Willebrand factor. In this test, the patient's plasma is tested against formalinized, normal platelets in the presence of ristocetin for its ability to agglutinate platelets. Ristocetin cofactor levels are normal in less than 10% of patients with von Willebrand's disease. In addition to being the most sensitive test, ristocetin cofactor activity levels have the best correlation with clinical bleeding and prolongation of the bleeding time. However, the correlation is still imperfect, and both clinical bleeding and prolongation of the bleeding time can be seen with normal levels of ristocetin cofactor, especially in variant von Willebrand's disease, after therapy with cryoprecipitate, and during pregnancy (see further on).

Ristocetin is also employed in a different test, ristocetin-induced platelet aggregation (RIPA).[13] In this test, the patient's platelet-rich plasma is tested in a standard system for platelet aggregation using ristocetin as the agonist. This test has largely been replaced by the ristocetin cofactor assay using patient plasma and normal platelets because it is much more sensitive. While less than 10% of patients with von Willebrand's disease have normal levels of ristocetin cofactor activity, the ristocetin-induced platelet aggregation test is normal in more than one third. However, the RIPA may be useful for diagnosis of one of the variants of von Willebrand's disease, type IIb.

In this disorder (described further on), platelets have increased sensitivity to ristocetin-induced aggregation and will aggregate at low concentrations of ristocetin that will not affect normal platelets.

The spectrum of circulating von Willebrand factor multimers can be examined immunologically using the technique of crossed immunoelectrophoresis (CIE).[3] In this test, patient plasma is put through electrophoresis in one dimension through an agarose gel to separate multimers according to molecular size. The proteins are then subjected to electrophoresis in a perpendicular direction into a gel impregnated with polyspecific antibody against factor VIII antigen. A precipitan arc will result that indicates the spectrum of sizes of multimer present in plasma. In the common type of von Willebrand's disease, which is a simple deficiency of a normal protein, the distribution of sizes of von Willebrand factor antigen are normal. In contrast, abnormalities in the CIE pattern are used to confirm a diagnosis of variant von Willebrand's disease. The CIE assay is available in many commercial laboratories.

The most recently described assay for von Willebrand factor, and one that has greatly enhanced our understanding of its physiology, is the assessment of the pattern of von Willebrand factor multimers on SDS-agarose gels.[9, 10] In this assay, patient plasma is applied to an SDS-agarose gel and electrophoresis is performed in one dimension to separate multimers of various sizes. The gel is then counterstained with a radiolabeled antibody to factor VIII antigen, and the pattern is developed by autoradiography. As in the CIE test, normal and common types of von Willebrand's disease are indistinguishable, whereas variant von Willebrand's disease gives a variety of abnormal patterns.

DIAGNOSIS

Although patients with von Willebrand's disease are classically described as having a positive family history, positive bleeding history, prolonged bleeding time, and prolonged partial thromboplastin time (PTT), the diagnosis is rarely this clear-cut. In fact, the majority of patients have neither a prolonged bleeding time nor a prolonged PTT, or they may have these abnormalities only intermittently and at different times.[14–16] The normal PTT in these patients is easily understood if it is appreciated that the PTT becomes prolonged only when factor VIII coagulant levels are lower than 25% to 30%. Since the normal level of factor VIII:C is greater than 45% to 50%, many patients with mildly reduced levels will not have a prolonged PTT. Similarly, the bleeding time is usually only prolonged when the ristocetin cofactor levels are lower than 30%, and consequently a patient can have a subnormal level without a prolonged bleeding time.

Both the clinical expression and laboratory parameters of von Willebrand's disease are notoriously variable for a given patient at different points in time.[17, 18] Patients observed longitudinally have widely fluctuating levels of all components of factor VIII, and the screening tests of bleeding time and PTT fluctuate in and out of the normal range. At any one given point in time, one may be unable to either confirm or exclude the diagnosis of von Willebrand's disease. Because the diagnosis is frequently not straightforward and because the laboratory evaluation is expensive, the history should be used as a guide to how extensive an evaluation for possible von Willebrand's disease should be. Patients who have had surgical or other challenges without incident have a low chance of being affected. However, the absence of a family history of bleeding disorders or the absence of bleeding in a patient who has not been seriously challenged does not exclude the diagnosis of a congenital bleeding disorder, even if the patient is well into adult life.

Patients suspected of having von Willebrand's disease should be screened with a bleeding time and PTT. If these tests are normal and one is still suspicious of the disorder, an aspirin challenge can be used to decide how likely the diagnosis is.[19] If a patient is given two tablets (600 mg) of aspirin and the bleeding time is checked two hours later, normal subjects will have minimal prolongation of bleeding time. Approximately 90% of patients with von Willebrand's disease will have significant prolongation of the bleeding time to levels that can be clearly differentiated from normal subjects. The precise diagnostic criteria used need to be established with normal controls in any given laboratory depending on how the bleeding time test is performed, but in general, a postaspirin bleeding time of more than 15 minutes is suggestive of von Willebrand's disease or another qualitative platelet disorder. It should be noted that an abnormal postaspirin bleeding time does not differentiate von Willebrand's disease from intrinsic qualitative platelet defects.

If a patient has abnormal screening laboratory tests or is still suspected of having von Willebrand's disease, the most sensitive test to perform is that of ristocetin cofactor activity. If this level is abnormal, the diagnosis of von Willebrand's disease is established. If the ristocetin cofactor level is normal and the patient has either a prolonged bleeding time or a prolonged postaspirin bleeding time, the most likely diagnosis is that of an intrinsic platelet defect. This possibility is best pursued by performing in vitro tests of platelet aggregation using collagen and ADP as agonists.

If the PTT is prolonged in a setting suspicious for von Willebrand's disease, the next step is to assay for factor VIII coagulant activity. A reduced factor VIII:C level (usually less than 30%) must be present if this is to explain the prolonged PTT. If the PTT is prolonged but the factor VIII:C level is normal, then the deficiency of factor IX or other coagulation factor must explain the prolonged screening test. If the factor VIII:C level is reduced, the patient may have either von Willebrand's disease or hemophilia. The level of factor VIII antigen should be used to differentiate between these two possibilities, since factor VIII antigen levels must be normal in patients with hemophilia, whereas they should be reduced in patients with von Willebrand's disease, the reduction generally being of a degree comparable to that of factor VIII:C.

In unusual cases, especially those of variant von Willebrand's disease, normal values for the bleeding time factor VIII:C level, factor VIII antigen, and ristocetin cofactor do not exclude the diagnosis of von Willebrand's disease. These tests may need to be performed serially to find fluctuating abnormal values or the qualitative aspects of von Willebrand factor may need to be examined by techniques such as CIE.

SUBTYPES OF VON WILLEBRAND'S DISEASE

Type I von Willebrand's Disease

The most common type of von Willebrand's disease, accounting for approximately 80% of all cases, is type I. The disorder is inherited as an autosomal dominant trait. All parameters of factor VIII activity are reduced to roughly the same extent, and the protein is qualitatively normal. Although usually mild, type I von Willebrand's disease can occasionally be severe, with factor VIII:C levels of less than 1%. The disorder is best explained as a quantitative deficiency of a normal protein.

Types IIa and IIb von Willebrand's Disease

Type IIa von Willebrand's disease is an autosomal dominant disorder that accounts for less than 10% of all cases.[20] It is characterized by a bleeding time that is almost always prolonged, but factor VIII:C and VIII antigen levels may be normal or only mildly reduced. The ristocetin cofactor level is almost always less than 1%, and the CIE shows a decrease in the large forms of von Willebrand factor. The larger physiologically functional multimers of von Willebrand factor are also absent in the platelet and endothelial cells. Type IIa von Willebrand's disease is best explained as a qualitative abnormality in the protein that prevents the large multimers from being formed.

Type IIb von Willebrand's disease is also an autosomal dominant disorder and accounts for approximately 5% of cases.[21] The bleeding time is almost always prolonged, but levels of factor VIII coagulant activity, antigen, and ristocetin cofactor may be normal or only moderately decreased. Accordingly, this is the most difficult of the variants to diagnose if only the preceding laboratory tests are available. The diagnosis can be made by demonstrating increased sensitivity of the patient's platelet-rich plasma to ristocetin-induced platelet aggregation, but the laboratory has to be specifically instructed to perform this test at lower concentrations of ristocetin than usual since, if only standard concentrations of this reagent are used, the result will appear normal. The diagnosis can be confirmed by performing a CIE test and demonstrating decreased large forms of von Willebrand multimers. Type IIb von Willebrand's disease appears to be caused by a qualitative abnormality in the protein that results in its being rapidly cleared from the circulation. When endothelial cells and platelets are examined, the large multimers of von Willebrand factor are present, indicating that they can be formed. In addition, when endothelial cells are stimulated with 1-disamino-8-D-arginine-vasopressin (DDAVP), large multimers are released into the circulation and then quickly cleared. The decrease in plasma von Willebrand factor activity thus appears to be related to rapid clearance from the plasma. Abnormally high avidity of IIb patient von Willebrand factor for normal platelets has been demonstrated.

Type III von Willebrand's Disease

Type III von Willebrand's disease is the rare autosomal recessive disorder characterized by absent factor VIII:C, factor VIII antigen, and ristocetin cofactor activity, absence of von Willebrand factor from tissue stores, and a severe bleeding disorder.[22]

Pseudo-von Willebrand's Disease

Pseudo-von Willebrand's disease (platelet type von Willebrand's disease) is usually indistinguishable from type IIb disease, except that mild thrombocytopenia is occasionally present.[23–25] The disorder appears to be caused by rapid clearance of von Willebrand factor from the circulation, but in contrast to type IIb disease in which the qualitative defect is in the patient's von Willebrand factor, the abnormality is caused by a platelet membrane that has increased avidity for von Willebrand factor. The only way to differentiate this disorder from type IIb von Willebrand's disease is to test patient platelets against normal plasma in a binding study and demonstrate increased avidity for normal factor VIII. In contrast, in type IIb von Willebrand's disease, normal platelets bind the patient's normal von Willebrand factor with increased avidity in a binding study. Such binding studies are performed only in research laboratories and are not generally available.

TREATMENT

In general, as in any patient with a hemostatic disorder, aspirin or nonsteroidal anti-inflammatory agents should be avoided because they exacerbate clinical bleeding. In addition, intramuscular injections or any invasive procedures should be avoided when possible.

The mainstay of treatment of von Willebrand's disease is replacement therapy using cryoprecipitate or normal plasma. Cryoprecipitate is preferred because the volume transfused is greatly decreased whereas the number of donor units the patient is exposed to is only slightly increased.[3, 26–27] Commercial concentrates of factor VIII (antihemophilic factor) are not suitable for treatment of von Willebrand's disease because, although these products contain factor VIII coagulant activity, during processing the von Willebrand factor activity necessary to support platelet adhesion is usually destroyed.[23–30] When cryoprecipitate is examined by SDS-agarose gels, it can be demonstrated that it contains the large multimers of von Willebrand factor that are physiologically active in supporting platelet adhesion, whereas commercial factor VIII concentrates contain only small multimers of factor VIII and will not improve platelet function.

In general, as with patients with factor VIII–deficient hemophilia, adequate surgical hemostasis is achieved by maintaining the factor VIII:C levels continuously higher than 30%. However, in von Willebrand's disease, simply achieving normal levels of factor VIII:C is not sufficient to produce normal hemostasis because the platelet dysfunction must also be corrected. Correction of platelet function generally requires achieving ristocetin cofactor levels higher than 30%. It should be noted that although the correlation between ristocetin cofactor level and the bleeding time is generally good in the resting state, discrepancies occur in certain situations such as following cryoprecipitate transfusion and during pregnancy.[31] In these situations, as in variant von Willebrand's disease, a normal level of ristocetin cofactor activity may not guarantee either a normal bleeding time or normal hemostasis. Although ristocetin cofactor activity is not synonymous with von Willebrand factor activity, it is still the best in vitro laboratory measure of this function.

To calculate the replacement dose of cryoprecipitate, several factors need to be taken into consideration. One bag (unit) of cryoprecipitate made from 200 ml of fresh frozen plasma generally contains 100 U of von Willebrand factor, since the yield after processing is approximately 50%. This concentration varies somewhat at different blood banks, and the local blood bank can be consulted to ascertain the level in the local product. The volume of distribution of von Willebrand factor is approximately equal that of the patient's plasma volume, 40 ml/kg body weight in the nonpregnant woman. The half-life of ristocetin cofactor activity is usually 8 to 12 hours, although the correction of bleeding time may be shorter.[32] Consequently, to maintain a level of ristocetin cofactor (R:RC) activity continuously higher than 30%, initially the levels should be raised to 60% and then half this amount should be replaced each half-life of the factor. To raise the level of R:RC to 60%, one would need 0.6×40 ml/kg, or 24 U/kg. Since cryoprecipitate contains 100 U/bag, approximately 0.24 bag/kg of cryoprecipitate will give the desired peak level. Following this, 0.12 bag/kg of cryoprecipitate should be administered every 12 hours. Table 9–1 provides the initial

Table 9–1. Dosage of Cryoprecipitate for Treating von Willebrand's Disease

	Initial Dose of Cryoprecipitate to Raise*	
Pregnancy State	**R:RC to 60% bag U/kg**	**Factor VIII:C to 60% bag U/kg**
Nonpregnant	0.24	0.36
1st trimester	0.28	0.42
2nd trimester	0.33	0.50
3rd trimester	0.39	0.59
Post partum	0.30	0.45

* Subsequent doses are half the initial dose given every 12 hours.

dose of cryoprecipitate during the various trimesters of pregnancy. In each instance, the maintenance doses are half the original, given every 12 hours. Usual doses for nonpregnant women thus will be 10–15 bags of cryoprecipitate followed by 5–8 bags every 12 hours.

Patients with von Willebrand's disease with reduced levels of factor VIII:C who require surgery should have the factor VIII:C levels maintained continuously at higher than 30%. To accomplish this, the level initially should be raised to 60% and then maintained above 30% with supplemental transfusions based on the half-life of the factor VIII:C. Since the volume of distribution of factor VIII coagulant activity is 50% greater than the patient's plasma volume, the number of bags of factor VIII:C required to reach a 60% level can be calculated as 0.6×40 ml/kg $\times$ 1.5, which calculates to approximately 36 U of factor VIII:C per kg body weight. Since cryoprecipitate contains approximately 100 U of factor VIII:C per bag, the appropriate dose of cryoprecipitate is 0.36 bag/kg. In patients treated for hemophilia A, the half-life of factor VIII:C is approximately 12 hours, and consequently approximately 0.18 bag of cryoprecipitate needs to be transfused every 12 hours to maintain a level continuously above 30%. However, patients with von Willebrand's disease have an unusual response in their factor VIII:C levels after transfusion with either plasma or cryoprecipitate. The initial plasma levels achieved are usually far greater than would be calculated on the basis of the amount infused. Furthermore, the half-life of factor VIII:C is greatly prolonged and is usually 36 to 48 hours. It appears that transfusion of cryoprecipitate in a patient with von Willebrand's disease increases both production and release of factor VIII:C by mechanisms that are still unclear. Because of the exaggerated rise in factor VIII:C levels and the prolonged half-life, supplemental doses of 0.1 to 0.2 bag/kg of cryoprecipitate are necessary every 36 to 48 hours. However, patients with von Willebrand's disease are quite heterogeneous in their response to transfusion, and patients with the severest forms of disease will frequently manifest the shortest half-lives of factor VIII:C, occasionally approximating those seen in patients with hemophilia. Consequently no detailed prescription for repeated doses of cryoprecipitate can be outlined in advance for patients who need supplemental doses of factor VIII:C; rather, patients need to be followed on an individual basis to determine their response to transfusion and their half-life of factor VIII:C. It should be noted that patients with severe von Willebrand's disease who have prolonged bleeding times will require supplemental doses of cryoprecipitate in a dose of 0.12 bag/kg body weight every 12 hours to maintain their ristocetin cofactor activity and improve platelet dysfunction. They will thereby receive the needed amount of factor VIII:C.

The appropriate dose and schedule of replacement therapy for patients of von Willebrand's disease vary according to different clinical circumstances and according to the nature of the patient's disease. Patients with mild disease who have normal bleeding times and normal PTTs at the time of surgery may not need any replacement. Patients undergoing difficult surgery in which extensive bleeding would normally be expected may need a higher dose or more frequent schedule than that outlined above. For example, patients undergoing extensive vascular surgery should have levels of factor VIII:C and ristocetin cofactor raised to 100% and maintained continuously above 50% for 10 to 14 days. This may necessitate doses of cryoprecipitate on the order of 30 U initially (0.4 bag/kg), followed by 15 U every 8 to 12 hours. It should also be noted that some patients with variant von Willebrand's disease (subtypes IIa, IIb, and pseudo-von Willebrand's disease) may have atypical responses to cryoprecipitate.[33, 34]

Treatment with DDAVP

Although replacement therapy using cryoprecipitate has been the mainstay of treatment for von Willebrand's disease, a new form of treatment has been described recently that is particularly effective in mildly affected patients and that may obviate the need for transfusion of blood products in patients undergoing surgery. The vasopressin analog, DDAVP (1-disamino-8-D-arginine-vasopressin), has been shown to cause release of von Willebrand factor from endothelial cells, where it is synthesized and stored.[35–37] Release of stored factor results in increased plasma levels of ristocetin cofactor activity and also of factor VIII:C; consequently it is of benefit for patients with von Willebrand's disease and hemophilia. Other as yet unidentified mechanisms may be involved, since DDAVP has benefited patients with bleeding disorders apparently unrelated to factor VIII.[38] Toxicity with this therapy has been minor. Occasional patients experience flushing and dizziness. There is a theoretical risk of water intoxication because of the vasopressin effect, but hyponatremia has not been observed with the currently employed dosage schedules. The recommended dose is an intravenous infusion of 0.3 μg/kg of DDAVP given over 30 minutes and an approximate total dose of 15 to 25 μg. Doses may be repeated every 12 to 24 hours.

In several studies,[39–47] in a total of 15 patients with mild type I von Willebrand's disease, factor VIII:C levels were observed to rise from a median level of 29% to 143%, more than a fourfold increase. All patients increased their levels to 250% of baseline, and this always resulted in peak factor VIII:C levels above 50%, provided that the patient's baseline was higher than 10%. The half-life of released factor VIII:C in the plasma is approximately six hours, less than after standard transfusion therapy.

The effect of DDAVP in improving the bleeding time is controversial. One author has reported seven cases with no improvement in the bleeding time,[39] but several others[38, 40, 41, 43–46] have reported a total of nine cases in which bleeding times were substantially improved after DDAVP. It is interesting that although the effect on the bleeding time is controversial, all authors agree that ristocetin cofactor levels in the plasma improve, although variably. In seven patients studied, mean ristocetin cofactor activity rose from 28% to 110%. The substantial rise in ristocetin cofactor activity with minimal effect on the bleeding time resulted in a marked discrepancy between ristocetin cofactor levels and their apparent physiologic result. However, despite the lack of improvement in bleeding time, all authors noted an improvement in clinical bleeding.

Although mild cases of von Willebrand's disease, especially common type I von Willebrand's disease, almost always improve following administration of DDAVP, the efficacy of DDAVP in treating variant von Willebrand's disease is unclear. Patients with type IIa disease do not have physiologically active large multimers of von Willebrand factor in their endothelial cells or platelets. Consequently, no benefit would be expected from releasing the small multimers present in storage sites. Mannucci and colleagues[39] have reported 11 cases of type IIa von Willebrand's disease treated with DDAVP and observed rises in factor VIII:C level from a mean level of 30% to 180%; they also observed a rise in ristocetin cofactor activity from a mean baseline of 0 to 14%. Bleeding times remained prolonged in these patients. Another author has reported two cases of type IIa von Willebrand's disease in which factor VIII:C levels rose substantially following DDAVP and remained elevated for more than six hours.[42]

Patients with type IIb von Willebrand's disease have large multimers of von Willebrand factor present in endothelial cells and platelets but are expected to clear this material rapidly after release.[47, 48] Four patients reported on in two separate studies showed substantial rises in factor VIII:C levels after treatment with DDAVP, and these increases were sustained for more than six hours.[42, 49] Two of two reported patients had rises in ristocetin cofactor activity and transient correction of markedly prolonged bleeding times. However, these prolonged bleeding times were normalized only for one to two hours.

Patients with severe autosomal recessive type III von Willebrand's disease would not be expected to benefit from DDAVP, since they have no von Willebrand factor or factor VIII:C to release, and this has been the experience in 10 reported cases.[39, 40, 43]

Overall, DDAVP can be recommended as a reasonable form of therapy in patients with mild von Willebrand's disease who need to undergo surgery or extensive dental procedures. In addition to the improvements in laboratory values described, patients have benefited clinically and been able to undergo surgical procedures without bleeding and without requiring replacement therapy. Patients with common type I von Willebrand's disease with baseline levels of factor VIII:C higher than 10% should have their levels raised over 25% and should achieve adequate hemostasis. The recommended dose of DDAVP is 0.3 $\mu g/kg$ intravenously every 12 hours. High doses of concentrated intranasal DDAVP have been effective, but this preparation is not currently available and absorption may be variable.[50] One limitation of therapy with DDAVP is that storage pools of von Willebrand factor may be exhausted after four to five doses, and tachyphylaxis has been observed. The effect of DDAVP may be prolonged by extending the dosage interval to every 24 hours, but this will leave gaps in the hemostatic coverage. Patients with severe von Willebrand's disease probably will not respond to DDAVP, and the response in variant von Willebrand's disease probably will be variable.

Curently there are no reports of the use of DDAVP during pregnancy, and its safety and efficacy in this setting are unknown. It is possible that DDAVP will be unable to raise factor VIII levels above the exaggerated levels these patients have already achieved based on the effects of pregnancy (see below).

FACTOR VIII IN PREGNANCY

During pregnancy, normal women experience a rise in factor VIII:C levels. These levels change little during the first trimester, but by five to six months they rise to approximately 160%. The levels then rise more, particularly during the eighth and ninth months, and at term mean levels of factor VIII:C in 84 women reported in seven different studies were 195%, with a range of 158% to 270%.[51–57] The values of factor VIII antigen and ristocetin cofactor are not as well studied, but in 36 reported normal women, levels at term were 204% for factor VIII antigen and 171% for ristocetin cofactor.[52] These levels then peak immediately following delivery, probably because of the effect of exercise and epinephrine, which are well known to result in rises in factor VIII levels.[53]

After delivery, normal women maintain their elevated factor VIII levels for at least five days and then experience a slow fall to baseline levels over four to six weeks. There is no transplacental transfer of any of the factor VIII activities. This has been documented both in normal women, whose twofold elevated levels are not seen in normal children, and in carriers of hemophilia, whose affected sons have very low levels of factor VIII at birth.

Estrogen is probably responsible for the rise in factor VIII levels seen during pregnancy. One author studying normal women has reported a rise in mean factor VIII levels from 115% to 209% for women on oral contraceptives.[58] This increase has not been confirmed by others.[59] Recent in vitro studies of cultured endothelial cells have documented that estradiol levels of 500 pcg/ml result in a 50% increase in in vitro synthesis of von Willebrand factor by endothelial cells.[60] Such levels of estradiol are achieved during pregnancy.

Women with von Willebrand's disease also experience a rise in factor VIII levels during pregnancy. In 11 studies, a total of 27 women were reported to have rises in factor VIII:C levels from a baseline of 16% to 67%.[54, 56, 57, 61–68] The bleeding time corrected substantially in 12 of 18 women in whom it was initially prolonged, and in 10 of 12 cases the bleeding time normalized.[56, 57, 61, 62, 64–68] As in normal women, the rise in factor VIII levels in women with von Willebrand's disease begins at five to six months, rises higher between the eighth and ninth months, and peaks immediately following delivery.

However, the degree of change in factor VIII levels in women with von Willebrand's disease depends to a large extent on the severity of the initial disease. Women with mild disease experience the most reliable changes in factor VIII levels. Women with factor VIII coagulation activity higher than 5% at baseline all had factor VIII levels higher than 25% at term. Of 17 women with baseline factor VIII:C levels higher than 10%, 15 of the 17 had rises at term to above 50%. Seven women with initial bleeding times prolonged to less than 20 minutes had complete normalization of bleeding time at term.

In contrast, patients with severe von Willebrand's disease may not benefit from the effects of pregnancy. Five women with baseline factor VIII:C levels of less than 5% have been reported, and three of these five failed to reach a level of 25% at term. Of 12 women with bleeding times of more than 20 minutes at baseline, bleeding times were normalized in only three at term and an additional three had some degree of improvement.

As with normal women, it is likely that estrogen effect is the major explanation for the changes in factor VIII levels in pregnancy. One author has reported three women with mild von Willebrand's disease who were able to undergo surgery after stimulation of their factor VIII levels with oral estrogens.[69] The factor VIII:C levels rose from a mean of 15% to 80%, and the bleeding times fell from approximately

20 minutes to 9 minutes. In another report, five of five women treated with oral estrogens appeared to benefit clinically with reduced bleeding.[70] Factor VIII:C levels rose in these women, and the bleeding time shortened. In this report, one male with severe von Willebrand's disease failed to benefit from estrogens, but it was not clear whether the lack of response was related to the severity of his disease or to his sex.

Although estrogen effect is probably the major explanation for the changes in factor VIII levels during pregnancy, it may not be the whole explanation. One carefully studied patient had impressive rises in her factor VIII–related activities between the eighth and ninth months of pregnancy, although her peak estradiol levels had already been reached by the seventh month.[68] The authors speculated that some additional factor was responsible for the rise in factor VIII activity close to term. It has already been demonstrated that women with von Willebrand's disease can experience a rise in their factor VIII levels in response to stress or exercise.[71]

Women with von Willebrand's disease, especially variant von Willebrand's disease, may develop marked discrepancies between their various factor VIII activities during pregnancy. Similar dissociations have been seen at baseline in variant von Willebrand's disease and following therapy with cryoprecipitate or DDAVP. In general, the bleeding time tends to correct to a lesser degree than the factor VIII coagulant levels. In one report of a woman who probably had variant von Willebrand's disease, the bleeding time at term remained prolonged at more than 30 minutes despite a rise to 140% in factor VIII antigen.[62] In another carefully studied case, at term a woman with type IIa von Willebrand's disease had a rise in ristocetin cofactor activity from 10% to 100% as well as partial correction of a prolonged bleeding time.[68] It is noteworthy that despite the substantial rise in ristocetin cofactor activity, the multimeric analysis of von Willebrand factor on SDS-agarose gel showed no change in the abnormal pattern and specifically did not show the presence of large multimers of von Willebrand factor at a time when ristocetin cofactor activity had normalized. This observation has been confirmed in a second report[72] in which R:RC activity in a pregnant woman with IIa von Willebrand's disease rose from 20% to 95%, with no improvement in multimer pattern. This phenomenon remains unexplained.

The rise in factor VIII activities at term in women with von Willebrand's disease is more short-lived than the rise seen in normal women.[61] Typically, the values fall by 50% in two days, fall significantly by five days post partum, and then fall slowly to baseline over the next six weeks. As in patients treated with cryoprecipitate transfusion, the increase in factor VIII:C levels above baseline lasts longer than other changes in factor VIII activities.

The duration of the increase in factor VIII activities appears to be related to the degree of severity of disease. One patient with mild disease had no drop in the elevated factor VIII levels two days post partum, and a second patient maintained an increased factor VIII:C level and a normal bleeding time for at least seven days.[65, 66] In contrast, patients with variant or severe von Willebrand's disease have a very short-lived increase in their factor VIII levels following delivery. One patient with severe von Willebrand's disease had correction of the bleeding time for less than one day.[66] A second patient had a substantial fall in factor VIII activities within two days.[63] One patient with type IIa von Willebrand's disease had a rapid drop in factor VIII activities following delivery, the ristocetin cofactor exhibiting a half-life of approximately six hours in contrast to the factor VIII:C levels, which exhibited a half-life of six days.[68] The bleeding time correction in this patient was quite transient.

CLINICAL COURSE DURING PREGNANCY

Women with von Willebrand's disease are at risk for bleeding during labor and following delivery. On occasion, bleeding episodes have been severe and rarely have been fatal.[61, 73–75] The availability of prophylactic treatment with cryoprecipitate should be able to reduce or eliminate significant postpartum bleeding, and many examples of successful prophylactic treatment have been reported.[61, 63, 64, 66, 73, 76, 79] Mildly affected women may need no treatment at the time of delivery, especially if their factor VIII levels have risen to the normal range at term. Nineteen women with mild von Willebrand's disease have been reported who had uneventful deliveries with no prophylactic transfusions.[61, 62, 65, 66, 68, 77, 78, 79] Eleven of these women had normal bleeding times, and in three other cases the bleeding times were only minimally prolonged. Five women with prolonged bleeding times did not experience bleeding following delivery, but in one of these cases a cesarean section was performed. When primary hemostasis can be achieved with suturing, the factor VIII coagulant level is more important for hemostasis than the bleeding time, and in this case the factor VIII:C level was 150%. Thirteen of the 19 women had factor VIII:C levels higher than 50%, and 16 had levels higher than 25%. However, although delivery is usually safe in women with mild von Willebrand's disease, unexpected bleeding may recur despite only mildly reduced levels.[75]

Patients with severe von Willebrand's disease are at substantial risk of bleeding. Of four women with factor VIII:C levels lower than 5%, two experienced significant postpartum hemorrhage, and one of these women with a level of 1% bled during labor. Of three women with bleeding times prolonged to over 20 minutes, two had significant postpartum hemorrhage. Postpartum bleeding seen in these cases may be delayed to 10 to 20 days after delivery. This is probably explained by the fall in factor VIII levels to the patient's baseline after transient improvement at the conclusion of pregnancy.

Treatment of Pregnant Women

Women with mild von Willebrand's disease who have a normal bleeding time and a factor VIII coagulant activity higher than 50% at term require no therapy and should be expected to do well.

Women with markedly prolonged bleeding times (more than 20 minutes) should receive prophylactic treatment with cryoprecipitate at the onset of labor. Cryoprecipitate should be given in an initial dose of 0.24 bag/kg and then 0.12 bag/kg every 12 hours for a total of seven days. The total doses involved are approximately 15 to 25 bags as an initial dose, followed by 7 to 12 bags twice a day for seven days. The bleeding time may not totally correct in these patients, but clinical bleeding should be reduced.

Similarly, women with factor VIII:C levels lower than 25% should be treated with prophylactic cryoprecipitate transfusion. The goal should be to maintain a factor VIII:C level continuously higher than 30%, and this should be done by initially raising the level to 60% and then giving supplemental cryoprecipitate transfusions every 12 hours. Therapy should be continued for at least seven days. The initial dose of cryoprecipitate should be 0.4 bag of cryoprecipitate/kg body weight, or approximately 20 to 30 bags of cryoprecipitate as a total dose. Although the half-life of factor VIII:C in patients with von Willebrand's disease treated with cryoprecipitate is usually longer than 12 hours, patients should receive 0.12 bag/kg of cryoprecipitate every 12 hours, because essentially all women with severely reduced factor VIII coagulant levels will also have reduced ristocetin cofactor levels and will need 12 hourly cryoprecipitate transfusions for correction of their platelet dysfunction.

For patients with mildly reduced factor VIII levels (factor VIII coagulant levels between 25% and 50% or bleeding times prolonged to less than 20 minutes), treatment recommendations are arbitrary. One reasonable approach is to withhold prophylactic transfusion but to have cryoprecipitate available in case the patient exhibits excessive bleeding. One should take into account the patient's bleeding history, particularly her experience with prior deliveries, and a woman who has had prior postpartum bleeding should be treated with prophylactic transfusions even if the laboratory values are only mildly abnormal.

These recommendations for cryoprecipitate transfusion entail exposing the women at risk to transfusion of blood products from more than 100 different donors. An effective vaccine has been developed that can protect transfused patients from transmission of hepatitis B virus. National guidelines for the use of the hepatitis B vaccine are currently being developed, but one could reasonably recommend its use in women who are certain to receive large amounts of blood products at delivery.[80, 81] This recommendation should be part of preconceptual counseling.

PRENATAL DIAGNOSIS OF VON WILLEBRAND'S DISEASE

Since most patients with von Willebrand's disease are only mildly affected, the need for prenatal diagnosis is very limited. However, in the rare instance when both parents are known to have the disease, the fetus would be at risk of having homozygous von Willebrand's disease, which could be as catastrophic as severe hemophilia. In these cases, one might consider prenatal diagnosis using fetoscopy to analyze fetal blood for the concentrations of factor VIII–related antigen and the factor VIII coagulant antigen.[82]

HEMOPHILIA A (FACTOR VIII DEFICIENCY)

Hemophilia A (factor VIII:C deficiency) is the most common severe congenital coagulation disturbance, with an incidence of approximately one case per 10,000 population. Since factor VIII:C is encoded by a gene on the long arm of the X chromosome, the disorder is transmitted as a classic X-linked recessive disorder; consequently disease expression is almost exclusively confined to males. However, there are several ways in which a woman can be clinically affected by hemophilia.[83] A woman may be homozygous for factor VIII deficiency if a carrier mother and a hemophiliac father both pass on their abnormal X chromosomes. A woman may also be severely affected if one X chromosome is affected and the other is either absent (Turner's syndrome) or structurally abnormal. Sporadic mutation could conceivably account for some cases, although spontaneous mutation of the factor VIII gene is quite uncommon. In one study of 41 men with no family history of hemophilia and apparently sporadic mutation, 39 could be documented to have carrier mothers.[84] Some women affected with hemophilia appear to have an autosomal dominant form of this disorder. Three families have been described in which several generations of women have been affected and in which the genetics can be explained only by an autosomal dominant pattern of inheritance.[85, 86] The nature of this disorder is unclear, but authors have suggested that the affected gene is one that controls factor VIII synthesis.

CLINICAL COURSE

The most common cause of clinically significant factor VIII deficiency in women (excluding von Willebrand's disease) is severe lyonization in a carrier woman. The Lyon hypothesis states that in any given cell, only one X chromosome is expressed. In heterozygote women, levels of factor VIII:C should be approximately 50% of normal. However, statistical analysis leads one to expect a broad range of factor VIII levels in heterozygote women, with some proportion of women having markedly reduced levels. Since the hemophilia carrier state is quite common, affecting three women per 10,000 population, if only 1% of carriers had factor VIII levels lower than 25%, then three women per million population would be clinically affected with hemophilia.[86]

Studies of hemophilia carriers have demonstrated that the carrier state is usually clinically silent. When the results of three recent studies are compiled, 204 carrier women had a mean factor VIII coagulant level of 56%.[87–89] Patients with 50% factor VIII:C levels are hemostatically normal and can undergo major surgery with no increased risk of bleeding. Women with factor VIII:C levels lower than 25% will be clinically affected, and women with levels less than 50% are at risk for surgical bleeding. The disease is clinically silent in the majority of these patients if not challenged by surgery or other invasive procedures. Ten women with hemophilia and factor VIII:C levels lower than 10% have been reported recently, and at least seven were severely lyonized carriers.[83] Two of six women had significant menorrhagia and one of four had significant postpartum bleeding.

CARRIER DETECTION AND PRENATAL DIAGNOSIS

The availability of prenatal diagnosis for hemophilia has made carrier detection even more important than previously. Mothers of males with hemophilia are obligate carriers, and sisters of male hemophiliacs have a 50% risk of being carriers. Measurement of factor VIII:C level is seldom helpful in making the diagnosis of the carrier state, because normal levels range from up to 45% to 145%, resulting in a large overlap between the usual carrier range and the normal range. Analysis of factor VIII:C level alone will document the carrier state only in the small percentage of women with factor VIII levels lower than 45%.[88]

Currently, the carrier state is best diagnosed by determining the ratio between factor VIII:C level and factor VIII antigen level in a given patient. Factor VIII antigen levels are determined by a gene on an autosomal chromosome and would not be expected to be affected by the hemophiliac carrier state. In several studies of obligate carriers, mean factor VIII:C levels were 56% and mean factor VIII antigen levels were 114% for a ratio of 0.49 compared with the normal ratio of 1.0.[87–89] Using discriminant analysis, the factor VIII coagulant-antigen ratio is 76% to 92% accurate in assigning carrier state. Although these results are far from ideal, the broad range of factor VIII expression precludes a higher sensitivity if normal women are not to be falsely identified as carriers.

Given the known changes in factor VIII levels with pregnancy, the question has been raised whether the factor VIII:C to antigen ratio can be used for carrier detection during pregnancy. One study of 23 obligate carriers suggests that the analysis can be used.[90] In this study, factor VIII:C levels during second trimester were 49% in the carriers and factor VIII antigen levels were 142%, allowing correct identification of all 23 obligate carriers. However, two of 34 normal women were falsely identified as carriers using this same analysis.

Once carriers of hemophilia are identified, families at risk have the option of prenatal diagnosis of hemophilia in fetuses at risk for the disease. It is very difficult to perform coagulation assays on fetal blood obtained by fetoscopy, because amniotic fluid contains a large amount of tissue factor that can cause spurious in vitro activation of coagulation, and even minute contamination of fetal blood samples with amniotic fluid can render coagulation assays inaccurate. Thus, until recently, assays of factor VIII coagulant activity in fetal blood samples had been unreliable. However, a radioimmunoassay is now available to measure the antigenic activity of the factor VIII coagulant protein.[91] This factor VIII coagulant antigen assay is very specific for the factor VIII coagulant protein and is distinct from the better known and widely available assays of factor VIII–related antigen. Fetal blood samples obtained at fetoscopy can be assayed for the immunologic levels of factor VIII coagulant antigen (VIIIC:Ag) and total factor VIII antigen (factor VIIIR:Ag), and these values can be compared with one another. Fetuses with severe hemophilia would be expected to have normal levels of total factor VIII antigen but very low or absent levels of factor VIII coagulant antigen, and the assay will not be confounded by activation of coagulation.[92] In one report, six fetuses at risk were successfully diagnosed, with three of the six correctly identified as having severe hemophilia.[93] At the present time, this method of measuring factor VIII coagulant antigen is the best available method of prenatal diagnosis of hemophilia. However, the factor VIII coagulant antigen assay is not widely available, and specimens must be sent by prior arrangement to the research laboratories involved. An additional potential drawback is that up to 10% of families with hemophilia have dysfunctional factor VIII:C rather than absent factor VIII:C and consequently immunologic factor VIII:C levels may be within the normal range in severely affected individuals. Before testing fetuses at risk, it must be determined whether affected individuals in that family have immunologically cross-reacting material.

One group of investigators has recently reported a new technique for measuring factor VIII coagulant levels in fetal blood, and this method appears to be accurate despite potential minute contamination with amniotic fluid.[94] However, these assays are not widely available.

In the immediate future, prenatal diagnosis of hemophilia will be available based on the analysis of DNA from cultured fetal fibroblasts obtained by amniocentesis. Such an approach offers advantages, since amniocentesis is a far easier and safer procedure than fetoscopy. Also, direct analysis of the gene encoding the proteins at interest is likely to be more accurate than protein analysis. Prenatal diagnosis of thalassemia and sickle cell anemia is currently available based on these techniques.[95, 96] The gene for factor IX has recently been sequenced and cloned and, given the rapid rate of progress in molecular biology, it can be expected that the factor VIII:C gene will soon be cloned as well.[97] Within several years, the focus of prenatal diagnosis of hemophilia will probably switch to analysis of the gene for factor VIII:C based on analysis of DNA from cultured fetal fibroblasts obtained at amniocentesis.

HEMOPHILIA A AND PREGNANCY

As in von Willebrand's disease, factor VIII:C levels rise during pregnancy in carriers of hemophilia. Four women have been described whose mean factor VIII:C levels rose from a baseline of 45% to a peak of 119% at term.[54] These four women maintained levels of factor VIII:C higher than 100% for more than two days after delivery. As in von Willebrand's disease, estrogen probably plays the major role in causing the rise in factor VIII levels, and three reports document rises in factor VIII:C levels in women with hemophilia after treatment with oral estrogen preparations.[70, 86, 98]

TREATMENT

Women with factor VIII levels lower than 25% at term are at risk for postpartum bleeding and should receive treatment with either cryoprecipitate or factor VIII concentrates. For women with mild disease who have infrequent need for transfusion during their lifetimes, cryoprecipitate has the advantage of exposing the women to fewer donors of blood products. As in other situations with hemophilia, adequate hemostasis is usually guaranteed by maintaining the factor VIII:C level continuously higher than 30%. This should be achieved by initially raising the factor VIII:C level to 60% and then repeating half the initial dose every 12 hours, since this is the approximate half-life of factor VIII:C after transfusion (see Table 9–1). Individuals vary in their half-life of factor VIII:C, and individual doses may be titrated based on analysis of levels in that individual following transfusion. Since factor VIII:C has a volume of distribution 50% higher than the plasma volume of the patient, and since the normal plasma volume in the nonpregnant individual is 40 ml/kg, the initial dose of factor VIII necessary to achieve a 60% level of approximately 0.6 x 40 ml/kg x 1.5 is 36 U/kg. Since cryoprecipitate contains approximately 100 U of factor VIII:C per bag, the initial dose is approximately 0.36 bag/kg, and this usually calculates to 20 to 25 bag for the average-sized nonpregnant woman. Factor VIII levels are then supplemented by transfusion of 0.18 bag/kg (10 to 12 U) of cryoprecipitate every 12 hours. Levels of factor VIII:C should be maintained continuously above 30% in this manner for seven days. The initial dose must be increased as pregnancy progresses, as outlined in Table 9–1.

If factor VIII concentrates are used instead of cryoprecipitate, the initial dose of 36 U of factor VIII/kg will require infusion of 2000 to 2500 U of factor VIII, with the units of Factor VIII:C in each vial marked on the container.

DDAVP, as discussed earlier in the section on von Willebrand's disease, has been shown to be of benefit for patients with mild hemophilia and results in transient increases in factor VIII:C levels in the plasma. Three studies have demonstrated both laboratory and clinical improvement for patients with mild hemophilia.[35, 40, 41] The factor VIII:C levels usually rise four- to fivefold at their peak and fall with a half-life of approximately eight to ten hours. As in von Willebrand's disease, the storage pools of factor VIII released during treatment with DDAVP can be exhausted with repeated doses, and tachyphylaxis does occur. DDAVP has not been used during pregnancy, and its safety and efficacy in this situation remain to be determined.

FACTOR IX DEFICIENCY (HEMOPHILIA B)

Factor IX deficiency (hemophilia B, Christmas disease) is approximately one seventh as common as factor VIII deficiency. The disease is transmitted as an X-linked recessive trait, and men are involved almost exclusively. Clinically, the disorder is indistinguishable from hemophilia A, and the diagnosis is made by specific factor analysis for factor IX. As with factor VIII deficiency, women carriers may be clinically affected if their levels are lower than 25%, and these clinically affected women are thought to be carriers victimized by severe lyonization. For reasons that are unclear, carriers of factor IX deficiency have lower factor levels than carriers of factor VIII deficiency. In contrast to the mean factor VIII levels of 56% in carriers of factor VIII, one study of 51 factor IX carriers demonstrated mean factor levels of 42%.[99] It has been estimated that 20% of factor IX carriers have levels of less than 25% and consequently may be clinically affected.

CLINICAL COURSE

Six factor IX carriers with levels lower than 10% have been reported.[83] One of four women had menorrhagia, and the only pregnant woman in this study had no difficulty with postpartum bleeding. However, women with low levels clearly are at risk for bleeding complications following delivery, and women with levels of factor IX lower than 25% at term should be treated prophylactically to prevent bleeding complications.[100, 101]

CARRIER DETECTION AND PRENATAL DIAGNOSIS

Carrier detection for factor IX carriers must rely on coagulation assays for factor IX. Carriers will overlap broadly into the normal range, which extends as low as 50%, but more than half of carriers can be identified by coagulation assays. Prenatal diagnosis of fetuses at risk for factor IX deficiency is not readily available, and only one reported technique has been able to overcome the problems of activation of coagulation in fetal blood samples caused by contamination by amniotic fluid.[94] This technique is not widely available. In the future, prenatal diagnosis for factor IX deficiency will probably be based on analysis of DNA from fetal fibroblasts cultured from amniotic fluid obtained by amniocentesis. The gene for factor IX has already been cloned, and attempts at prenatal diagnosis using molecular biology techniques will probably be reported soon.[97]

TREATMENT

As with factor VIII, adequate hemostasis is usually ensured by maintaining a factor IX level continuously higher than 30%. The factor IX level should initially be raised to 60%, and half of the initial dose should be given every half-life of factor IX. In contrast to factor VIII:C, the volume of distribution of factor IX is twice the calculated plasma volume, and the half-life of factor IX is 18 hours. Cryoprecipitate and factor VIII concentrates do *not* contain factor IX and cannot be used for treatment of factor IX deficiency. The volumes of fresh-frozen plasma necessary to achieve adequate factor IX levels are usually prohibitive. Consequently, the treatment of factor IX deficiency is based on the use of factor IX concentrates (Konyne, Proplex).

To achieve an initial level of 60%, the appropriate dose of factor IX for a non-pregnant woman is 0.6 x 40 ml/kg x 2, or 50 U/kg of factor IX. This usually calculates to 2500 to 3000 U of factor IX as an initial dose, followed by infusion of 1200 to 1500 U every 18 hours. The half-life of factor IX varies in individual patients, and these dosage schedules may be modified based on analysis of factor IX levels after transfusion in any given patient.

FACTOR XI DEFICIENCY

Factor XI deficiency is an autosomal recessive disorder seen primarily in families of Ashkenazic Jewish descent. Affected individuals usually have markedly prolonged

PTTs. The effective hemostatic level of factor XI is approximately 25%, and factor XI has a plasma half-life of approximately two days. Patients are treated with fresh-frozen plasma, with an initial dose of 20 ml/kg followed by 5 ml/kg/day.

AFIBRINOGENEMIA AND DYSFIBRINOGENEMIA

Afibrinogenemia is an autosomal recessive disorder. Patients usually have incoagulable blood and the PT and PTT are infinitely prolonged. Levels of 50 mg/dl of fibrinogen are sufficient to protect against spontaneous bleeding, and levels of 100 mg/dl are effective for surgical hemostasis. The plasma half-life of fibrinogen is approximately four days. Patients undergoing surgery are treated with cryoprecipitate, with an initial dose of 0.4 bag/kg of cryoprecipitate followed by 0.1 bag/kg cryoprecipitate every two days.

Dysfibrinogenemia, or qualitatively abnormal fibrinogen, is an autosomal dominant disorder. Affected women may have recurrent spontaneous abortions. The PTT is variably prolonged, and the diagnosis is made by demonstrating a prolonged thrombin time with a normal immunologic fibrinogen level. Patients are treated as for afibrinogenemia. A recent report by Ness and colleagues details the association of repeated placental abruption with hypo- or dysfibrinogenemia.[102]

OTHER PLASMA FACTOR DISORDERS

Congenital deficiency of factors II, V, VII, and X is extremely rare. Factors II, VII, and X are replaced using factor IX concentrates, and patients with factor V deficiency are treated with fresh-frozen plasma. Platelets contain factor V in their α-granules, and some patients with factor V deficiency have been treated with platelet transfusion, since factor V appears to exert its physiologic role by accelerating the conversion of prothrombin to thrombin on the platelet surface.[103]

DISORDERS OF FIBRINOLYSIS

The hemostatic mechanism is a dynamic state in which formation of fibrin is counterbalanced by dissolution of these clots by the fibrinolytic mechanism that culminates in the formation of plasmin. The fibrin clot initially formed by the action of thrombin on fibrinogen is unstable and may be readily dissolved. The clot is usually stabilized by the action of activated factor XIII. Activated factor XIII is a transglutaminase that cross-links adjacent fibrin strands by forming a covalent bond between lysine and glutamine residues.

Factor XIII deficiency is an autosomal recessive disorder.[104] Affected patients almost always have neonatal bleeding from the umbilical cord stump and later in life have a bleeding diathesis, poor wound healing, and spontaneous abortions. Bleeding is characteristically delayed and presents in a slow, oozing fashion. All standard coagulation tests are normal in these individuals. The screening test for severe factor XIII deficiency is the clot solubility test in 5 M urea. Normal fibrin clots formed from plasma will not dissolve overnight when incubated in this milieu, whereas the unstable clots formed in the absence of factor XIII will be dissolved. Only 5% of normal factor XIII levels are necessary for effective hemostasis, and factor XIII has a half-life of approximately six days. Consequently patients can be treated with fresh-frozen plasma in a dose of 3 ml/kg.

Other congenital disorders of fibrinolysis are very difficult to diagnose because the necessary laboratory tests are not widely available. Bleeding due to excessive fibrinolysis should be suspected when patients present with slow, delayed bleeding. Rare patients are affected by deficiency of α-$_2$-antiplasmin inhibitor.[105] Some abnormal fibrinogens appear to be extremely sensitive to plasmin. Patients with excessive fibrinolysis should be treated in consultation with a hematologist. ϵ-Amino-caproic acid (EACA, Amicar) may be used for treatment in a dose of 2 g every two hours initially, followed by 2 to 4 g every four hours for a total dose of 12 g to 24 g a day for ten days.

CONGENITAL DISORDERS OF PLATELET FUNCTION

Formation of a platelet plug at a site of vascular injury is the initial step in hemostasis. Following exposure to subendothelial components, platelets initially adhere to the site of injury via von Willebrand factor and its specific receptor on the platelet membrane. Following stimulation, platelets undergo shape change and express fibrinogen receptors on their surface. These receptors are composed of glycoproteins IIb and IIIa of the platelet membrane and are the anchors by which fibrinogen links platelets to one another to form a platelet aggregate. With further activation, platelets secrete their α-granules and dense bodies. α-Granules contain proteins such as von Willebrand factor, fibrinogen, factor V, platelet factor 4, β-thromboglobulin, and platelet-derived growth factor. The dense granules contain calcium, serotonin, ADP, and ATP. With sufficient platelet secretion, enough platelets are recruited to form a platelet aggregate. Congenital disorders of all of these types of platelet function have been described.[105–107]

Patients with mild qualitative platelet disorders will be clinically silent unless challenged by surgery. Moderately affected patients experience mucosal bleeding such as epistaxis, menorrhagia, and gastrointestinal bleeding. Severely affected patients may experience spontaneous petechiae in addition to mucosal and surgical bleeding.

Qualitative platelet disorders are diagnosed by the presence of a prolonged bleeding time and a normal platelet count. Von Willebrand's disease is excluded by analysis of ristocetin cofactor activity and other measurements of factor VIII activity described earlier. The diagnosis of intrinsic platelet abnormality is confirmed by performing in vitro tests of platelet aggregation using calcium, ADP, thrombin, and ristocetin as agonists.

Patients with mild abnormalities of platelet function frequently do not require any treatment, but those with severe qualitative platelet abnormalities require treatment with platelet transfusions. The degree of prolongation of the bleeding time correlates fairly well with clinical bleeding, and the decision to use platelet transfusions should be based on the patient's history and the degree of prolongation of bleeding time. In general, patients with bleeding times in excess of 20 minutes are at serious risk of surgical bleeding. The transfusion of 10 bags of random donor platelets should be expected to raise the platelet count by approximately 100,000/mm^3. Transfused platelets usually have a survival of three to five days, unless other factors such as sepsis or disseminated intravascular coagulation are present. Patients who require repeated platelet transfusion will eventually become alloimmunized to HLA antigens present on the platelet surface. In these situations, HLA-matched platelets may provide adequate hemostasis when random donor platelets fail. Patients may be alloimmunized to antigens other than the HLA complex, and in situations in which HLA-matched platelets fail to improve clinical bleeding, those from family members, especially siblings, may be of benefit. Patients with Glanzmann's thrombasthenia have a particularly high risk of alloimmunization because glycoproteins IIb and IIIa appear to be potent immunogens in patients lacking these antigens.

For unclear reasons, some patients with storage pool disease will respond to transfusion of cryoprecipitate[108] and DDAVP.[38]

SPECIFIC QUALITATIVE PLATELET DISORDERS

The Bernard-Soulier syndrome is a rare autosomal recessive disorder that may be severe. It is caused by absence of glycoprotein I on the platelet membrane. Since glycoprotein I is the platelet receptor for von Willebrand factor, these platelets cannot adhere to subendothelial components. The diagnosis may be suspected because of the presence of giant platelets on the peripheral blood smear. It is confirmed by normal in vitro platelet aggregation in response to agonists such as ADP or collagen but absent platelet agglutination in response to ristocetin. Plasma assays for von Willebrand factor activity are normal. Patients are treated with platelet transfusions.

Glanzmann's thrombasthenia is a rare autosomal recessive disorder caused by absence of glycoproteins IIb and IIIa of the platelet membrane. Since these glycoproteins form the fibrinogen receptor and since it is fibrinogen that links platelets to one another and leads to platelet aggregation, Glanzmann's platelets cannot aggregate in response to any physiologic stimulus. The disorder is often very severe, and fatal bleeding may occur. The diagnosis is confirmed by absent platelet aggregation in response to agonists such as collagen, ADP, and thrombin but normal agglutination in response to ristocetin. Clot retraction is absent in this disorder. Severely affected patients are treated with platelet transfusion, but ultimately many become completely refractory to this form of therapy because of the development of alloantibodies against the missing glycoproteins.

Storage pool disease is a common mild bleeding disorder with heterogeneous clinical expression. The disease is clinically silent in most patients unless surgically challenged. It is caused by a decrease in dense bodies in the platelet. Consequently, although platelets undergo shape change and initial secretion in response to a stimulus, the quantity of ADP they secrete is insufficient to recruit enough platelets to form a large platelet aggregate and effective platelet plug. The diagnosis is made using in vitro tests of platelet aggregation in response to ADP. In response to stimulation, platelets undergo an initial phase of aggregation, but this is reversible, and the secondary or complete form of platelet aggregation fails to occur. When patients are severely affected clinically, they should be treated with platelet transfusions.

Pseudo-von Willebrand's disease (platelet-type von Willebrand's disease) is discussed in the preceding section on von Willebrand's disease. It is an autosomal dominant disorder caused by an as yet uncharacterized abnormality in the platelet membrane that results in increased avidity of the platelet for plasma von Willebrand factor. Because of rapid clearance from the plasma, circulating levels of von Willebrand factor are reduced and the condition manifests as variant von Willebrand's disease.

Other rare types of congenital platelet disorders include the gray platelet syndrome, characterized by a decrease in platelet α-granules, and deficiency in platelet procoagulant activity caused by a decrease in factor V binding sites.

REFERENCES

1. Rapaport, S.I.: Preoperative hemostatic evaluation: Which tests if any? Blood *61*:229, 1983.
2. Silwer, J.: von Willebrand's disease in Sweden. Acta Pediatr Scand *238* (Suppl): 80, 1973.
3. Zimmerman, T.S., and Ruggieri, Z.M.: von Willebrand's disease. Prog Hemost Thromb *6*:203, 1982.

4. Bloom, A.L.: The von Willebrand syndrome. Sem Hematol *17*:215, 1980.
5. Ahr, D.J., Rickles, F.R., Hoyer, L.W., O'Leary, D.S., and Conrad, M.E.: von Willebrand's disease and hemorrhagic telangiectasia: Association of two complex disorders of hemostasis resulting in life-threatening hemorrhage. Am J Med *62*:452, 1977.
6. Weinstein, D., Rabinowitz, R., Malach, D., Mor-Yosef, S., Eldor, A., and Schenker, J.G.: Ovarian hemorrhage in women with von Willebrand's disease: A report of two cases. J Reprod Med *28*:500, 1983.
7. Tresch, D.D., Halverson, G., Blick, M., and Keelan, M.H.: Ovarian (corpus luteum) hemorrhage during anticoagulation therapy. Ann Int Med *88*:642, 1978.
8. Hoyer, L.W.: The factor VIII complex: Structure and function. Blood *58*:1, 1981.
9. Ruggieri, Z.M., and Zimmerman, T.S.: The complex multimeric composition of factor VIII/von Willebrand factor. Blood *57*:1140, 1981.
10. Hoyer, L.W., and Shainoff, J.R.: Factor VIII-related protein circulates in normal human plasma as high molecular weight multimers. Blood *55*:1056, 1980.
11. Meyer, D., Obert B., Pietu G., Lavergne J.M., and Zimmerman T.S.: Multimeric structure of factor VIII/von Willebrand factor in von Willebrand's disease. J Lab Clin Med *95*:590, 1980.
12. Weiss, H.J., Sussman, I.I., and Hoyer, L.W.: Stabilization of factor VIII in plasma by the von Willebrand factor. J Clin Invest *60*:390, 1977.
13. Weiss, H.J.: Abnormalities of factor VIII and platelet aggregation—use of ristocetin in diagnosing the von Willebrand syndrome. Blood *45*:403, 1975.
14. Italian Working Group: Spectrum of von Willebrand's disease: A study of 100 cases. Br J Haematol *35*:101, 1977.
15. Shoa'i, I., Lavergne J.M., Ardaillou, N., Obert, B., Ala, F., and Meyer, D.: Heterogeneity of von Willebrand's disease: Study of 40 Iranian cases. Br J Haematol *37*:67, 1977.
16. Larrieu, M.J., Caen, J.P., Meyer, D.O., Vainer, H., Sultan, Y., and Bernard, J.: Congenital bleeding disorders with long bleeding time and normal platelet count. II Von Willebrand's disease (report of 37 patients). Am J Med *45*:354, 1968.
17. Abildgaard, C.F., Simone, J.V., Honig, G.R., Forman, E.N., Johnson, C.A., and Seeler, R.A.: von Willebrand's disease: A comparative study of diagnostic tests. J Pediatr *73*:355, 1968.
18. Abildgaard, C.F., Suzuki, Z., Harrison, J., Jefcoat, K., and Zimmerman, T.S.: Serial studies in von Willebrand's disease: Variability versus "variance." Blood *56*:712, 1980.
19. Stuart, M.J., Miller, M.L., Davey, F.R., and Wolk, J.A.: The post-aspirin bleeding time: A screening test for evaluating hemostatic disorder. Br J Haematol *43*:649, 1979.
20. Ruggieri, Z.M., and Zimmerman, T.S.: Variant von Willebrand's disease: Characterization of two subtypes by analysis of multimeric composition of factor VIII/von Willebrand factor in plasma and platelets. J Clin Invest *65*:1318, 1980.
21. Ruggieri, Z.M., Pareti, F.I., Mannucci, P.M., Ciavarella, N., and Zimmerman, T.S.: Heightened interaction between platelets of factor VIII/von Willebrand factor in a new subtype of von Willebrand's disease. N Engl J Med *302*:1047, 1980.
22. Zimmerman, T.S., Abildgaard, C.F., and Meyer, D.: The factor VIII abnormality in severe von Willebrand's disease. N Engl J Med *301*:1307, 1979.
23. Weiss, H.J., Meyer, D., Rabinowitz, R., et al.: Pseudo von Willebrand's disease: An intrinsic platelet defect with aggregation by unmodified human factor VIII/von Willebrand factor and enhanced adsorption of its high molecular weight multimers. N Engl J Med *306*:326, 1982.
24. Miller, J.L., and Castella, A.: Platelet type von Willebrand disease: Characterization of a new bleeding disorder. Blood *60*:790, 1982.
25. Gralnick, H.R., Williams, S.B., Shafer, B.C., and Corash, L.: Factor VIII/von Willebrand factor binding to von Willebrand's disease platelets. Blood *60*:328, 1982.
26. Perkins, H.A.: Correction of the hemostatic defects in von Willebrand's disease. Blood *30*:375, 1967.
27. Weiss, H.J., and Rogers, T.: Correction of the platelet abnormality in von Willebrand's disease by cryoprecipitate. Am J Med *53*:734, 1972.
28. Chediak, J.R., Telfer, M.C., and Green, B.: Platelet function and immunologic parameters in von Willebrand's disease following cryoprecipitate and factor VIII concentrate infusion. Am J Med *62*:369, 1977.
29. Green, D., and Potter, E.V.: Failure of AHF concentrate to control bleeding in von Willebrand's disease. Am J Med *60*:357, 1976.
30. Blatt, P.M., Brinkhous, K.M., Culp, H.R., Krauss, J.S., and Roberts H.R.: Antihemophilic factor concentrate therapy in von Willebrand's disease: Dissociation of bleeding time factor and ristocetin cofactor activities. JAMA *236*:2770, 1976.
31. Weiss, H.J.: Relation of von Willebrand factor to bleeding time. N Engl J Med *291*:420, 1974.
32. Ober, J., Sixma, J.J., Bouma, B.N., Bolhuis, P.A., Vlooswijk, R.A., and Beeser-Visser, N.H.: Survival of ^{125}I-labeled factor VIII in patients with von Willebrand's disease. J Lab Clin Med *97*:332, 1981.
33. Weinger, R.S., Cimo, P.L., Moake, J.L., Olson, J.D., and Heller, M.S.: Type IIb von Willebrand's disease: Unusual response to cryoprecipitate infusion. Ann Int Med *94*:47, 1981.

34. Krizek, D.M., Rick, M.E., Williams, S.B., and Gralnick, H.R.: Cryoprecipitate transfusion in variant von Willebrand's disease and thrombocytopenia. Ann Int Med *98*:484, 1983.
35. Mannucci, P.M., Paretti, F.I., Ruggieri, Z.M., and Capitanio, A.: 1-D-amino-8-D-arginine vasopressin: A new pharmacological approach to the management of hemophilia and von Willebrand's disease. Lancet *i*:869, 1977.
36. Ruggieri, Z.M., Mannucci, P.M., Lombardi, R., Federici, A.B., and Zimmerman, T.S.: Multimeric composition of factor VIII/von Willebrand factor following administration of DDAVP: Implications for pathophysiology and therapy of von Willebrand's disease subtypes. Blood *59*:1271, 1982.
37. Mannucci, P.M., Canciani, M.T., Rota, L., and Donovan, B.S.: Response of factor VIII/von Willebrand factor to DDAVP in healthy subjects and patients with hemophilia A and von Willebrand's disease. Br J Haematol *47*:283, 1981.
38. Kobrinsky, N.L., Gerrard, J.M., Watson, C.M., et al.: Shortening of bleeding time by 1-D-amino-8-D-arginine vasopressin in various bleeding disorders. Lancet *i*:1145, 1984.
39. Mannucci, P.M., Pareti, F.I., Holmberg, L., Nilsson, I.M., and Ruggieri, Z.M.: Studies on the prolonged bleeding time in von Willebrand's disease. J Lab Clin Med *88*:662, 1976.
40. Ludlam, C.A., Peake, I.R., Allen, N., Davies, B.L., Furlong, R.A., and Bloom, A.L.: Factor VIII and fibrinolytic response to D-amino-8-D-arginine vasopressin in normal subjects and dissociate response in some patients with hemophilia and von Willebrand's disease. Br J Haematol *45*:499, 1980.
41. Ockelford, P.A., Menon, N.C., and Berry, E.W.: Clinical experience with arginine vasopressin (DDAVP) in von Willebrand's disease and mild hemophilia. N Engl J Med *92*:375, 1980.
42. McCarroll, D.R., Ruggieri, Z.M., and Montgomery, R.R.: The effect of DDAVP on plasma levels of von Willebrand antigen II in normal individuals and patients with von Willebrand's disease. Blood *63*:532, 1984.
43. Nilsson, I.M., Holmberg, L., Aberg, M., and Vilhardt, H.: The release of plasminogen activator and factor VIII after injection of DDAVP in healthy volunteers and in patients with von Willebrand's disease. Scand J Hematol *24*:351, 1980.
44. Menon, C., Berry, E.W., and Ockelford, P.: Beneficial effect of DDAVP on bleeding time in von Willebrand's disease. Lancet *ii*:743, 1978.
45. Isola, L., Forster, A., and Aledort, L.M.: Desamino-D-arginine vasopressin and bleeding time in von Willebrand's disease. Ann Int Med *101*:719, 1984.
46. Mannucci, P.M., Ruggieri, Z.M., Pareti, F.I., and Capitano, A.: DDAVP in hemophilia. Lancet *ii*:1171 (Letter), 1977.
47. Ruggieri, Z.M., Lombardi, R., Gatti, L., Bader, R., Valsecchi, C., and Zimmerman, T.S.: Type IIb von Willebrand's disease: Differential clearance of endogenous versus transfused large multimer von Willebrand's factor. Blood *60*:1453, 1982.
48. Holmberg, L., Nilsson, I.M., Borge, L., Gunnarson, M., and Sjorin, E.: Platelet aggregation induced by 1-desamino-8-D-arginine vasopressin (DDAVP) in type IIb von Willebrand's disease. N Engl J Med *309*:1816, 1983.
49. Takahashi, H.: Studies on pathophysiology and treatment of von Willebrand's disease. V. Properties of factor VIII after DDAVP infusion in variant von Willebrand's disease. Thromb Res *21*:357, 1981.
50. Garcia, V.V., Silva, I.A., and Borrasca, A.L.: Response of factor VIII/von Willebrand factor to intranasal DDAVP in healthy subjects and mild hemophiliacs (with observations in patients with combined deficiency of factors V and VIII). Thromb Haemost *48*:91, 1982.
51. Nossel, H.L., Lanzkowsky, P., Levy, S., Mibshan, R.S., and Hansen, J.D.: A study of coagulation factor levels in women during labor and in their newborn infants. Thromb Diath Haemor *16*:185, 1966.
52. Fournie, A., Monrozies, M., Pontonnier, G., Boneu B., and Bierme, R.: Factor VIII complex in normal pregnancy, pre-eclampsia and fetal growth retardation. Br J Obstet Gynecol *88*:250, 1981.
53. Bennett, B., and Ratnoff, O.D.: Changes in anti-hemophilic factor procoagulant activity and AHF-like antigen in normal pregnancy, and following exercise and pneumoencephalography. J Lab Clin Med *80*:256, 1972.
54. Kasper, C.K., Hoag, M.S., Aggeler, P.M., and Stone, S.: Blood clotting factors in pregnancy: Factor VIII concentrations in normal and AHF-deficient women. Obstet Gynecol *24*:242, 1964.
55. Preston, A.E.: The plasma concentration of factor VIII in the normal population. I. Mothers and babies at birth. Br J Haematol *10*:110, 1964.
56. Strauss, H.S., and Diamond, L.K.: Elevation of factor VIII (anti-hemophilic factor) during pregnancy in normal persons and in a patient with von Willebrand's disease. N Engl J Med *269*:1251, 1963.
57. Bennett, B., Oxnard, S.C., Douglas, A.S., and Ratnoff, O.D.: Studies on antihemophilic factor (AHF) (factor VIII) during labor in normal women, in patients with premature separation of the placenta, and in a patient with von Willebrand's disease. J Lab Clin Med *84*:851, 1974.
58. Crowell, E.B., Clatanoff, D.V., and Kiekhofer, W.: The effect of oral contraceptives on factor VIII levels. J Lab Clin Med *77*:551, 1971.
59. Ygge, J., Brody, S., Korsna-Bengtsen, K., and Nilsson, L.: Changes in blood coagulation and fibrinolysis in a woman receiving oral contraceptives. Am J Obstet Gynecol *104*:87, 1969.

60. Harrison, R.L., and McKee, P.A.: Estrogen stimulates von Willebrand factor production by cultured endothelial cells. Blood *63*:657, 1984.
61. Noller, K.L., Bowie, E.J.W., Kempers, R.D., and Owen, C.A.: Von Willebrand's disease in pregnancy. Obstet Gynecol *41*:865, 1973.
62. Krishnamurty, M., and Miotti, A.B.: Von Willebrand's disease and pregnancy. Obstet Gynecol *49*:244, 1977.
63. Lipton, R.A., Ayromlooi, J., and Coller, B.S.: Severe von Willebrand's disease during labor and delivery. JAMA *248*:1355, 1982.
64. Adashi, E.Y.: Lack of improvement in von Willebrand's disease during pregnancy. N Engl J Med *303*:1173 (Letter), 1980.
65. Leone, G., Monetta, E., Paparatti, G., and Boni, P.: Von Willebrand disease in pregnancy. N Engl J Med *293*:456 (Letter), 1975.
66. Walker, E.H., and Dormandy, K.M.: The management of pregnancy in von Willebrand's disease. J Obstet Gynecol Br Comm *75*:459, 1968.
67. Hagedorn, B.: Von Willebrand's disease. JAMA *216*:991, 1971.
68. Hanna, W., McCarroll, D., McDonald, T., et al.: Variant von Willebrand's disease and pregnancy. Blood *58*:873, 1981.
69. Alperin, J.B., Estrogens and surgery in women with von Willebrand's disease. Am J Med *73*:367, 1982.
70. Glueck, H.I., and Flessa, H.C.: Control of hemorrhage in von Willebrand's disease and a hemophiliac carrier with norethynodrel-mestranol. Thromb Res *1*:253, 1972.
71. Biggs, R., and Matthews, J.M.: The treatment of hemorrhage in von Willebrand's disease and the blood level of factor VIII (AHG). Br J Haematol *9*:203, 1963.
72. Takahashi, H.: Studies on the pathophysiology and treatment of von Willebrand's disease. VI. Variant von Willebrand's disease complicating placenta previa. Thromb Res *31*:285, 1983.
73. Hill, C., and Taylor, J.J.: Von Willebrand's disease in obstetrics and gynecology. J Obstet Gynecol Br Comm *75*:453, 1968.
74. Nilsson, I.M., and Blomback, M.: Von Willebrand's disease in Sweden: Occurrence, pathogenesis and treatment. Thromb Diath Hemorr *9* (Suppl 2):103, 1963.
75. Punnonen, R., Nyman, D., Gronroos M., and Wallen O.: Von Willebrand's disease and pregnancy. Acta Obstet Gynecol Scand *60*:507, 1981.
76. Evans, P.C.: Obstetric and gynecologic patients with von Willebrand's disease. Obstet Gynecol *38*:37, 1971.
77. Levine, N.M.: Von Willebrand's disease during pregnancy: Review and case report. JAMA *79*:520, 1980.
78. Gelman, S.R., O'Leary, J.A., and Feldman, M.: Von Willebrand's disease and pregnancy. South Med J *65*:897, 1972.
79. Telfer, M.C., and Chediak, J.: Factor VIII-related disorders and their relationship to pregnancy. J Reprod Med *19*:211, 1977.
80. Szmuness, W., Stevens, C.E., Harley, E.J., et al.: Hepatitis B vaccine: Demonstration of efficacy in a controlled clinical trial in a high risk population in the United States. N Engl J Med *303*:833, 1980.
81. Sacks, H.S., Rose, D.N., and Chalmers, T.C.: Should the risk of acquired immunodeficiency syndrome deter hepatitis B vaccination? A decision analysis. JAMA *252*:3375, 1984.
82. Hoyer, L.W., Lindsten, J., Blomback, M., et al.: Prenatal evaluation of fetus at risk for severe von Willebrand's disease. Lancet *ii*:191 (Letter), 1979.
83. Lusher, J.M., and McMillan, C.W.: Severe factor VIII and IX deficiency in females. Am J Med *65*:637, 1978.
84. Biggs, R., and Rizza, C.R.: The sporadic case of hemophilia A. Lancet *ii*:431, 1976.
85. Graham, J.B., Barrow, E.S., Roberts, H.R., et al.: Dominant inheritance of hemophilia A in three generations of women. Blood *46*:175, 1975.
86. Eyster, M.E., Ladda, R.L., and Bowman, H.S.: Carrier with excessively low factor VIII procoagulant activity (VIII AHF): A study of two unrelated families with mild hemophilia A. Blood *49*:607, 1977.
87. Klein, H.G., Aledort, L.M., Bouma, B.N., Hoyer, L.W., Zimmerman, T.S., and DeMets, D.L.: A cooperative study for the detection of the carrier state of classic hemophilia. N Engl J Med *296*:959, 1977.
88. Ratnoff, O.D., and Jones, P.A.: The laboratory diagnosis of the carrier state of classic hemophilia. Ann Int Med *86*:521, 1977.
89. Rizza, C.R., Rhymes, I.L., Austen, D.E.G., Kernoff, P.B.A., and Aroni, S.A.: Detection of carriers of hemophilia: A "blind" study. Br J Haematol *30*:447, 1975.
90. Hoyer, L.W., Carta, C.A., and Mahoney, M.J.: Detection of hemophilia carriers during pregnancy. Blood *60*:1407, 1982.
91. Lazarchick, J., and Hoyer, L.W.: Immunoradiometric measurement of the factor VIII procoagulant antigen. J Clin Invest *62*:1048, 1978.
92. Peake, I.R., and Bloom, A.L.: Immunoradiometric assay of procoagulant factor VIII antigen in

plasma and serum and its reduction in hemophilia: Preliminary studies on adult and fetal blood. Lancet *i*:473, 1978.
93. Firshein, S.I., Hoyer, L.W., Lazarchick, J., et al.: Prenatal diagnosis of classic hemophilia. N Engl J Med *300*:937, 1979.
94. Mibashan, R.S., Thumpston, J.K., Singer, J.D., et al.: Plasma assay of fetal factors VIII:C and IX for prenatal diagnosis of hemophilia. Lancet *i*:1309, 1979.
95. Wong, V., Ma, H.K., Todd, D., Golbus, M.S., Dozy, A.M., and Kan, Y.W.: Diagnosis of homozygous alpha-thalassemia in cultured amniotic fluid fibroblasts. N Engl J Med *298*:669, 1978.
96. Chang, J.C., and Kan, Y.W.: Antenatal diagnosis of sickle cell anaemia by direct analysis of the sickle mutation. Lancet *ii*:1127, 1981.
97. Giannelli, F., Choo, K.H., Rees, D.J.G., Boyd, Y., Rizza, C.R., and Brownlee, G.G.: Gene deletions in patients with hemophilia B and anti-factor IX antibodies. Nature *303*:181 (Letter), 1983.
98. Schiffman, S., and Rapaport, S.I.: Increased factor VIII levels in suspected carriers of hemophilia taking contraceptives by mouth. N Engl J Med *275*:599, 1966.
99. Kasper, C.K., Osterud, B., Minami, J.Y., Shonick, W., and Rapaport, S.I.: Hemophilia B: Characterization of genetic variants and detection of carriers. Blood *50*:351, 1977.
100. Kitchens, C.S., Levin, J., and Smith, W.K.: Hemorrhagic diathesis in a carrier of hemophilia B. Am J Med *60*:138, 1976.
101. Rust, L.A., Goodnight, S.H., Freeman, R.K., and Johnson, C.S.: Pregnancy and delivery in a woman with hemophilia B. Obstet Gynecol *46*:483, 1975.
102. Ness, P.M., Budzynski, A.Z., Olexa, S.A., et al.: Congenital hypofibrinogenemia and recurrent placental abruption. Obstet Gynecol *61*:519, 1983.
103. Chediak, J., Ashenhurst, J.B., Garlick, I., and Desser, R.K.: Successful management of bleeding in a patient with factor V inhibitor by platelet transfusions. Blood *56*:835, 1980.
104. Kitchens, C.S., and Newcomb, T.F.: Factor XIII. Medicine *58*:413, 1979.
105. Aoki, N., Saito, H., Kamiya, T., Koie, K., Sakata, Y., and Kobakura, M.: Congenital deficiency of $alpha_2$-plasmin inhibitor associated with severe hemorrhagic tendency. J Clin Invest *63*:877, 1979.
106. George, J.N., Nurden, A.T., and Phillips, D.R.: Molecular defects in interactions of platelets with the vessel wall. N Engl J Med *311*:1084, 1984.
107. Shattil, S.J., and Bennett, J.S.: Platelets and their membranes in hemostasis: Physiology and pathophysiology. Ann Int Med *94*:108, 1980.
108. Gerritsen, S.W., Akkerman, J.N., and Sixma, J.J.: Correction of the bleeding time in patients with storage pool deficiency by infusion of cryoprecipitate. Br J Haematol *40*:153, 1978.

Chapter 10

ACQUIRED COAGULATION DISORDERS

Russell K. Laros, Jr.

DISSEMINATED INTRAVASCULAR COAGULATION

Disseminated intravascular coagulation (DIC) is really a syndrome produced as part of an underlying disease that in some way leads to activation of the coagulation mechanism.[1-3] Many of the conditions associated with DIC are listed in Table 10–1. In obstetrics and gynecology, DIC is seen in association with placental abruption,[4] the dead fetus syndrome,[5-7] amniotic fluid embolism,[8] gram-negative sepsis,[9] saline-induced abortion,[10] and severe pre-eclampsia and eclampsia.[11]

PATHOPHYSIOLOGY

There are two animal models of DIC. In the first, procoagulant materials such as thrombin, thromboplastin, or serum are slowly infused into an animal. Slow infusion creates a state of hypercoagulability that may or may not be associated with fibrin deposition. However, if venous stasis is created or if hepatic circulation is occluded, extensive disseminated thrombosis will result and rapidly lead to death.

In the second model the generalized Shwartzman reaction is induced by two intravenous injections of endotoxin administered 8 to 24 hours apart. This leads to fibrin deposition in the glomerular capillaries, with bilateral renal necrosis. In this model both endotoxin damage to platelets and capillary endothelium and inhibition of fibrinolysis appear to be important factors in the pathogenesis.

One result of DIC is a disturbance of the coagulation mechanism. This results from both the consumption of plasma factors and the production of anticoagulants by the fibrinolytic system. The coagulation factors consumed are platelets, prothrombin, factor V, and factor VIII. The body has a limited capacity to produce circulating plasma factors and platelets necessary for clot formation. When the available plasma factors are consumed by DIC, the circulating blood becomes deficient in these factors, and a severe diathesis may occur. Activation of the fibrinolytic system produces fibrin-fibrinogen degradation products (FDP), which serve to further interfere with the clotting mechanism. This pathophysiology is summarized in Figure 10–1.

A second major result of DIC is the presence of small clots in the microcirculation. These clots can cause plugging of small vessels and ischemia of various organs. DIC occurs when the coagulation mechanism is inappropriately triggered by any of several underlying disease processes.

Disease entities associated with DIC fall into three major groups, based on the mechanism by which the primary disease initiates intravascular clotting. The underlying mechanism in the first group is the intravascular infusion of tissue thrombo-

Table 10–1. Some Clinical Conditions Associated with DIC

Acute	Subacute	Chronic
Acute intravascular hemolysis	Aortic aneurysm	Allergic vasculitis
Acute liver disease	Disseminated malignancy	Certain local carcinomas
Acute pulmonary embolism	Giant hemangioma	Ischemic enterocolitis
Amniotic fluid embolism	Promyelocytic leukemia	Liver disease
Burns	Retained dead fetus	Myocardial infarction
Cardiac arrest		Paroxysmal nocturnal hemoglobinuria
Extensive trauma		Pre-eclampsia/eclampsia
Heat stroke		Renal disease
Placental abruption		Sarcoidosis
Saline-induced abortion		Systemic lupus erythematosus
Septicemia		
Shock		
Snake bite		

plastins. Placental abruption and the dead fetus syndrome fall into this category. They differ in that in cases of abruption, consumption is rapid and fulminant, while in the dead fetus syndrome consumption is very slow, occurring over a period of days to weeks. Some authors have suggested that the fall in plasma coagulation factors is explained on the basis of consumption in the retroplacental clot. However, neither the magnitude of the decrease nor the presence of FDP can be accounted for by this mechanism. Rather, material from the placenta itself or serum derived from the retroplacental clot enters the maternal circulation, where it causes activation of the coagulation system.[4] With fetal death, tissue thromboplastins are progressively released into the amniotic fluid and slowly cross into the maternal circulation. Additionally, fetal death appears to enhance the rate of transport of thromboplastin from the fetal

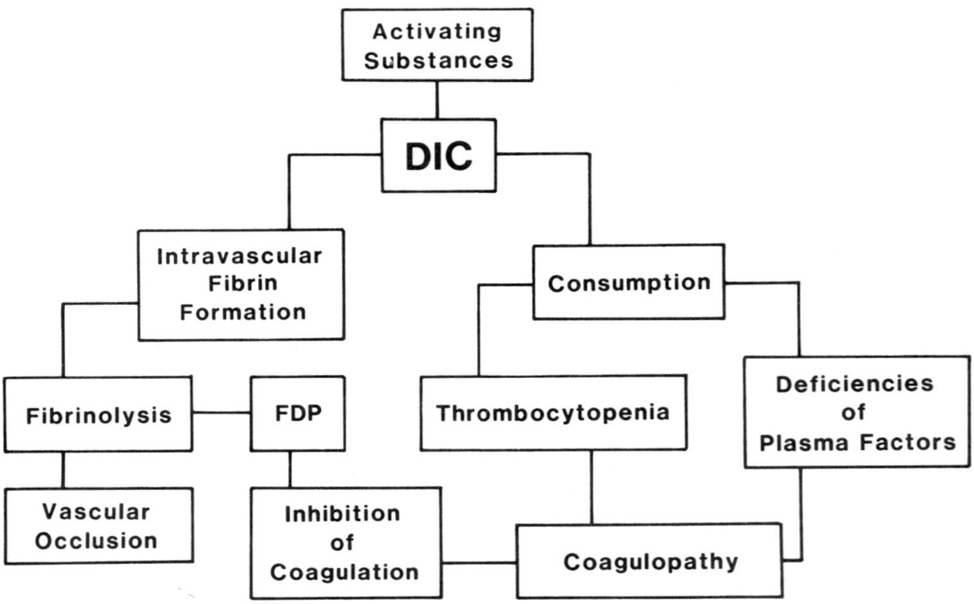

Figure 10–1. Pathophysiology of disseminated intravascular coagulation.

to the maternal compartment.[12] Until recently, all the cases of the dead fetus syndrome have been reported in association with a single fetus. There are now reports of the syndromes occurring in cases of multiple gestation in which only one of the fetuses has died.[7]

A second group of pathologic conditions causing DIC includes those associated with endothelial damage. Both the extrinsic and intrinsic pathways are activated by endothelial damage. Eclampsia/pre-eclampsia is felt to fall into this category.[13] In an extensive study by Pritchard and colleagues, thrombocytopenia was identified in 29%, a prolonged thrombin time (TT) in 50%, and increased FDP's in 3% of 95 patients.[14] The incidence of DIC appears to be lower in cases of pre-eclampsia,[15, 16] except when the toxemia also produces liver dysfunction or hemolysis or both.[17–20] In these cases, the degree of thrombocytopenia generally correlates directly with the degree of liver dysfunction. Additionally, one study has shown mild platelet dysfunction in cases of pre-eclampsia.[21]

A third group of conditions associated with DIC encompasses nonspecific or indirect effects of certain diseases. This group includes amniotic fluid embolism (AFE), gram-negative sepsis, and saline abortion. The detailed studies of Phillips and Davidson indicate that the amount of procoagulant activity in amniotic fluid is insufficient to cause significant intravascular coagulation.[8] It may be that the DIC is secondary to the profound shock seen with AFE or to secondary platelet aggregation and plasma factor consumption in the obstructed pulmonary capillary bed. Peterson and Taylor observed that in nine cases of hemorrhage not associated with placental abruption, bleeding did not occur immediately but from 30 minutes to 4 hours after the acute embolic episode.[22] This latent period militates against the amniotic fluid's initiating the DIC.

The prototype for sepsis causing DIC is meningococcal bacteremia, in which profound shock, cutaneous petechiae, and autopsy evidence of small vessel occlusion by thrombi occur. While it is tempting to attribute the DIC seen with other organisms causing gram-negative sepsis to a Shwartzman-like reaction caused by endotoxin, proof of this pathogenic mechanism is lacking.

Finally, the mechanism by which saline abortion causes DIC also is not understood. Coagulation changes of DIC are seen frequently, and it has been suggested that the mechanism must be similar to that seen in the dead fetus syndrome, i.e., disrupted fetal tissues producing thromboplastins that make their way into the maternal circulation.[10, 23] However, the studies of Laros and Penner failed to demonstrate any change in the thromboplastic activity of amniotic fluid after instillation of hypertonic saline.[24]

SIGNS AND SYMPTOMS

In DIC, the signs and symptoms are basically those of the underlying disease with the addition of hemorrhage, thrombosis, or both hemorrhagic and thrombotic manifestations. Acute DIC is more often associated with a hemorrhagic presentation, while chronic DIC evidences more thrombotic complications. Both the thrombotic and hemorrhagic presentations of DIC may assume a wide variety of clinical presentations. Hemorrhagic presentations include dermatologic conditions such as ecchymoses, petechiae, and oozing from venipuncture sites. Epistaxis and gingival bleeding are further evidence of DIC's affecting the mucous membranes. Intracranial hemorrhage, gastrointestinal bleeding, and hematuria also may occur. Thrombotic presentations may be neurologic, with multifocal seizures, delirium, or coma, or dermatologic, with focal ischemia and superficial gangrene. Renal manifestations of a thrombotic presentation are cortical necrosis with renal failure. Acute ulceration with bleeding is an example of a gastrointestinal thrombotic presentation. Infarcts and emboli represent pulmonary vascular obstruction, while phlebitis and peripheral gangrene are the result of thrombotic effects within peripheral vessels.

LABORATORY DIAGNOSIS

While the laboratory diagnosis of full-blown DIC is relatively easy to make (Table 10–2), low-grade DIC can produce confusing findings. Generally all the routine laboratory tests of coagulation yield grossly abnormal results. The platelet count is almost invariably decreased or falls progressively, the fibrinogen level is low, and circulating FDPs are increased.[2] Several measures of circulating split products are available, including the TT, ethanol gelation, protamine precipitation test, and latex agglutination test. The prothrombin time (PT) and activated partial prothrombin time (aPTT) may be normal, prolonged, or shortened. Indirect evidence of obstructed microcirculation can be found by examining a peripheral blood smear. As normal red cells are forced through the obstructed microcirculation, they tend to fragment. Bizarre cell forms called schistocytes and helmet cells are formed and are readily identifed. If the rate of red cell destruction is brisk, the patient may show evidence of intravascular hemolysis by the appearance of an elevated plasma hemoglobin level and hemoglobinuria.

TREATMENT

The most important step in treating DIC is the recognition and treatment of the underlying disease process. In the obstetric situation especially, treatment of the underlying process is all that is necessary. Several questions must be answered in order to determine whether replacement therapy with procoagulants is needed and if interruption of the DIC with heparin is warranted.[3]

1. Are the levels of platelets, fibrinogen, and other clotting factors low, and if so is the patient bleeding actively?

If the answer to the second part is no and the patient does not require surgery, replacement therapy is usually not necessary. In contrast, if the patient is actively bleeding or surgical intervention is required or both, replacement therapy with appropriate agents should be started. It is important not to consider the uterine bleeding seen with placental abruption as bleeding requiring procoagulant therapy. This hemorrhage is caused by the mechanics of the placental separation and not by the co-

Table 10–2. Laboratory Findings in DIC

Laboratory Study	Finding
Platelet count	Decreased
Fibrinogen	Decreased
Prothrombin time (PT)	Variable
Activated partial thromboplastin time (aPTT)	Variable
Fibrinogen-fibrin degradation products (FDP)	Increased

agulation disorder. Furthermore, the intramyometrial bleeding seen in the Couvelaire uterus is not by itself evidence of the need for procoagulant therapy.

2. Is there evidence of thrombotic vascular obstruction?

If the answer is yes, active inhibition of thrombin with heparin is indicated.[25–27] Another condition in which heparin therapy is indicated is the dead fetus syndrome.[7, 28, 29] The availability of prostaglandins for the induction of preterm labor and an aggressive attitude toward the termination of pregnancy after intrauterine fetal death have made the occurrence of the dead fetus syndrome very rare. However, when the physician is confronted by DIC in these circumstances, anticoagulation with heparin is begun, and the procoagulant levels are allowed to return to normal before labor is induced. Normalization can usually be accomplished in three to five days. Romero and his associates describe heparin therapy in a case of DIC in association with the death of one of a set of twins.[7] Two courses of heparin therapy were required between the 26th and 34th weeks of gestation, after which procoagulant levels remained normal.

Procoagulant Therapy

It is important to administer enough platelets to keep the count above 50×10^9/L and enough cryoprecipitate to achieve a fibrinogen level of over 150 mg/dl.

Platelet Transfusions

Platelet transfusions can be accomplished with either platelet-rich plasma or platelet concentrates. Each unit increases the platelet count by approximately 5×10^9, and the number of units requested should be predicated on the patient's pretransfusion platelet count. The survival of the transfused platelets will depend both on the freshness of the platelets and on the rate of consumption resulting from the DIC.

Cryoprecipitate and Fresh or Frozen Plasma

Fresh or frozen plasma provides slightly lower concentrations than are found in a similar volume of whole blood. Cryoprecipitate is made by freezing and then thawing fresh plasma. The small volume of protein precipitated is rich in both fibrinogen and factor VIII and is present in a total reconstituted volume of only 40 ml. Either source of fibrinogen should be given in sufficient volume to achieve rapid normalization of the fibrinogen level. Appropriate dosages for fresh or frozen plasma are 10 to 20 ml/kg, and for cryoprecipitate 1 to 2 bags/10 kg.

Heparin Therapy

The patient should receive a loading dose of 2500 to 5000 U followed by 5 to 10 U/kg/hr. The dosage should be adjusted based on clinical and laboratory parameters. Laboratory control may be difficult if the fibrinogen level is very low. However, an adequate endpoint can usually be obtained and consists of a prolongation of the aPTT or TT to 1½ times control. It is essential to assure a platelet count of 50×10^9/L or higher with platelet transfusions when heparin is used.

Fortunately, in obstetric practice those diseases associated with DIC are usually cured by delivery. Therefore, specific treatment for the coagulopathy produced by the DIC is also limited in scope in pregnant patients. After delivery, the DIC will ameliorate and the coagulation abnormalities will return to normal. Because of the enormous capacity of the healthy liver to produce procoagulant, the plasma factors will normalize within 24 hours of cessation of DIC. The return of the platelet count to normal will be slower (five to seven days) because of the time required for a generation, maturation, and release of new platelets by the bone marrow.

IMMUNE THROMBOCYTOPENIC PURPURA

During the three decades since Harrington's classic experiment demonstrating the immune nature of idiopathic thrombocytopenic purpura (ITP), great advances have been made in our understanding of the pathophysiology of the disease. Harrington and coworkers noted that mothers with ITP often delivered children with transient thrombocytopenia.[30] The possibility of placental transfer of a humoral factor prompted Harrington's famous experiment, which established the immunologic nature of ITP. He infused plasma from patients with ITP into several normal recipients, including himself. All recipients developed thrombocytopenia that resolved in 4 to 6 days.[31] Shortly thereafter, Shulman and associates demonstrated that the factor responsible for platelet destruction had many characteristics of an antibody. It was in the 7S gamma globulin faction of serum, it was absorbed by human platelets, it was species-specific, and it affected both autologous and homologous platelets.[32]

PATHOPHYSIOLOGY

The details of the pathophysiology of ITP are presented in several recent publications and will only be summarized here.[33, 34] In ITP platelet destruction is caused by an antiplatelet antibody that results in the removal of platelets by the reticuloendothelial system. In most patients the antibody is of the IgG class and is directed against a platelet-associated antigen.[35] While the spleen is usually the major site of antibody production, bone marrow cells of patients with ITP also have been shown to be able to synthesize antiplatelet IgG.

Most evidence suggests that antiplatelet IgG binds directly to platelet antigens. Nevertheless, circulating immune complexes have been demonstrated in patients with ITP. Additionally, there are data that suggest a role for complement (C3) in the pathogenesis of thrombocytopenia in some patients.[36–38] Most patients with ITP have increased levels of platelet-associated IgG (PA-IgG), and an inverse relationship exists between the PA-IgG level and the platelet count.[37–39] Another group of patients have activated C3, causing elevated levels of both IgG and C3.[36, 37] A third group of patients, constituting 10 to 30% of cases of ITP, has normal levels of PA-IgG but elevated levels of PA-C3.[37, 39]

The reticuloendothelial system, including the spleen, liver, and bone marrow, is responsible for platelet destruction. The spleen is the primary site for antibody production and is also the main site for platelet destruction. After splenectomy, the bone marrow is also capable of intramedullary platelet destruction and is probably the major site of antibody production. The liver's major function is phagocytic; it also produces small amounts of antibody. The pathophysiology of ITP is summarized in Figure 10–2.

Techniques are now available for measuring antiplatelet antibodies.[37, 40] In the direct test the patient's platelets are incubated with ^{125}I-labeled anti-IgG, and the platelet-associated radioactivity is measured after washing. This test is the platelet equivalent of the direct Coombs' test for detecting red cell antigen–antibody reactions. In the indirect test, normal platelets are incubated with the patient's plasma, washed, and

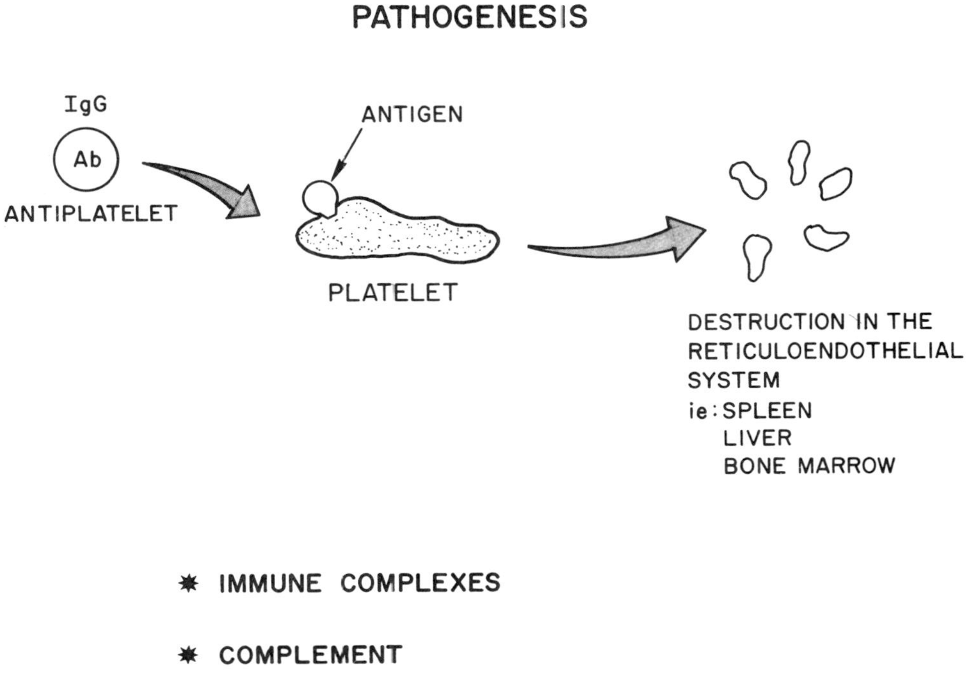

Figure 10–2. Pathophysiology of idiopathic thrombocytopenic purpura.

then the radioactivity is measured as in the direct technique. This study is analogous to an indirect Coombs' test. A similar procedure is carried out for the measurement of C3. An increase in direct PA-IgG has been reported in the majority of patients with ITP. The direct assay usually correlates well with the clinical picture, and an inverse relationship is noted with the patient's platelet count. Because the indirect assay does not correlate well with the clinical status, it is of limited use. Cines and associates have recently reported a correlation between circulating PA-IgG (indirect test) and the presence and extent of neonatal thrombocytopenia.[40]

SIGNS AND SYMPTOMS

The diagnosis of ITP is made according to the criteria listed in Table 10–3.[41, 42] Most patients have a history of easy bruising. Physical examination is normal except for ecchymoses, petechiae, and mucosal bleeding. Many women will be seen first by the physician because of menorrhagia. Generally the platelet count is less than 30 to $50 \times 10^9/L$ when capillary bleeding or purpura appears.

ITP can be classified on the basis of acuity. The acute disorder mostly affects children and generally follows an acute viral illness. The usual interval between the illness and purpura is two weeks. Males and females are affected with equal frequency. The acute form is generally a milder disease, but approximately 7 to 28% of children go on to develop the chronic form. The intermediate form can occur at any age and is characterized by intervals when the platelet count and platelet survival are normal. The chronic variety most often affects adults and is long-lasting. Platelet counts usually remain low, and remission refers to absence of purpura rather than normalcy of the

Table 10–3. Criteria for the diagnosis of ITP

Normal blood count except for thrombocytopenia
Increased platelet volume
Normal bone marrow with adequate or increased megakaryocytes
Normal RBC and WBC morphology
Normal clotting studies except for those affected by thrombocytopenia
No other obvious cause for thrombocytopenia

platelet count. This form tends to be more common in women with a female-male ratio of 2–4:1.[33]

TREATMENT

The goal of treatment of ITP is remission, not necessarily cure.[43] Thus, a step-wise approach is ideal: corticosteroids, then splenectomy, and last, immunosuppression or other modalities such as androgen or immunoglobulin therapy.

Corticosteroids

The major effect of corticosteroids is the blunting of reticuloendothelial function, with consequent reduction of platelet destruction. Additionally, corticosteroids diminish immunoglobulin synthesis and reduce capillary fragility.

Some platelet response will be seen in 70 to 90% of patients with chronic ITP and in 15 to 60% of those with the acute form of the disease.[43, 44] Prednisone is started in a dose of 40 to 60 mg per day (1 mg/kg/day in children) and continued for three to six weeks. The dose is then reduced gradually and stopped. A response is usually seen in a matter of days. While short-term use of corticosteroids is relatively safe, long-term complications can be very serious. Thus, initial therapy should not be continued for more than six to eight months.

Splenectomy

Splenectomy is usually indicated in patients who fail to achieve a clinical remission with corticosteroids. It removes both the major site of platelet destruction and the main site of antibody production. A positive response to splenectomy of 50 to 85% has been reported in various series.[43, 44] Although splenectomy may produce a clinical remission with normal platelet counts, patients may still produce large amounts of PA-IgG. This is of importance in considering the management of the pregnant patient.[40]

Immunosuppressive Therapy

Immunosuppression has generally been reserved for patients who are refractory to corticosteroids or splenectomy or both. The primary agents used have been azathioprine, cyclophosphamide and the vinca alkaloids. A favorable response has been reported in 20 to 55% of cases.[33, 35, 43–45] Approximate dosages are as follows: cyclophosphamide, 50 to 200 mg/day orally; azathioprine, 50 to 200 mg/day orally; vincristine, 0.025 mg/kg (not > 2 mg). While there is a substantial experience in renal transplant patients indicating the safety of azathioprine during pregnancy, its use should be limited to patients who have failed to respond to corticosteroids and splenectomy and who continue to have purpura.

Danazol

Ahn and associates reported a series of 22 patients treated with danazol after failing to obtain a clinical remission with corticosteroids or splenectomy or both.[46] Danazol was used in a dose of 200 mg two to four times daily. Sixty-eight percent of cases improved, and in 50% a sustained remission was obtained. Because of the androgenic properties of danazol, it should not be used in pregnancy if the fetus is female.

High-Dose Intravenous Gamma Globulin

There are several reports of successful treatment of refractory ITP with high-dose intravenous gamma globulin.[47–52] The gamma globulin is thought to interfere with phagocytic Fc receptor–mediated immune clearance. Furthermore, platelets in ITP treated with immunoglobulin are fully hemostatic.[47] Eighty percent of patients have obtained clinical remission after receiving immune globulin in a dose of 400 mg/kg/day for five days. Response is prompt and appears to be long-lasting. Two cases of successful treatment during pregnancy have been reported.[50, 52]

PREGNANCY CONSIDERATIONS

The management of ITP in pregnancy requires special consideration because the human placenta is known to have receptors for the Fc portion of the IgG molecule.[53] Active transport of IgG from mother to fetus can occur, leading to neonatal thrombocytopenia.[54] Even women in remission may still have circulating PA-IgG and thus deliver a thrombocytopenic newborn.[37, 54–56] Neonatal thrombocytopenia affects 50 to 70% of newborns.[55–60] O'Reilly and Taber's review of the literature indicated an overall incidence of neonatal thrombocytopenia of 44%[61]

While some authors have reported an increased incidence of spontaneous abortion in women with ITP, recent data do not find an increase compared with normal women.[34]

Maternal Morbidity

In general, pregnancy has no effect on the course of ITP. However, some patients may show a slight deterioration in platelet count.[59–62] The overall mortality during pregnancy is low. O'Reilly and Taber reported a 4% incidence of maternal death prior to 1976, with the last death occurring in 1951.[61] Noriega-Guerra has subsequently reported one maternal death from hemorrhage.[56]

Varying degrees of maternal morbidity have been reported, primarily the result of maternal hemorrhage. Postpartum hemorrhage from the placental site is unusual because bleeding from decidual vessels is controlled mechanically primarily by myometrial contraction. Of greater concern is bleeding from operative sites. Episiotomies and lacerations may require platelet transfusions for primary hemostasis. The overall incidence of puerperal hemorrhage is reported as 5 to 25%.[34] Adherence to meticulous surgical technique is of prime importance. If an operative delivery is indicated and the platelet count is less than $50 \times 10^9/L$, platelet transfusions should be given to minimize maternal hemorrhage.

We have managed 19 pregnancies in patients with ITP during pregnancy. Although nine (47%) were thrombocytopenic at the time of delivery, none experienced significant bleeding relating to their deliveries or, in two instances, to their postpartum tubal ligations.[59, 60]

Similarly, antepartum hemorrhage from placental abruption and placenta previa does not occur more frequently in women with ITP than in the general pregnant population.[34]

Management

Most obstetricians and hematologists would agree that the overall management of pregnant women with ITP should be similar to that of the nonpregnant individual. The major controversy revolves around the mode of delivery. Prior to the mid-1970s, little thought was given to the route of delivery as a possible cause of morbidity and mortality for infants of mothers with ITP. In 1973, Territo and associates suggested that the maternal platelet count correlated with the neonatal count and advocated cesarean section for all women whose platelet counts were lower than $100 \times 10^9/L$ at the onset of labor.[55] This recommendation spread quickly in both the general medical and hematologic literature despite the lack of data to support it. While some authors have supported this approach,[63–65] others have questioned its validity.[51, 56, 60, 61, 66] Table 10–4 summarizes data on 165 cases reported over an 11-year period. Series were included if the data were sufficient to allow evaluation of the method of delivery, neonatal platelet count, and neonatal outcome. Cases in which fetal death occurred prior to labor were excluded because the method of delivery no longer influenced their outcomes. Of the 134 infants delivered vaginally, 50 (37%) either had or developed platelet counts below $100 \times 10^9/L$, and 28 (21%) had counts below $30 \times 10^9/L$. Only one infant was described as having severe bleeding; this was intracranial but nonfatal.[67] By contrast, 17 (55%) of the 31 infants delivered by cesarean section had counts below $100 \times 10^9/L$ and 9 (29%) below $30 \times 10^9/L$. There were three serious hemorrhages, one of which was intracranial and occurred on the third day of life.[55] These data do not support the premise that delivery by cesarean section prevents intracranial bleeding in thrombocytopenic infants.

If cesarean section is ever demonstrated to be beneficial for fetuses, it will only be so for those who are in fact thrombocytopenic. Territo and associates' suggestion that the fetal platelet count correlates with the maternal count has not been supported by other studies.[40, 56, 60, 68] Several authors have demonstrated the correlation between fetal scalp blood platelet counts obtained during labor and the platelet count obtained from the newborn immediately after delivery.[68, 71] This technique allows identification of those fetuses who are actually thrombocytopenic.

Another method proposed for identifying fetuses with thrombocytopenia involves measurement of the maternal level of PA-IgG. Cines and associates found no correlation between Pa-IgG (direct assay) and the fetal platelet count.[40] However, the

Table 10–4. Neonatal Status in Infants of Mothers with ITP According to Mode of Delivery*

Method of Delivery	Number of Cases	Lowest Neonatal Platelet Count ($\times 10^9/L$) <100	<50	<30	Neonatal Hemorrhage Any	Serious	Treatment
Vaginal	134	50	38	28	21	1	18
Cesarean section	31	17	15	9	6	3	4

* Data from references 55, 56, 60, 61, 63, and 67–70.

level of circulating antibody as measured by the indirect method did correlate with the occurrence of neonatal thrombocytopenia. Similarly, Kelton and associates found the maternal antibody levels (direct assay) highly predictive of neonatal thrombocytopenia.[70] However, the levels of maternal PA-IgG did not predict the severity of fetal thrombocytopenia.

Therapeutic Regimen

The therapeutic regimen used at our institution is outlined in Figure 10–3. We define a remission as a platelet count of 50 to 100 × 10^9/L without bleeding manifestations. At 37 weeks, betamethasone is substituted for prednisone, in a dosage of 0.6 mg equaling 5 mg. Betamethasone is used because it crosses the placenta and, in theory, should improve the fetal platelet count and platelet survival. If splenectomy is required, ideally it should be performed prior to 32 weeks of gestation because of the technical difficulties encountered thereafter. If the course of the disease does not allow this timing (i.e., onset in the third trimester), cesarean section and splenectomy should be performed together if the clinical situation requires intervention—that is, a platelet count lower than 20 × 10^9/L or a higher count with bleeding. Other modes of therapy (gamma globulin, danazol, immunosuppression) should be considered in selected cases.

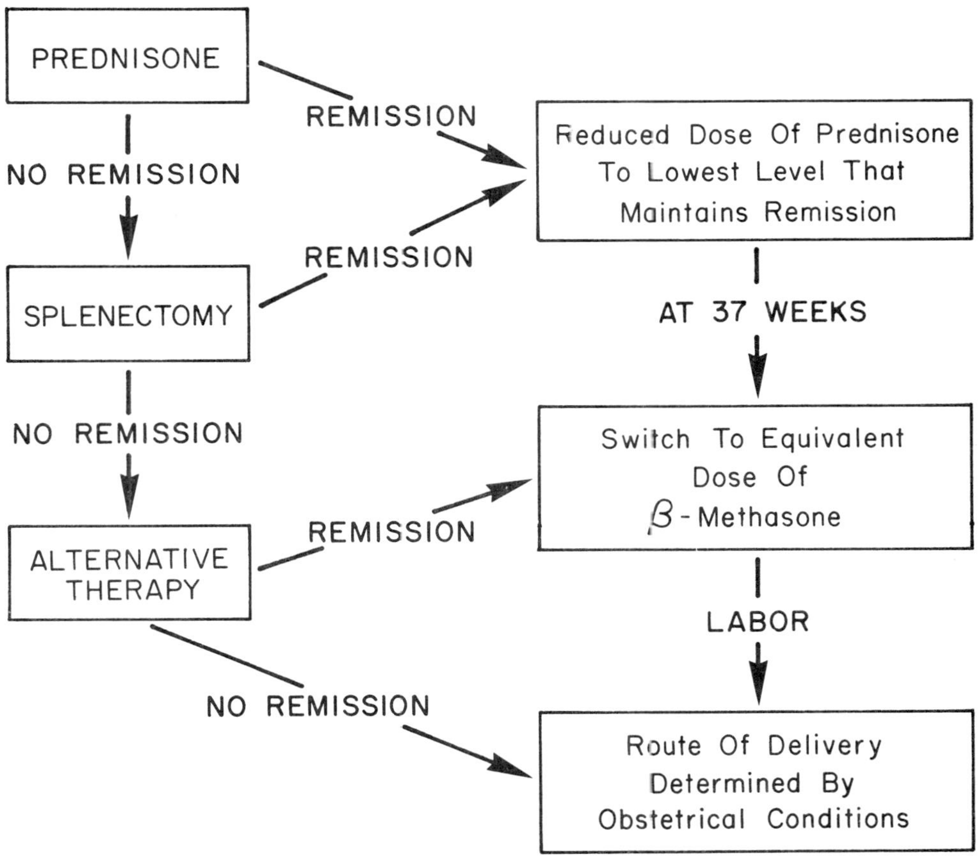

Figure 10–3. Schema for the management of immune thrombocytopenic purpura during pregnancy.

THROMBOTIC THROMBOCYTOPENIC PURPURA

Thrombotic thrombocytopenic purpura (TTP) was first described in 1924 by Moschkovitz as a syndrome characterized by a pentad of symptoms, including thrombocytopenia, microangiopathic hemolytic anemia, neurologic manifestations, renal failure, and fever. Until recently the outcome generally was fatal. However, advances in therapy have resulted in a marked improvement in survival.

PATHOPHYSIOLOGY

The pathophysiology of TTP is controversial and not well defined. A constant feature of the disease is platelet aggregates in small vessels. Whether these aggregates occur because of damage to the vessel wall or because of an intrinsic abnormality in platelet function is unclear. Factors proposed as contributory to the pathophysiology include (1) direct damage to the vessel wall by a virus or the deposition of immune complex, (2) decreased plasmogen activator in the vessel wall, (3) the presence of an abnormal plasma factor that initiates platelet aggregation, (4) the deficiency of a normally present plasma factor that inhibits platelet aggregation, (5) decreased circulating PGI_2 activity or a stimulator of such activity, and (6) the presence of a plasma factor that inhibits PGI_2 activity.[72–74] Although some data have been presented to support each of these factors, it is far from clear what if any role each plays in the pathophysiology of TTP.

SIGNS AND SYMPTOMS

There is a striking female preponderance in all but the first decade of life, with women accounting for over 70% of cases. More than 50 cases have now been reported during pregnancy or the puerperium.[75–78] The onset of symptoms is abrupt, with more than one half of patients presenting with neurologic manifestations. The most common neurologic symptoms are changes in mental status, paresis, paresthesias, headache, aphasia, seizures, dysarthria, visual changes, and coma. Malaise, weakness, fatigue, and abdominal pain are also present in one quarter of patients. Fever, nausea, vomiting, headache, jaundice, and pallor occur at some time during the course of illness in most patients but are not usually presenting signs and symptoms.

LABORATORY DIAGNOSIS

The characteristic findings in TTP include thrombocytopenia, a low hematocrit reading, reticulocytosis, and a normal PT and aPTT. The peripheral smear shows microangiopathic changes, including fragmented cells, nucleated RBCs, and polychromasia. The serum bilirubin and lactate dehydrogenase values are almost always elevated, and hematuria and proteinuria occur in the majority of cases. Some patients have slight elevations in the level of FDPs. The serum creatinine level is variably elevated, depending on the degree of renal dysfunction.

Pathologic findings are distinctive and consist of occlusive hyaline thrombi composed primarily of platelets filling the lumina of capillaries and small arterioles. Overt evidence of vasculitis is usually absent. These findings are present in the bone marrow in 50% of cases and in gingival biopsy material in similar frequency.

TREATMENT

The most effective therapeutic agents appear to be (1) plasma, (2) vincristine, (3) corticosteroids, and (4) oral antiplatelet agents.[75–82] Therapy should be sequential and if response is not achieved with the preceding, splenectomy and PGI_2 infusion should be tried. Ten to 20 U of plasma should be infused as rapidly as the patient's cardiovascular status can tolerate. Alternatively, plasma exchange can be carried out and should be a 1.0 to 1.5 volume exchange with fresh frozen plasma (85 to 90%) and 5% albumin (10 to 15%).[75] During pregnancy, the second modality of treatment should be high dose cortocosteroids followed by aspirin (600 mg every 12 hours) and dipyridamole (200 mg every 12 hours). Vincristine is then added if these agents fail to achieve a remission. The dosages for both corticosteroids and vincristine are the same as discussed earlier in the treatment of ITP.

HEMOLYTIC-UREMIC SYNDROME

The hemolytic-uremic syndrome (HUS) shares many of the clinical and laboratory features of TTP.[72, 73] However, it occurs primarily in children and produces a paucity of neurologic symptoms and a far greater degree of renal dysfunction. Table 10–5 contrasts the clinical and laboratory findings in TTP, HUS, DIC, and pre-eclampsia-eclampsia. Management remains controversial; however, there is general agreement that dialysis is indicated. A sequential approach identical to that described for TTP should be used. Unfortunately, data supporting efficacy are largely lacking.

OTHER DISORDERS

ISOIMMUNE NEONATAL THROMBOCYTOPENIA

Isoimmune neonatal thrombocytopenia (INT) is analogous to Rh disease in that it occurs when a mother who lacks a specific platelet antigen carries a fetus who has inherited that paternal antigen. The Pl^{A1} platelet antigen is present on the platelets of all but 2 to 3% of individuals and is usually responsible for sensitization.[83] Several other antigens, including Pl^{E2}, Bak^a, and HLA antigens, also can be involved. The alloantibodies are IgG and mostly of the IgG1 subclass. This disorder differs strikingly from Rh disease in that it occurs in the first pregnancy in almost one half of the reported cases.

An affected newborn is usually the product of an uncomplicated pregnancy and shows no evidence of hemorrhage at birth. However, within several hours the platelet count begins to drop, and clinical evidence in the form of petechiae and ecchymoses

Table 10–5. Clinical and Laboratory Findings in Thrombotic Thrombocytopenic Purpura (TTP), Hemolytic-Uremic Syndrome (HUS), Disseminated Intravascular Coagulation (DIC), and Pre-eclampsia/Eclampsia (PE/E)

	Disease			
Findings*	**TTP**	**HUS**	**DIC**	**PE/E**
Neurologic findings	+	±	±	±
Fever	+	±	±	−
Hypertension	±	+	±	+
Renal dysfunction	±	+	±	+
Thrombocytopenia	+	+	+	±
Hemolytic anemia	+	+	±	±
Elevated plasma FDPs	±	±	+	±
Low plasma fibrinogen	−	−	+	±

* (+) usually present; (±) variably present; (−) absent.

begins to appear. Serous bleeding can occur, and the neonatal mortality rate has been reported as high as 15% with intracranial hemorrhage being the most common cause of death.

In addition to neonatal thrombocytopenia, both direct and indirect PA-IgG can be demonstrated in the newborn's blood and indirect PA-IgG in the maternal blood.[84] Therapy consists of corticosteroids, platelet transfusions, and exchange transfusion.[84–86] The ideal platelet donor is the mother herself. In mothers who have delivered one infant with INT, there is a dual problem of determining whether or not the fetus is at risk in a subsequent pregnancy and choosing the best route of delivery, as in cases of ITP. Kelton and colleagues have presented some data suggesting the value of PA-IgG studies.[84] While some authors[85, 86] have advocated elective cesarean section to avoid the cranial trauma associated with vaginal delivery, there are again no data to support this recommendation, and we prefer vaginal delivery unless there is an obstetric indication for cesarean section.

LIVER DISEASE

Both severe, acute hepatitis and cirrhosis can be accompanied by severe hemorrhagic manifestations. Platelets, plasma factors, and circulating FDPs all can be affected.[87–89] A careful screening of the coagulation system should be done and should include a platelet count, PT, aPTT, plasma fibrinogen, and some measure of plasma FDPs.

Treatment consists of both vitamin K administration and procoagulant replacement therapy. Vitamin K can be administered as vitamin K_1 in a dose of 50 mg intramuscularly and will produce improvement in approximately 30% of patients with liver disease. Replacement therapy is accomplished with fresh frozen plasma in a dose of 10 to 20 ml/kg.

REFERENCES

1. Deykin, D.: The clinical challenge of disseminated intravascular coagulation. N Engl J Med *283*:636, 1970.
2. Ockelford, P.A., and Carter, C.J.: Disseminated intravascular coagulation: The application and utility of diagnostic tests. Semin Thromb Hemost *8*:198, 1982.
3. Feinstein, D.I.: Diagnosis and management of disseminated intravascular coagulation: The role of heparin therapy. Blood *60*:284, 1982.
4. Sutton, D.M.C., Hauser, R., Kulaping, S., et al.: Intravascular coagulation in abruptio placentae. Am J Obstet Gynecol *109*:604, 1971.
5. Phillips, L.L., Skrodelis, V., and Kers, T.A.: Hypofibrinogenemia and intrauterine fetal death. Am J Obstet Gynecol *89*:907, 1964.
6. Jimenez, J.M., and Pritchard, J.A.: Pathogenesis and treatment of coagulation defects resulting from fetal death. Obstet Gynecol *32*:449, 1968.
7. Romero, R., Duffy, T.P., Berkowitz, R.L., et al.: Prolongation of a preterm pregnancy complicated by death of a single twin in utero and disseminated intravascular coagulation. N Engl J Med *310*:772, 1984.
8. Phillips, L.L., and Davidson, E.C.: Procoagulant properties of amniotic fluid. Am J Obstet Gynecol *113*:911, 1972.
9. Phillips, L.L., Skrodilis V., and Quigley, H.J.: Intravascular coagulation in septic abortion. Obstet Gynecol *30*:350, 1967.
10. Laros, R.K., Penner, J.A., Collins, J., et al.: Coagulation changes in saline induced abortion. Am J Obstet Gynecol *116*:277, 1973.
11. Davidson, E.C., and Phillips, L.L.: Coagulation changes in hypertensive toxemias of pregnancy. Am J Obstet Gynecol *113*:905, 1972.
12. Courtney, L.D., Boxall, R.R., and Child, P.: Permeability of membranes of the dead fetus. Br J Med *1*:492, 1971.
13. MacKay, D.: Hematologic evidence of disseminated intravascular coagulation in eclampsia. Obstet Gynecol Surv *27*:399, 1972.
14. Pritchard, J.A., Cunningham, F.G., and Mason, R.A.: Coagulation changes in eclampsia: Their frequency and pathogenesis. Am J Obstet Gynecol *124*:855, 1976.

15. Kitzmiller, J.L., Lang, J.E., Yelenosky, P.F., et al.: Hematologic assays in pre-eclampsia. Am J Obstet Gynecol *118*:362, 1974.
16. Starkie, C.M., Harding, L.K., Fletcher, D.J., et al.: Intravascular coagulation and abnormal lung scans in pre-eclampsia and eclampsia. Lancet *2*:889, 1971.
17. Scott, R., Gordon, S., Schatz, A., et al.: Acute hemolysis and thrombocytopenia in eclampsia. Obstet Gynecol *36*:128, 1970.
18. Killam, A.P., Dillard, S.H., Patton, R.C., et al.: Pregnancy-induced hypertension complicated by acute liver disease and disseminated intravascular coagulation. Am J Obstet Gynecol *123*:823, 1975.
19. Weinstein, L.: Syndrome of hemolysis, elevated liver enzymes, and low platelet count: A severe consequence of hypertension in pregnancy. Am J Obstet Gynecol *142*:159, 1982.
20. Thiagarajah, S., Bourgeois, F.J., Habert, G.M., et al.: Thrombocytopenia in pre-eclampsia: Associated abnormalities and management principles. Obstet Gynecol *150*:1, 1984.
21. Whigham, K.A.E., Howie, P.W., Drummond, A.H., et al.: Abnormal platelet function in pre-eclampsia. Br J Obstet Gynaecol *85*:28, 1978.
22. Peterson, E.P., and Taylor, H.B.: Amniotic fluid embolism. Obstet Gynecol *35*:787, 1970.
23. Talbert, L.M., Adcock, D.F., Weiss, A.E., et al.: Studies on the pathogenesis of clotting defects during salt-induced abortions. Am J Obstet Gynecol *115*:656, 1973.
24. Laros, R.K., and Penner, J.A.: Pathophysiology of disseminated intravascular coagulation in saline-induced abortion. Obstet Gynecol *48*:353, 1976.
25. Spicer, T.E., and Tan, J.M.: Purpura Fulminans. Am J Med *61*:566, 1976.
26. Mant, M.J., and Kink, E.G.: Severe acute disseminated intravascular coagulation. A reappraisal of its pathophysiology, clinical significance and therapy based on 47 patients. Am J Med *67*:557, 1979.
27. Thragarajah, S., Wheby, M.S., Jarn, R., et al.: Disseminated intravascular coagulation in pregnancy. The role of heparin. J Reprod Med *25*:17, 1981.
28. Gallup, D.G., and Lucas, W.E.: Heparin treatment of consumption coagulopathy associated with intrauterine fetal death. Obstet Gynecol *22*:889, 1970.
29. Howie, P.W., Prentice, C.R.M., and Forbes, C.D.: Failure of heparin therapy to affect the clinical course of severe pre-eclampsia. Br J Obstet Gynaecol *82*:711, 1975.
30. Harrington, W.J., Minnich, V., and Arimura, G.: The autoimmune thrombocytopenia. Prog Hematol *1*:166, 1956.
31. Harrington, W.J., Minnich, V., Hollingsworth, J.W., et al.: Demonstration of a thrombocytopenic factor in the blood of patients with thrombocytopenic purpura: J Lab Clin Med *9*:44, 1950.
32. Shulman, N.R., Marder, V.J., and Weinrach, R.S.: Similarities between known antiplatelet antibodies and the factor responsible for thrombocytopenia in idiopathic thrcmboctopenic purpura: Physiologic, serologic and isotopic studies. Ann NY Acad Sci *124*:499, 1965.
33. Karpatkin, S.: Autoimmune thrombocytopenic purpura. Blood *56* 329, 1980.
34. Kagan, R., and Laros, R.K.: Immune thrombocytopenia. Clin Obstet Gynecol *26*:537, 1983.
35. McMillan, R.: Chronic idiopathic thrombocytopenic purpura. N Engl J Med *304*:1135, 1981.
36. Hauch, T.W., and Rosse, W.F.: Platelet-bound complement (C_3) in immune thrombocytopenia. Blood *50*:1129, 1977.
37. Cines, D.B., and Schreiber, A.D.: Immune thrombocytopenia: Use of a Coombs' antiglobulin test to detect IgG and C_3 on platelets. N Engl J Med *300*:106, 1979.
38. Dixon, R., Rosse, W., and Ebbert, L.: Quantitative determination of antibody in idiopathic thrombocytopenic purpura: Correlation of serum and platelet-bound antibody with clinical response. N Engl J Med *292*:230, 1975.
39. Myers, T.J., Kim, R., Syeiner, M., et al.: Platelet associated complement C_3 in immune thrombocytopenic purpura. Blood *59*:1023, 1980.
40. Cines, D., Dussk, B., Tomaski, A., et al.: Immune thrombocytopenic purpura and pregnancy. N Engl J Med *306*:826, 1982.
41. Baldini, M.: Idiopathic thrombocytopenic purpura. N Engl J Med *274*:1245, 1966.
42. Baldini, M.: Idiopathic thrombocytopenic purpura and the ITP syndrome. Med Clin North Am *56*:47, 1972.
43. Ahn, Y.S., and Harrington, W.J.: Treatment of idiopathic thrombocytopenic purpura (ITP). Annu Rev Med *28*:299, 1977.
44. Pizzuto, J., and Ambriz, R.: Therapeutic experience of 934 adults with idiopathic thrombocytopenic purpura: Multicentric trial of the cooperative Latin America Group on Hemostasis and Thrombosis. Blood *64*:1179, 1984.
45. Cervantes, F., Monserrat, E., Rozman, C., et al.: Low dose vincristine in the treatment of corticosteroid-refractory immune thrombocytopenic purpura in non-splenectomized patients. Postgrad Med *56*:711, 1980.
46. Ahn, Y.S., Harrington, W.J., Simon, S.R., et al.: Danazol for the treatment of idiopathic thrombocytopenic purpura. N Engl J Med *308*:1396, 1983.
47. Fehr, J., Hofmann, V., and Kappeler, U.: Transient reversal of thrombocytopenia in idiopathic thrombocytopenic purpura by high-dose intravenous gamma globulin. N Engl J Med *306*:1245, 1982.

48. Bussel, J.B., Kimberly, R.P., Inman, R.D., et al.: Intravenous gamma globulin treatment of chronic idiopathic thrombocytopenic purpura. Blood *62*:480, 1983.
49. Carrol, R.R., Noyes, W.D., and Kitchen, C.S.: High-dose intravenous immunoglobulin therapy in patients with immune thrombocytopenic purpura. JAMA *249*:1748, 1983.
50. Tchernia, G., Dreyfus, M., Laurian, Y., et al.: Management of immune thrombocytopenia in pregnancy: Response to infusion of immunoglobulins. Am J Obstet Gynecol *148*:225, 1984.
51. Adderley, R.J., Rogers, P.C.J., Shaw, D., et al.: High-dose intravenous therapy with immune globulin before delivery for idiopathic thrombocytopenic purpura. Can Med Assoc J *130*:894, 1984.
52. Mizunuma, H., Taguchi, H., Morita, K., et al.: A new approach to idiopathic thrombocytopenic purpura during pregnancy by high-dose immunoglobulin G infusion. Am J Obstet Gynecol *148*:218, 1984.
53. Kohler, P.F., and Farr, R.S.: Elevation of cord maternal IgG immunoglobulins: Evidence for an active placental IgG transport. Nature *210*:1070, 1966.
54. Kernoff, L., Malan, E., and Gunston, K.: Neonatal thrombocytopenia complicating autoimmune thrombocytopenia in pregnancy. Ann Intern Med *90*:55, 1979.
55. Territo, M., Finklestein, J., Oh W., et al.: Management of autoimmune thrombocytopenia in pregnancy and in the neonate. Obstet Gynecol *41*:579, 1973.
56. Noriega-Guerra L., Aviles-Miranda, A., de la Cadena, O.A., et al.: Pregnancy in patients with autoimmune thrombocytopenic purpura. Am J Obstet Gynecol *133*:439, 1979.
57. Tancer, M.L.: Idiopathic thrombocytopenic purpura and pregnancy. Am J Obstet Gynecol *79*:148, 1960.
58. Jones, W.: Tissue specific autoimmune disease in pregnancy. Clin Obstet Gynecol *6*:473, 1979.
59. Laros, R.K., and Sweet, R.L.: Management of idiopathic thrombocytopenic purpura during pregnancy. Am J Obstet Gynecol *122*:182, 1975.
60. Laros, R.K., and Kagan, R.: Route of delivery for patients with immune thrombocytopenic purpura. Am J Obstet Gynecol *148*:901, 1984.
61. O'Reilly, R.A., and Taber, B.Z.: Immunologic thrombocytopenic purpura and pregnancy: Six new cases. Obstet Gynecol *51*:590, 1978.
62. Zilliacus, H.: Thrombocytopenia in pregnancy. Clin Obstet Gynecol *2*:404, 1964.
63. Murray, J.M., and Harris, R.E.: The management of the pregnant patient with idiopathic thrombocytopenic purpura. Am J Obstet Gynecol *126*:449, 1976.
64. Carloss, H.W., McMillan, R., and Crosby, W.H.: Management of pregnancy in women with immune thrombocytopenic purpura. JAMA *244*:2756, 1980.
65. McMillan, R.: Chronic idiopathic thrombocytopenic purpura. N Engl J Med *304*:1135, 1981.
66. Goodhue, P.A., and Evans, T.S.: Idiopathic thrombocytopenic purpura during pregnancy. Obstet Gynecol *18*:671, 1963.
67. Jones, R.W., Asher, M.I., Rutherford, C.J., et al.: Autoimmune (idiopathic) thrombocytopenic purpura in pregnancy and the newborn. Br J Obstet Gynaecol *84*:679, 1977.
68. Scott, J.R., Cruikshank, D.P., Kochenour, N.K., et al.: Fetal platelet counts in the obstetric management of immunologic thrombocytopenic purpura. Am J Obstet Gynecol *136*:495, 1980.
69. Karpatkin, M., Porges, R., and Karpatkin, S.: Platelet counts in infants of women with autoimmune thrombocytopenia. N Engl J Med *305*:936, 1981.
70. Kelton, J.C., Inwood, M.J., Barr, R.M., et al.: The prenatal prediction of thrombocytopenia in infants of mothers with clinically diagnosed immune thrombocytopenia. Am J Obstet Gynecol *144*:449, 1982.
71. Ayromlooi J.: A new approach to the management of immunologic thrombocytopenic purpura in pregnancy. Am J Obstet Gynecol *130*:235, 1978.
72. Kwaan, H.C. (ed): Management of thrombotic thrombocytopenic purpura. Semin Thromb Hemost *7*:1, 1981.
73. Kwaan, H.C. (ed): Thrombotic thrombocytopenic purpura. Semin Thromb Hemost *6*:328, 1980.
74. Moake, J.L., Rudy, C.K., Troll, J.H., et al.: Unusually large plasma factor VIII: von Willebrand factor multimers in chronic relapsing thrombotic thrombocytopenic purpura. N Engl J Med *307*:1432, 1982.
75. Caggiano, V., Fernando, L.P., Schneider, J.M., et al.: Thrombotic thrombocytopenic purpura: Report of fourteen cases—occurrence during pregnancy and response to plasma exchange. J Clin Apher *1*:71, 1983.
76. Davies, G.: Thrombotic thrombocytopenic purpura in pregnancy with maternal survival. Br J Obstet Gynaecol *91*:396, 1984.
77. Vanderckhove, F., Noens, L., Cloardyn, F., et al.: Thrombotic thrombocytopenic purpura mimicking toxemia of pregnancy. Am J Obstet Gynecol *150*:320, 1984.
78. Blakowski, S.A., Zacharski, L.R., Telfer, M.C., et al.: Pregnancy complicated by thrombotic thrombocytopenic purpura with fetal sparing. Arch Intern Med *143*:2207, 1983.
79. Byrnes, J.J., and Khurana, M.: Treatment of thrombotic thrombocytopenic purpura with plasma. N Engl J Med *297*:1386, 1977.
80. Gutterman, L.A., and Stevenson, T.D.: Treatment of thrombotic thrombocytopenic purpura with vincristine. JAMA *247*:1433, 1982.

81. Evans, T.L., Winkelstein, A., Zeigler, Z.R., et al.: Thrombotic thrombocytopenic purpura. Am J Hematol *17*:401, 1984.
82. Crain, S.M., and Choudury, A.M.: Thrombotic thrombocytopenic purpura—a reappraisal. JAMA *246*:1243, 1981.
83. Von dem Borne, A.E.G.K., van Leeuwen, E.F., von Riesz, L.E., et al.: Neonatal alloimmune thrombocytopenia: Detection and characterization of the responsible antibodies by the platelet immunofluorescent test. Blood *57*:649, 1981.
84. Kelton, J.G., Blanchette, V.S., Wilson, W.E., et al.: Neonatal thrombocytopenia due to passive immunization. N Engl J Med *302*:1401, 1980.
85. Sitarz, A.L., Driscoll, J.M., and Wolff, J.A.: Management of isoimmune neonatal thrombocytopenia. Am J Obstet Gynecol *124*:39, 1976.
86. Pochedly, C., Merson, E.J., and Fotino, M.: Isoimmune neonatal purpura. J Reprod Med *6*:212, 1970.
87. Roberts, H.R., and Cederbaum, A.I.: The liver and blood coagulation: Physiology and pathology. Gastroenterology *63*:297, 1972.
88. Straub, P.W.: Diffuse intravascular coagulation in liver disease. Semin Thromb Hemost *4*:29, 1977.
89. Palascak, J.E., and Martinez, J.: Dysfibrinogenemia associated with liver disease. J Clin Invest *60*:89, 1977.

Chapter 11
TRANSFUSION THERAPY

Harold A. Oberman

Blood transfusion had its origins in the 17th century, coincident with the description of the circulation of blood by William Harvey. However, such early efforts uniformly consisted of transfusion of animal blood. Samuel Pepys, in his diary, described transfusion of blood from a dog, while other early transfusions utilized lamb's blood. As would be expected, there was considerable risk to the blood recipient in such situations, and a hemolytic reaction following a transfusion in Paris caused the practice to fall into disrepute by the latter part of that century.[1] Transfusion of human blood did not take place until early in the 19th century when an obstetrician, James Blundell, conceived of it as rational treatment for postpartum hemorrhage. British obstetricians played a leadership role in the resurgence of interest in this therapeutic technique and performed most of the transfusions in the first half of that century.

Therefore it is appropriate from a historical standpoint and because obstetricians frequently use the blood bank that a discussion of blood transfusion practices be included in this text. Blood bank support plays an important role in many aspects of obstetric care. Not only are blood transfusions of obvious significance in operative obstetrics but also the serologic studies performed in a blood bank are necessary for proper management of the antepartum and postpartum patient at risk of having an infant with hemolytic disease.

The following discussion elaborates the role of the blood bank in current obstetric practice. A survey of pretransfusion and antenatal serologic testing sets the framework for discussions of the use of blood components, transfusion of massive amounts of blood, and adverse reactions to transfusion.

PRETRANSFUSION AND ANTENATAL SEROLOGIC TESTING; RED CELL TYPING; SCREENING FOR UNEXPECTED ANTIBODIES

Blood transfusion is associated with many possible adverse consequences. Most feared is the hemolytic transfusion reaction, and most such fatal reactions are related to ABO incompatibility. Therefore, accurate determination of the ABO type of the patient and the donor is of critical importance. Sensitization of the blood recipient is a second concern, as it can lead to subsequent transfusion reactions, result in difficulty in providing blood for transfusion, or provide the setting for subsequent hemolytic disease of the newborn. Because of its immunogenicity, particular care must be taken in typing both donor and recipient blood for the D antigen. Serologic testing of the patient's red cells for other Rh antigens or for antigens such as Kell or Duffy is not routinely performed both because of their antigenicity and because of their relatively frequent occurrence in the patient and donor populations.

All donated units of blood are typed for ABO and $Rh_o(D)$. A pilot tube or segment of donor's blood, filled during the donation procedure, is used for testing, thereby assuring the constancy of identity of the specimen. Red cells from the segment are tested against known reagent antibody to define the ABO type, and a sample of serum from the pilot tube is reacted against red cells of known ABO type, thereby constituting a confirmatory test. Similarly, testing for the D antigen is performed with appropriate controls. Units of blood found negative for the D antigen are considered Rh negative. It must be appreciated that an Rh-negative unit of blood may test positively for C or E antigens.

Weak expressions of the D antigen, considered D variants, are designated D^u. Red cells with such weak expressions of the D antigen are not agglutinated by appropriate antiserum unless antiglobulin reagent is added to the reaction mixture. Such units of blood are considered Rh-positive and may result in sensitization of an Rh-negative patient. However, there is little risk of patients with this blood type forming anti-D through exposure to the D antigen by transfusion or pregnancy.

Recipient blood also is tested for ABO and Rh, using confirmatory techniques. As with donor blood, designation of Rh-positive is based upon the reaction of the red cells with anti-D typing serum. This determines whether the recipient should receive Rh-positive or Rh-negative blood. In contrast to testing of donor blood, testing for D^u is not performed when testing recipient red cells.

Both donor and recipient blood are "screened" for unexpected antibodies, i.e., antibodies to antigens other than ABO. These antibodies are considered "naturally occurring" in patients' or donors' blood. Antibody screening is performed by reacting the serum with red cells of known antigen specificities. In most instances such red cells are commercially provided, and test cells contain antigenic specificities corresponding to clinically significant antibodies. Such testing is more important when testing recipient blood than donor blood, because the presence of such an antibody in the patient may result in lysis of transfused red cells when the corresponding antigen is present on the transfused red cells. In contrast, the presence of antibodies in donor blood is of much less concern because of their dilution after transfusion.

When the findings of the screening test for unexpected antibodies are positive, it is necessary to define the cause. This involves identification of the antibody by mixing the suspect serum with a panel of reagent red cells that contain a varying distribution of antigenic specificities. Through the process of elimination, recognizing which cells react with the serum, and using the optimum temperature and medium for reactions, the antibody specificity can be defined. Subsequent red blood cell transfusions must then lack the corresponding antigen. Depending upon the characteristics of the antibody and the possible presence of mixtures of antibodies, such identification procedures require time intervals varying from one to many hours.

The frequency of occurrence of a positive screening test for unexpected antibodies depends upon the patient population. A patient who has had the opportunity for sensitization is far more likely to have these antibodies than is a patient who has never been pregnant or transfused. At one time, group O, Rh-negative blood was considered universal donor. This is an improper assumption because such units may contain antigenic specificities other than ABO or Rh that may be incompatible with antibodies in the patient's serum.

Because of the antigenic profile of the red cells used in the screening procedure in contrast to the unpredictable antigenic profile of donor red cells used in the crossmatch test, the screening test is more likely to detect clinically significant antibodies that may interfere with transfusion. In contrast to the crossmatch, the screening test for unexpected antibodies may be performed well in advance of the transfusion. This facilitates provision of compatible blood for a subsequent operation, since crossmatch tests performed for additional units of blood unexpectedly required in the course of an operation for a patient with a nonreactive pretransfusion screening test are more likely to prove compatible.

THE CROSSMATCH

The final test performed before transfusion of blood is the crossmatch. It serves as a final check on ABO compatibility and may also detect unexpected antibodies in recipient serum that were not recognized by the pretransfusion antibody screening test.

At one time both major and minor crossmatch tests were performed. In the major crossmatch the patient's serum and the donor's red cells are mixed to determine the presence of agglutination or lysis. In contrast, the minor crossmatch procedure is a mixture of the donor's serum and the patient's red cells. Over the past 25 years it has become evident that the minor crossmatch is unnecessary.[2] Transfusion reactions related to antibodies in the donor unit are rarely of clinical significance. The frequency of "minor side" reactions has been further reduced by the increased tendency to transfuse red blood cells rather than whole blood.

At the present time only a test between the patient's serum and red cells from the transfused unit is performed. This test is performed at 37°C, thereby recognizing clinically significant antibodies. In most instances the crossmatch procedure is augmented by use of potentiating solutions such as albumin or low ionic strength saline. The mixture is incubated for at least 10 minutes and antihuman globulin serum is added before interpretation. Recently there has been interest in abbreviating the procedure.[3] Such a proposed modification would eliminate incubation at 37°C and also would not include the antiglobulin phase of the reaction. While an occasional unexpected antibody may be overlooked by such testing, it would confirm ABO compatibility, the most important function of the crossmatch.

Provided that ABO typing has been accurately performed and that the pretransfusion screening test for unexpected antibodies is nonreactive, the major crossmatch usually will prove compatible. On rare occasions (approximately 0.03%) a clinically significant antigen will be evident solely with the crossmatch.[3] This may be related to improper performance of the screening test for unexpected antibodies, a dosage effect manifested by the antibody wherein the screening cells lack homozygous antigenic representation, or laboratory error in the interpretation of the pretransfusion screening test. Nevertheless, the most important reason for performance of the crossmatch is the verification of ABO compatibility. It must be recognized that the most common cause of severe hemolytic transfusion reactions is ABO incompatibility, and this is usually the result of human error. This may occur when the recipient's blood sample is collected, during processing in the blood bank, or at the time of the transfusion. Therefore, compulsive adherence to procedure is necessary at all steps.

PRENATAL TESTING

Serologic testing is performed during the antenatal period for two reasons. (1) Detection of the antibodies in the maternal serum is necessary for the diagnosis of possible hemolytic disease of the newborn in the fetus. (2) Furthermore, determination of the ABO and Rh types, as well as detection of unexpected antibodies in the maternal serum, is necessary for meeting possible postpartum transfusion requirements. Postpartum verification of Rh type is necessary to assure proper administration of Rh immune globulin.

Determination of the ABO and Rh types, as well as performance of a screening test for unexpected antibodies, should be carried out during the first trimester of pregnancy. Testing is comparable to that described for prospective transfusion recipients. A positive result of the screening test for unexpected antibodies must occasion additional testing to identify the antibody. The clinical significance of such antibodies must be taken into consideration in terms of subsequent management of the patient. For example, many antibodies are not known to cause hemolytic disease of the newborn in the fetus, whereas others may result in red cell coating by antibody but no clinically evident disease.

If no unexpected antibodies are detected during the first trimester, especially if the patient is Rh_o(D)-negative, testing should be repeated during the third trimester. The later test may reveal sensitization, reflecting either primary sensitization caused by small intrapartum fetal-maternal hemorrhage or possibly an anamnestic response of an antibody whose titer was too low for detection earlier in pregnancy. Since antenatal serologic testing is often performed in laboratories unrelated to the hospital where delivery will occur, it is important that ABO and Rh typing and screening for unexpected antibodies be repeated during the admission for delivery. It is important to appreciate that anti-D detected at this time may reflect sensitization or passive administration of antibody during the third trimester of pregnancy.

While it may not be necessary to crossmatch blood for the delivery, such testing is a logical precaution to facilitate blood transfusion in case unexpected hemorrhage occurs. In many institutions an emergency supply of O, Rh-negative red blood cells is maintained in or near the delivery unit for patients who may have unexpected postpartum hemorrhage. It is always preferable to provide the patient with type-specific blood rather than to rely on O, Rh-negative red blood cells. If it is necessary to transfuse the patient with O, Rh-negative red blood cells in an emergency, the blood bank should determine the patient's ABO and Rh type and provide antigen-negative, crossmatch-compatible blood as soon as possible.

Clinically significant antibodies identified during the antenatal period should be titered. As discussed in Chapter 7, this information may augment the findings from spectrophotometric examination of the amniotic fluid in predicting hemolytic disease of the newborn. It is important that samples of serum be frozen and preserved for parallel tests with subsequent serum samples later in the pregnancy. Without such comparative samples the accuracy of changes in titer is questionable.

Rh_o(D) IMMUNE GLOBULIN (RhIG)

Rh_o(D)-negative patients who lack anti-D in their serum must receive RhIG in proximity to fetal-maternal hemorrhage to forestall primary sensitization. In most instances the preparation is given within 72 hours after abortion or delivery. It may also be administered in other potentially sensitizing situations, such as amniocentesis, transfusion of red cell–containing blood products, or during the third trimester of pregnancy. The last usually implies administration of the product at or around the

28th week of pregnancy. Patients who receive antenatal RhIG also must receive the postpartum treatment.

The standard dose of RhIG contains 300 μg of anti-D. This will neutralize approximately 15 to 17 ml of D-positive red cells. A test must be performed to determine the presence of a larger fetomaternal hemorrhage that would necessitate a higher dose of RhIG. In contrast, the small fetomaternal hemorrhage that may be associated with a first trimester abortion can be treated with a 50 μg dose of RhIG.

It is essential that the Rh type of all women who are pregnant, have recently delivered, or who have recently had an abortion be determined so as to ensure that all eligible patients receive this product. While an erroneous designation of an Rh-negative patient as Rh-positive is quite serious in that such a patient might not receive RhIG, there is little evidence of harm from administration of RhIG to an Rh-positive patient. Therefore, the need for typing at the time of delivery, especially confirmatory typing, is most important for patients who were previously typed as Rh-positive. It also must be recognized that, in the event of a large fetal-maternal hemorrhage from an Rh-positive fetus, there may be sufficient numbers of Rh-positive red cells in the maternal circulation to result in an improper designation of the patient as Rh-positive. Since it is unnecessary to administer RhIG to patients previously sensitized to the D antigen, tests for anti-D should be performed on a serum sample obtained at the time of delivery or abortion from all Rh-negative women or women whose Rh type is unknown.

Patients who receive RhIG during the third trimester of pregnancy may manifest reactive screening tests for unexpected antibodies because of the passively administered anti-D, but they must also receive the usual postpartum dose. If the delivering hospital is not alerted to this situation, it is possible that the detection of anti-D at the time of delivery may result in the patient's not being considered a candidate for the additional RhIG. It is a good idea to provide a patient with a card indicating that she has received this product, whether ante partum or post partum. It is not possible to determine whether or not primary immunization has occurred following delivery until the passively administered anti-D is no longer detectable. Anti-D detected six months post partum may be assumed to be present on the basis of primary immunization. Attempts to determine the presence of primary sensitization at an earlier time are inappropriate.

TRANSFUSION OF BLOOD COMPONENTS AND DERIVATIVES

The major change in the practice of blood transfusion over the past two decades has been the advent of blood component therapy. This allows transfusion of the specific component required by the patient rather than the use of whole blood. In most instances, patients require replacement of only a specific fraction of whole blood, thereby permitting a single blood donation to serve the needs of more than one patient. A single unit of whole blood, consisting of approximately 500 ml of blood and anticoagulant, can provide red cells for the anemic patient, platelet concentrates for the thrombocytopenic patient, cryoprecipitated factor VIII for the hemophiliac, and plasma as a volume expander for the hypovolemic patient. Moreover, further processing of the plasma on a commercial basis can yield human serum albumin, clotting factor concentrates, or immune serum globulin. Therefore, transfusion therapy has become focused and, at the same time, safer and more efficient.

Plasmapheresis has greatly expanded the ability to collect large volumes of plasma for use either as components or for subsequent processing. This procedure involves collection of a unit of blood, centrifugation, return of the red cells to the donor, and harvesting of the plasma. Whereas the blood donor can donate whole blood or red blood cells only five times per year, with plasmapheresis a donor may provide up to a liter of plasma every week. This is based upon the greater rapidity of replacement of serum proteins than red cells in the circulation.

CELLULAR COMPONENTS

WHOLE BLOOD

Although not a component, it is important that we review some aspects of whole blood, which serves as the basis for all blood component preparation. It represents the initial product collected, whether for unmodified use in subsequent transfusion or as the "raw material" for further component preparation. Blood is collected in an anticoagulant solution (currently CPDA-1) that allows it to be stored for 35 days when refrigerated at 1° to 6°C. This storage interval is based upon a minimum 24-hour post-transfusion survival of 70% of the transfused red cells. However, the quantitative survival of the transfused red cells does not necessarily reflect their functional integrity.

Red cells are transfused to enhance the oxygen-carrying capacity of the patient, and this is best reflected by levels of intracellular 2,3-diphosphoglycerate (2,3-DPG). Although 2,3-DPG is depleted in storage, it is rapidly reconstituted after transfusion. When 2,3-DPG is depleted in blood, there is increased affinity of hemoglobin for oxygen, thereby compromising the ability of the red cell to deliver oxygen to tissues. Levels of 2,3-DPG remain relatively normal for the first seven to ten days of storage and then decrease during the remainder of the storage interval. However, transfusion of 2,3-DPG–depleted red cells is followed by a rapid return to nearly normal intracellular levels. Approximately half of the 2,3-DPG is reconstituted within four hours, and normal levels are restored within 24 hours.[4] In most instances this transient in vitro lesion is of no consequence.

There are many other alterations in blood during storage.[5] For example, the platelets in whole blood become rapidly depleted. Therefore, whole blood, regardless of its age, is not an adequate source of platelets. The changes in blood during storage are termed "the storage lesion," yet they usually are of little consequence for the recipient. Among these changes are increases in plasma potassium, ammonia, and hemoglobin concentrations resulting from the movement of these constituents from an intracellular to an extracellular location. Leakage of potassium from red cells is related to thermal inhibition of membrane ATPase.[6] Similarly, as lactic acid increases from red cell metabolism, the pH of the blood falls to approximately 6.5 by 21 to 35 days. At that time plasma hemoglobin may be as high as 100 mg/ml. The labile plasma clotting factors, factors V and VIII, also become depleted quite rapidly in blood during storage. Both factors manifest a biphasic depletion curve, with loss of approximately 50% of activity during the first 24 to 48 hours of storage.

This raises the question of the appropriateness of transfusion of "fresh blood." It is doubtful that there are any clinical situations in which "fresh" whole blood is necessary.[7] The availability of specific blood components has obviated the need for this product. In most instances, requests for "fresh blood" reflect an uncertainty on the part of the physician as to the appropriate means of treating a bleeding patient. For example, if this request is prompted by a need for clotting factors that become depleted during storage of blood, these labile factors can best be replaced through specific component therapy. The electrolyte changes in blood during storage are of little consequence to most patients. At one time it was thought that patients undergoing cardiopulmonary bypass operations should receive freshly drawn blood. However, it has been demonstrated that this is unnecessary and that these patients can be managed satisfactorily with blood of any age. Two exceptions might pertain in this regard. Patients who require frequent transfusions for chronic anemia may realize a reduction in transfusion frequency if they receive blood less than 10 days old, since they are thereby receiving a greater percentage of viable red cells per transfusion. Similarly, the neonatal patient is best managed with blood less than one week old in order to avoid the transient electrolyte and pH changes that might occur with transfusion of older blood.

Which patients should receive whole blood? It is generally agreed that no more than 30% of collected blood should be in the form of whole blood. In most hospitals red cells for transfusion are provided in the form of red blood cells ("packed cells"). In our institution, whole blood is reserved for patients who have experienced an acute blood loss of at least 1000 ml. The first two units of blood provided for all adult patients undergoing operative procedures is in the form of red blood cells, and subsequent transfusions may be provided as whole blood.

RED BLOOD CELLS

Most patients requiring replacement of red cells should receive this component. The various blood components available are summarized in Table 11–1. Red blood cells are prepared through either centrifugation or sedimentation of whole blood, resulting in a product with a maximum hematocrit value of 80%. Like whole blood, its shelf life is 35 days. The product can be prepared either at the time of donation or the time of transfusion. It must be appreciated that the "storage lesion" of the red cells referred to earlier is also manifested in this product. When the component is prepared at the time of donation, the concentration of electrolytes in the supernatant plasma will be proportionately higher than in whole blood because of the greater dilution in whole blood. However, the total quantity of electrolytes is the same, as the source is from the impaired integrity of the red cell membrane. Although it is inconvenient for the blood bank, when the product is prepared at the time of transfusion there is a considerable reduction in supernatant plasma electrolyte and hemoglobin concentrations.

The primary function of transfused red cells is enhancement of tissue oxygenation. Therefore the usual indication for transfusion of red blood cells is correction of symptomatic oxygen-carrying deficits. One unit of this component has the same red cell mass as a unit of whole blood and thereby provides the same oxygen-carrying capacity with corresponding reduction in plasma volume. The decreased plasma volume minimizes the risk of circulatory overload and also allows for more efficient correction of the red cell deficit.

Isotonic saline may be added to units of red blood cells to facilitate transfusion. This is the only acceptable diluent electrolyte solution for this purpose, although some balanced electrolyte solutions are being assessed and may prove suitable. In some

Table 11–1. Summary Chart of Blood Components

Component	Contents	Indications for Use	Approximate Volume	Risk of Hepatitis	Shelf Life of Product
Red cells	Red cells, some plasma, few WBCs	Increase patient red cell mass	250–350 ml	2*	21 days
Frozen red cells	Red cells—no plasma, minimal WBC and platelets	Increase red cell mass, prevent tissue antigen sensitization, prevent febrile or anaphylactic IgA reaction, provide rare bloods	200 ml	3*	3 yr frozen, 24 hr thawed
Leukocyte-poor blood	Red cells, some plasma, few WBCs	Prevent febrile reactions from leukoagglutins	200–250 ml	2	21 days, closed, 24 hr open
Platelets	Platelets, few WBCs, some plasma	Bleeding due to thrombocytopenia	30–50 ml	2	6–72 hours, depending on storage
Concentrated leukocytes	WBCs, few platelets	Agranulocytosis	Variable, 50–100 ml	2	12 hours
Single donor plasma	Plasma—no labile coagulation factors	Blood volume expansion	220–250 ml	2	5 yr
Fresh frozen plasma	Plasma—all coagulation factors, no platelets	Treatment of coagulation disorders	220–250 ml	2	2 hr thawed, 12 mo frozen
Cryoprecipitate	Coagulation factors I and VIII	Hemophilia and von Willebrand's disease, fibrinogen deficiency	10–25 ml	2	4–6 hr thawed, frozen
Plasma substitutes	Electrolytes and macromolecular substances	Blood volume expansion	As stated	3	NA
Plasma protein fraction (PPF)	PPF-albumin α- and β-globulin	Blood volume expansion	230 ml	3	3–5 yr

* 1 = greater than whole blood; 2 = same as whole blood; 3 = less than whole blood.

situations reconstitution of units of red blood cells through administration of plasma is practiced. Lactated Ringer's solution, or 5% dextrose in water, is incompatible with blood. Not only is it inappropriate to instill these solutions into the unit of red blood cells but also they should not come in contact with the red cells in the drip chamber of the transfusion set.

FROZEN RED BLOOD CELLS

Through use of cryoprotective agents such as glycerol, red blood cells can be stored at −70°C or below for many years. When needed for transfusion the cells are thawed, deglycerolized through serial washings, and resuspended in saline solution. This results in a product with oxygen-delivering capacity comparable to the original unit of red blood cells, but, because the bag has been entered, it has a shelf life of only 24 hours. The potential clinical indications for this product are comparable to those for liquid-stored red blood cells; however, its utilization has remained limited because of delay in availability due to processing, short shelf life, and high cost.

At the present time frozen red blood cells serve as a source of blood lacking high-incidence antigens for patients with corresponding antibodies. They also allow for long-term preservation of autologous units of blood, especially for patients with antibodies to high-incidence antigens who anticipate future operative procedures or pregnancies. Finally, since this product is relatively poor in leukocytes, and the washed component is free of plasma proteins, frozen red blood cells may be used for management of patients who have febrile responses to transfusion and also for patients who have anti-IgA and manifest anaphylaxis when transfused with blood or plasma containing IgA. It should be noted that the optional product for the latter patients is blood or plasma obtained from donors who lack IgA.

LEUKOCYTE-POOR RED BLOOD CELLS

This component is appropriate for transfusion in patients who manifest febrile transfusion reactions related to antibodies against donor leukocyte antigens. The role of antibodies vis-à-vis leukocyte antigens in the causation of these febrile reactions has been recognized for many years, and the intensity of the reactions appears related to the absolute quantity of transfused granulocytes.[8] Although these reactions may be reduced by premedication with antipyretics or steroids, in some individuals the severity of the reaction requires the use of a leukocyte-poor component. There are a variety of methods for preparation of this product, and all require retention of at least 70% of the original red cells and removal of at least 70% of the leukocytes in the unit.

Leukocyte-poor red blood cells can be prepared through washing of the unit of blood in a mechanical cell washer with resuspension in saline. Frozen, deglycerolized red blood cells also can serve as a leukocyte-poor product. At one time units of blood were inverted and centrifuged, with the lower two thirds of the red cell mass removed through the adjacent outlet into an attached satellite bag; however, this method has the obvious disadvantage of reduced therapeutic effectiveness related to loss of potentially transfusable red cells.

AUTOLOGOUS BLOOD

Autologous transfusion may involve predeposit or intraoperative methodology. The latter requires use of mechanical devices in the operating room that process blood aspirated from body cavities. Patients for whom transfusion is anticipated for a subsequent elective operation or delivery, and who have an acceptable hemoglobin level, are effectively managed through blood donation prior to the time of anticipated transfusion.[9] Because of its source, such blood has several advantages over homologous transfusion, including freedom from risk of incompatibility, hepatitis, and antigenic stimulation. The limitation on frequency of autologous donation is the donor's hemoglobin level. A minimum donor hemoglobin level of 11 g/dl must be maintained. Therefore, it is feasible to obtain several units of blood during the month before the anticipated requirement. The number of units collected may be expanded by storage in the frozen state.

While autologous blood is ideal for transfusion in patients who have antibodies to high-incidence red cell antigens in whom compatible blood would be difficult to locate, it should find greater use in routine transfusion because of the preceding advantages. Unfortunately, the special arrangements required for collection and storage of such blood products prove somewhat cumbersome for clinician, patient, and blood bank, thereby precluding optimal utilization of the product.

PLATELET CONCENTRATES

One of the most significant advances in blood component therapy in recent years is the expanded use of platelet concentrates for prevention or control of hemorrhage in patients with thrombocytopenia or qualitative platelet dysfunction. Such concentrates may be obtained from units of whole blood at the time of red blood cell preparation. In this instance they are termed "random donor" platelet concentrates. They also may be obtained through plateletpheresis of a donor using automated equipment ("single-donor" platelet concentrates). A random donor concentrate contains a minimum of 5.5×10^{10} platelets suspended in 50 to 70 ml of plasma, and a single-donor concentrate contains a minimum of 30×10^{10} platelets. Random donor concentrates are stored at room temperature with constant agitation and have a shelf life of five days. Because they are prepared in an "open" system, single-donor concentrates become outdated in 24 hours.

While thrombocytopenia is the principal indication for transfusion of platelet concentrates, the cause of the thrombocytopenia must still be defined. For example, patients with immune thrombocytopenic purpura who have antibody-mediated platelet destruction are best treated with steroids rather than platelet concentrates. Similarly, patients with thrombocytopenia associated with disseminated intravascular coagulation do not uniformly benefit from administration of platelet concentrates.

The dose of platelets needed to provide hemostasis varies with the clinical condition. The effectiveness of platelet concentrates may be impaired by infection, splenomegaly, fever, or antiplatelet antibodies in the recipient.[10] In general, a random donor platelet concentrate should increase the platelet count of a 70-kg adult by 7500/μl. In most instances patients are not treated with a single such concentrate; rather, several concentrates are pooled into a single container before transfusion and administered as rapidly as is practical through a standard blood filter.

Indications for treatment depend upon the level of thrombocytopenia. In general, surgical patients manifest hemostasis with platelet levels above 60,000 to 80,000/μl. In contrast, patients with thrombocytopenia caused by inadequate platelet production, as in leukemia or aplastic anemia, may not require treatment until platelet counts fall below 10,000 to 20,000/μl.[11] Lack of correlation between the platelet count and hemorrhagic tendency is seen in patients with a platelet dysfunction, aspirin-induced injury, or inherited qualitative platelet disorders. Patients receiving massive blood transfusions related to surgical or traumatic blood loss may develop dilutional thrombocytopenia and occasionally require platelet transfusions to restore normal hemostasis.

The effectiveness of platelet transfusions is best determined through assessment of a pretransfusion platelet count followed by a post-transfusion count, usually obtained at one and 24 hours. Similar information may be obtained through use of a bleeding time determination. Patients who fail to respond to adequate platelet transfusions probably are refractory because of antiplatelet antibodies. This is a most frustrating situation and may be managed through use of single-donor platelets from compatible donors. Although other systems may be involved, concentrates compatible in the human leukocyte antigen (HLA) system are most effective for such patients. Unfortunately, it is difficult to locate HLA-matched donors to provide these single-donor platelets.

Platelet concentrates contain sufficient numbers of red cells to cause alloimmunization to red cell antigens. Therefore, if Rh-positive platelet concentrates are transfused to an Rh-negative patient, it may be appropriate to treat the patient within the following 72 hours with Rh-immune globulin. Since a single 300-μg dose of Rh-immune globulin is sufficient to prevent immunization by 15 to 17 ml of red cells, and since it is uncommon for a single platelet concentrate to contain more than 0.3 ml of red cells, one dose of Rh-immune globulin should be adequate to treat a patient who has received many units of concentrates.

GRANULOCYTE CONCENTRATES

This component is prepared by leukapheresis, involving automated separation of blood into its components with retrieval of the granulocyte layer. Each concentrate contains approximately 6 to 10 $\times$ 10^9 granulocytes. Administration of this product can effectively augment antibiotic treatment in patients with profound neutropenia associated with life-threatening bacterial infection. Clinical studies have shown that transfusion of granulocyte concentrates in appropriate amounts (at least 1 $\times$ 10^{10}) to such patients can reduce mortality, especially when there is likelihood of bone marrow recovery.[12]

In general, granulocyte concentrates are prepared from donors whose ABO type is compatible with that of the patient. Since there is considerable red cell contamination of these units, sensitization to other blood group antigens can occur. Furthermore, this component carries the risks associated with transfusion of other blood components.

Granulocyte concentrate transfusions usually are reserved for patients with profound neutropenia whose granulocyte counts are lower than 500 cells per μl and who have a documented bacterial infection that has failed to respond to appropriate antibiotic treatment administered for at least 48 hours.

The usual course of treatment with granulocyte concentrates entails transfusion of one unit of granulocytes per day for at least four consecutive days, and treatment is continued until clinical improvement is noted, as indicated by defervescence or bone marrow recovery. Absence of a therapeutic effect after 14 days should prompt consideration of discontinuing treatment because of clinical unresponsiveness. Several questions remain to be resolved with respect to granulocyte concentrates. The optimum therapeutic course has yet to be defined, and the need for compatibility testing and HLA matching and the degree of risk for both donor and recipient have yet to be resolved. Finally, the expense of this component in relationship to the uncertainty of long-term benefit has led to additional debate.

PLASMA COMPONENTS

Plasma can be transfused either as single-donor plasma (SDP) or as fresh frozen plasma (FFP). The only difference between the two products is the manner of preparation. Single-donor plasma is separated from whole blood at any time during its shelf life, whereas FFP is separated within the first few hours of collection and is preserved at a temperature below −30°C. FFP contains the labile clotting factors V and VIII. However, this potential advantage of FFP must be tempered by the realization that patients requiring factor VIII replacement are best treated with cryoprecipitated factor VIII or with commercial factor VIII concentrates. Isolated factor V deficiency is exceedingly rare, although it can be treated with FFP. Most patients who require plasma replacement should receive SDP, thereby conserving the factor VIII in FFP for production of factor VIII concentrates. Regardless of duration of storage, the stable clotting factors are present in normal amounts during the acceptable shelf life of SDP. The two products have comparable risk of transmitting hepatitis to the patient in that both are prepared as single-donor products.

The use of plasma as a source of colloid for patients requiring volume expansion has been largely replaced by crystalloid solutions, hydroxyethyl starch of dextran, or hepatitis-free plasma derivatives such as albumin or plasma protein fraction (PPF). Electrolyte solutions have proved suitable both for initial resuscitation in massive hemorrhage and for adjusting plasma volume loss. However, their effect is somewhat more transient than that of plasma because of the relatively rapid equilibration of electrolytes and water between the intravascular and extravascular compartment.

Cryoprecipitated factor VIII is prepared from fresh frozen plasma as a concentrate of factor VIII. It contains the small amount of protein that precipitates when the plasma from a unit of whole blood is frozen and then thawed at refrigerator temperatures. This precipitate is rich in factor VIII, containing approximately 80 to 100 U of antihemophilic factor activity in less than 10 ml of plasma as well as approximately 200 mg of fibrinogen.

Cryoprecipitated factor VIII has the disadvantage of requiring storage at −30°C. This is inconvenient for the hemophilic patient. Therefore, in many instances its use has been supplanted by commercial factor VIII preparations that may be stored at refrigerator temperatures, or, in some instances, at room temperature. Cryoprecipitated factor VIII has the advantage of being a single-donor product. Therefore, there is reduction in the risk of transmission of hepatitis when it is used as a source of factor VIII. It also finds widespread use as a source of fibrinogen, since lyophilized fibrinogen concentrates are no longer available because of their high risk of hepatitis. Ten units of cryoprecipitated factor VIII can provide 2 g of fibrinogen in approximately 100 ml of plasma volume. Fibrinogen is also present in SDP and FFP.

PLASMA DERIVATIVES

The two most commonly used plasma derivatives are albumin and plasma protein fraction (PPF). These are chemically treated derivatives of pooled plasma that have been heated to inactivate hepatitis virus. The difference between the two relates to the somewhat lesser purification of albumin in PPF. Both products are more expensive than SDP or FFP of comparable oncotic activity. Moreover, in contrast to plasma, they contain very little immunoglobulin and no clotting factors. The safety of these products and their ready availability have contributed to their excessive use by physicians.

Albumin is available as a 5% or 25% salt-poor solution. Since these products move fluid from the extravascular compartment into the intravascular one, there is a resultant increased intravascular volume with the potential for hemodilution. Therefore, caution must be exercised to avoid fluid overload and subsequent congestive heart failure.

Moreover, in the presence of dehydration, additional fluids must be used in conjunction with these derivatives to avoid tissue damage caused by extravascular water depletion. Neither albumin nor PPF is appropriate for treatment of chronic hypoproteinemia with edema, as in cirrhosis or chronic renal failure. In these situations albumin produces only a transient elevation of serum protein levels. Because of its ability to bind bilirubin, albumin has been suggested for use in exchange transfusion of patients with hemolytic disease of the newborn. However, there has not been general acceptance of this form of treatment.

BLOOD SUBSTITUTES

There is no substitute for blood. For the most part, so-called blood substitutes supplant the oxygen-carrying capacity of red cells yet do not provide the other attributes of whole blood.

One of the first oxygen transport solutions was stroma-free hemoglobin.[13] Hemoglobin preparations free of insoluble red cell stroma have greatly reduced the renal damage associated with earlier hemoglobin-plasma products.

A more recent approach is the use of perfluorochemicals. It has been shown that "bloodless" animals can be maintained for many hours with such preparations. Perfluorochemicals are chemically inert and are not metabolized. Although some are stored in the tissues, most leave the body rapidly, principally through the lungs. Most recently perfluorodecalin has been mixed with other perfluorochemicals to provide a relatively stable emulsion for intravenous injection.[14]

While there may be great potential use for these products in the future, at present they must be considered experimental. They require high levels of oxygen for efficacy and are of questionable benefit, even in patients with profound anemia. They have been used with success for severely anemic patients who have religious objections to blood transfusion; however, uncertainty over potential toxicity continues to inhibit more widespread use of these products, and safety must be demonstrated before they can be generally recommended.

MASSIVE TRANSFUSION

While massive replacement of blood may prove life-saving, it may also occasion complications related, in part, to the administration of stored blood lacking platelets and labile clotting factors. A massive transfusion is generally defined as the equivalent of total blood replacement (transfusion of at least 10 U of blood to an adult patient within 24 hours).[15] In addition to coagulation abnormalities related to massive blood replacement, other adverse effects may result from electrolyte imbalance, administration of large volumes of citrate, and transfusion of a refrigerated product. Finally, there is the potential for selective depletion of a blood bank's inventory of compatible blood.

After the patient has received a massive transfusion, his or her blood volume is largely that received through transfusion. Therefore, the routine practice of crossmatching may be inappropriate. We commonly only perform a test for direct agglutination between donor red cells and patient's serum to ensure ABO compatibility. There is no need to expend the time or reagents for incubation of the reaction mixture or for performance of the antihuman globulin reaction; however, any clinically significant unexpected antibodies detected in pretransfusion tests necessitate administration of blood lacking corresponding antibodies. This abbreviated crossmatch is implemented after the patient has received the equivalent of total replacement and facilitates the ability of the laboratory to respond rapidly to the patient's blood loss.

Since it may not be possible to meet the patient's transfusion requirement with blood of the same ABO and Rh type, it may prove necessary to provide blood of a differing type that is compatible with the patient. In deciding which blood to provide, one must relate the potential need for blood to its availability. For example, an A, Rh-positive patient can receive both Rh-positive and Rh-negative blood. Moreover, this patient can be transfused with type A whole blood or red blood cells, or with type O red blood cells. Therefore, approximately 87% of a laboratory's inventory will be compatible with this patient in an emergency situation. If large volumes of red blood cells are transfused, it may be necessary to replace lost plasma volume. This can be accomplished in several ways. Type A, and, if available, type AB plasma can be administered with the red blood cells. Such plasma should be in the form of single-donor plasma, since fresh frozen plasma usually is unnecessary. In addition, electrolyte solutions can be administered in a Y-type set with the red blood cells, or through a separate port. It is important that only solutions compatible with blood be infused. Volume expanders such as albumin, plasma protein fraction, or dextran also can be used.

Patients receiving massive transfusions may sustain a coagulation defect related to transfusion of stored blood. The most common problem is that of platelet depletion. Although platelets may be reduced during massive transfusion, platelet counts usually do not fall below hemostatic levels, even with replacement of several blood volumes. The recommendation that "freshly drawn" units of blood be transfused on an empiric basis periodically during a massive transfusion for provision of platelets cannot be supported. Such a practice is both impractical and wasteful. It is best that platelet levels be monitored during the transfusion and that platelet concentrates be provided in adequate amounts if warranted by a bleeding tendency associated with thrombocytopenia. It is important to emphasize that a hemolytic transfusion reaction in an anesthetized patient may present as a bleeding tendency resulting from disseminated intravascular coagulation. This should be considered before assuming that generalized oozing of blood in such a patient is related to thrombocytopenia from use of stored blood.

No strict guidelines for transfusion of platelet concentrates during the massive blood replacement can be provided. It is most important to provide the platelet concentrates at the time the patient manifests a bleeding tendency. It is uncommon for this to occur until at least the equivalent of two blood volumes has been transfused.[16] Moreover, the platelet concentrates are most useful when provided as an aggregate of 6 to 12 concentrates, at the conclusion of the operative procedure. Labile clotting factors are provided in the plasma used for suspension of platelet concentrates. Approximately 50 ml of plasma are present in each concentrate. Therefore, it usually is unnecessary to issue FFP for such patients. Stable clotting factors are present in the stored blood or SDP being transfused.

Surprisingly few complications attributable to the use of stored blood are associated with massive transfusion.[17] Among these is hypothermia resulting from transfusion of refrigerated blood. If time permits, the transfused blood may be warmed with an in-line warming device. Unfortunately, many such instruments impede the flow of blood, thereby mitigating their effectiveness in patients requiring rapid blood replacement. Similarly, microaggregates, consisting of fibrin, leukocytes, and platelets, are a presumed cause of respiratory insufficiency when transfusing stored blood that is older than seven to ten days. Microaggregate filters have been advocated for removal of these particles. However, these filters reduce the ability to transfuse blood rapidly. Even more important, recent studies have cast doubt on the benefit of such filtration.[18]

More in theory than in practice, calcium depletion is considered a complication of transfusion of large amounts of citrate in stored blood. Although hypocalcemia may result from rapid transfusion, clinically significant effects are most unusual in this situation. Hypocalcemia is best detected by noting delayed cardiac electrical conduction. Laboratory measurement of total calcium usually requires too much time to be useful; moreover, it does not reflect changes in ionized calcium in the face of normal total calcium. Administration of calcium is potentially more dangerous than transient hypocalcemia in that calcium may result in potentially dangerous ventricular arrhythmias.[19] Supplementation of ionized calcium in these patients is rarely necessary. Patients receiving extremely rapid and massive blood replacement may experience decreased cardiac output. This may result from a synergistic effect between high potassium and low ionized calcium in producing patient morbidity.[20] Transfusion of one unit of blood in 20 minutes results in little alteration of either serum potassium or calcium level, and a rate of transfusion of one unit in ten minutes should be tolerated. Even transfusion of large volumes of anticoagulant solution alone, not as banked blood, does not result in citrate intoxication.[21]

The elevated concentration of potassium in the plasma of stored blood in massive transfusions may be associated with transient hyperkalemia in the patient. However, this does not reflect an increased potassium load in these patients.[17] The source of the potassium in the transfused blood is from intracellular depletion of potassium during red cell storage. These patients, even those with compromised renal function, usually adjust to the transiently elevated potassium levels without complication, as the potassium rapidly resumes its intracellular location after transfusion.

In some instances massively transfused patients have reduced fibrinogen levels. Since fibrinogen is relatively stable in bank blood, severe hypofibrinogenemia may indicate the presence of disseminated intravascular coagulation.

ADVERSE REACTIONS TO TRANSFUSION

While procedural standardization, quality control programs, educational efforts, and improvements in reagents have enhanced the safety of blood transfusion in recent years, the procedure continues to be associated with patient morbidity and mortality. The variety of reactions that may occur are related in part to the heterogeneity of blood and its components. Some of these reactions are antibody-mediated, representing a reaction between recipient antibody and donor blood, while others are of a mechanical or physiologic nature. In addition, blood may represent a vehicle for the transmission of disease, especially hepatitis.

HEMOLYTIC TRANSFUSION REACTIONS

Reactions between antibody in the patient and antigens on donor red cells may vary greatly in intensity, depending upon the specificity of antigen and antibody and the titer of antibody in the recipient plasma.

Immediate hemolytic transfusion reactions result from acute destruction of transfused red cells through a reaction between preformed serum antibody in the patient and corresponding antigenic determinants on the donor red cells. Such reactions most often are a result of human error at some level of the transfusion process. This may include misidentification or mislabeling of the patient blood specimen, selection of the improper unit of blood in the blood bank, or administration of the unit of blood to the wrong patient.

The conscious patient receiving a unit of incompatible blood, with resultant destruction of the transfused red cells, usually experiences a burning sensation in the arm receiving the transfusion, chills, fever, shortness of breath associated with tightness in the chest, lumbar pain, and diaphoresis. The patient also will manifest tachycardia and tachypnea, may be hypotensive, and, in severe reactions, may experience vascular collapse. In contrast, as noted earlier, a bleeding tendency may be the only sign of such a reaction in the anesthetized patient.

Immediate hemolytic reactions result from an antigen-antibody reaction involving red cell stroma and usually are related to ABO incompatibility. Hemoglobin liberated from the destroyed red cells does not play a significant role in the clinical manifestations of the reaction. In general, the intensity of the reaction is in proportion to the volume of incompatible blood transfused. Severe reactions are uncommon with administration of less than 50 ml of incompatible red cells.

It is of extreme importance that the blood transfusion be discontinued immediately when signs or symptoms suggestive of a hemolytic reaction occur. The transfusion should not be reinstituted until it is certain that the patient is not experiencing intravascular hemolysis. The following procedure indicates whether the transfusion has caused intravascular hemolysis:

1. The label on the container of blood or blood product, as well as the patient's identifying wrist band, must be examined to verify that the proper unit of blood has been transfused to the intended patient.
2. Avoiding hemolysis, a sample of blood must be obtained from the patient and sent to the blood bank with the transfusion set and any attached intravenous solutions.
3. The blood bank must immediately compare the patient's prereaction serum or plasma with the postreaction specimen for the presence of hemolysis and also must perform a direct antiglobulin test on the patient's red cells.
4. On the basis of this evaluation, as well as the clinical findings, initial evaluation of the patient also may include repeating the ABO typing of patient and donor blood and the crossmatch and screening tests for recipient serum antibodies. Determination of levels of serum bilirubin, haptoglobin, and urine hemoglobin or hemoglobin breakdown products is not of value in the immediate assessment of the patient.

Treatment of hemolytic transfusion reactions is directed at prevention of acute renal failure and disseminated intravascular coagulation. Renal ischemia appears to result from a combination of thrombosis and stasis in the renal circulation. Mannitol has been used to increase urinary output in this situation, but furosemide not only promotes diuresis but also enhances renal blood flow. The patient also should be provided with intravenous fluids to promote diuresis. A urinary output of 1 ml per minute is desired; however, if fluid loading does not result in diuresis within two hours, further fluid administration may prove harmful. Anticoagulant therapy, especially heparin, has been advocated to counteract disseminated intravascular coagulation.[22] Not only may this prevent the hemorrhagic diathesis but it may also prevent further red cell destruction through its anticomplementary effect. However, heparin is not without risk and should be restricted to those patients in whom a severe reaction has been confirmed.

The patient with a delayed hemolytic transfusion reaction usually presents with unexpected anemia one to three days after transfusion associated with a positive direct antiglobulin test. In this situation the patient has formed an antibody, usually to antigenic determinants in the Rh, Kell, or Kidd systems, from previous transfusion or pregnancy; however, the antibody titer is too low to be detectable in pretransfusion tests. The offending antibody manifests an anamnestic response to the corresponding antigen in the transfused blood and is detectable at the time of the reaction in eluates prepared from the patient's red cells and in the patient's serum. The patient may have few other clinical findings, although some have hemoglobinemia, hemoglobinura, and elevated bilirubin levels. In most patients with such reactions, no specific treatment is necessary other than use of compatible blood for subsequent transfusions, thereby avoiding the offending antibody. Since such antibodies may again become undetectable over a period of several years, it is important that the patient be apprised, preferably both verbally and in writing, of the presence of the antibody so that future reactions may be avoided.

FEBRILE TRANSFUSION REACTIONS

The most common adverse reaction to blood transfusion is a febrile response, usually representing a reaction to transfused leukocyte antigens. These reactions may occur during the transfusion or within the first few hours following transfusion and may be associated with shaking chills. While self-limited, they may occasion considerable discomfort. It is essential to exclude a hemolytic reaction by the method described previously. The transfusion must be temporarily discontinued during this evaluation until intravascular hemolysis has been excluded as a possibility.

Treatment of such reactions is symptomatic, consisting of administration of antipyretics. In general, the intensity of these reactions is related to the dose of leukocyte antigen transfused. The patient who manifests multiple febrile reactions should receive leukocyte-poor red blood cells to mitigate such responses. There are a variety of ways of achieving such leukocyte antigenic reduction, including use of washed red cells, frozen and deglycerolized red cells, or leukocyte-poor red cells prepared by differential centrifugation. A relatively easy way to achieve this result is to prepared "spin-filtered" red cells.[23] This involves centrifugation of a unit of red blood cells immediately before transfusion and administration of the blood through a microaggregate filter.

On occasion the patient will manifest not only fever but also hypotension and dyspnea, with leukocyte antibody-induced reactions. Pulmonary infiltrates may be evident on chest roentgenograms; these are indicative of noncardiogenic edema and present clinically as adult respiratory distress syndrome. Such reactions have been associated with HLA-specific leukocyte antibodies in recipient serum, and, more often, in donor plasma. Treatment involves cessation of the transfusion, diuresis, and other supportive measures. The condition usually resolves within a day or two.

ALLERGIC TRANSFUSION REACTIONS

These reactions are quite common, occurring in association with approximately 1% of transfusions. Although urticaria rarely may accompany other symptoms of hemolytic transfusion reactions, when present as an isolated finding it is not a result of a red cell antigen–antibody reaction. Urticaria may occur during the transfusion or within the first few hours post transfusion, and, on occasion, it may be accompanied by other manifestations of histamine release, such as bronchospasm. After assurance that the allergic manifestations are the only adverse response to the transfusion, the patient is best treated symptomatically with antihistamines.

The most severe allergic reactions are anaphylactic responses to transfused blood, which are almost always a result of incompatibility of IgA in donor blood and IgG antibodies in the patient directed to IgA antigen.[24] Such reactions usually occur in patients who lack IgA and who develop class-specific antibodies to this immunoglobulin. These reactions are extremely rare and are related to the fact that approximately one in 700 persons lacks IgA and thereby has the potential for sensitization; however, only rarely do such individuals actually form the antibody. Demonstration of the antibody is not necessary for inferential diagnosis, since the presence of an anaphylactic relation in a patient lacking IgA is sufficient. Management of such reactions corresponds to the treatment for any anaphylactic reaction but also includes avoidance of future transfusion with any blood products containing IgA.

POST-TRANSFUSION PURPURA

Acute, severe thrombocytopenia may occur within a week after transfusion of blood. This is an extremely rare complication and indicates that an antibody present in the patient's plasma reacts with platelet antigen in the transfused blood product. Destruction of donor platelets and of autologous platelets occurs, probably related to release of incompatible platelet antigen from the donor platelets or to antigen-antibody complexes absorbed on recipient platelets.[25] The thrombocytopenia persists for as long as one month and usually does not respond to treatment with corticosteroids; however, there have been reports of successful treatment by plasma exchange.

CIRCULATORY OVERLOAD

This complication usually occurs in patients who receive excessive fluid through transfusion in the presence of pulmonary, renal, or cardiac disease. Treatment is that of management of congestive heart failure; on occasion, plasmapheresis or phlebotomy may be required. This is a preventable complication of transfusion in that patients with chronic anemia who have a normal plasma volume should not be transfused with whole blood but should receive red blood cells.

BACTERIAL CONTAMINATION

With the advent of plastic blood transfusion equipment, bacterial contamination has become an extremely uncommon complication. Gram-negative organisms implicated in such reactions are psychrophilic and usually are capable of utilizing citrate as a sole source of carbon. Such organisms may contaminate the unit of blood during collection as a result of donor bacteremia or ineffective antisepsis of donor skin. The clinical response is related to contamination of blood by endotoxin and may be associated with vascular collapse and even death. Prevention of these reactions is based on collection of blood using strict asepsis and on outdating units of blood after 24 hours if the container has been entered. Furthermore, avoidance of prolonged transfusion should be practiced; all transfusions should be completed within four hours.

TRANSMISSION OF DISEASE

The most important post-transfusion disease is hepatitis. The incidence of post-transfusion hepatitis has been reduced over the past decade through implementation of an all-volunteer blood donor program and mandatory testing for hepatitis B surface antigen. Most cases of post-transfusion hepatitis at the present time are related to non-A, non-B disease.[26, 27] Hepatitis A does not play a significant role in post-transfusion hepatitis. Unfortunately, there is no test for detection of the causative agent(s) of non-A, non-B hepatitis.

While units of whole blood and of all blood components are potentially capable of transmitting hepatitis, pooled products, such as commercial clotting factor concentrates, are particularly dangerous in this regard because they compound the risk. In contrast, albumin and plasma protein fraction are heat-treated to eliminate the possibility of transmission of hepatitis.

Hepatitis B immune globulin may be used for prevention of hepatitis B after recent exposure to infected blood, either through transfusion or through accidental injection. In addition, a vaccine has recently been introduced to confer active immunity against hepatitis B.[28] This may be appropriate for administration to health care workers who have a high risk of acquiring the disease and also for patients receiving multiple transfusions over an extended period of time.

In addition to hepatitis, other diseases may be transmitted through transfusion. Most are uncommon; however, cytomegalovirus (CMV) infection probably plays a significant role in post-transfusion disease, especially in neonatal patients or recipients with immunologic deficiency syndromes. It appears likely that the risk of such infection may be reduced by testing donor blood for antibody to CMV before transfusing susceptible patients.[29] The risk of this infection also may be lessened through the use of frozen, deglycerolized red blood cells.

REFERENCES

1. Oberman, H.A.: The history of blood transfusion. *In* Clinical Practice of Blood Transfusion. Edited by S.N. Swisher and L.D. Petz. New York Churchill Livingstone, 1981.
2. Jennings, E.R., and Hindmarsh, C.: The significance of the minor crossmatch. Am J Clin Pathol *30*:302, 1958.
3. Oberman, H.A., Barnes, B.A., and Steiner, E.A.: Role of the crossmatch in testing for serologic incompatibility. Transfusion *22*:12, 1982.
4. Beutler, E., and Wood, L.: The in vivo regeneration of red cell 2,3-diphospholglyceric acid (DPG) after transfusion of stored blood. J Lab Clin Med *74*:300, 1969.
5. Limbird, T.J., and Silver, D.: Sequential changes observed in blood preserved with citrate-phosphate-dextrose. Surg Gynecol Obstet *138*:401, 1974.
6. Wood, L., and Beutler, E.: Temperature dependence on sodium-potassium activated erythrocyte adenosine triphosphatase. J Lab Clin Med *70*:287, 1974.
7. Oberman, H.A.: The indications for transfusion of freshly drawn blood. JAMA *199*:129, 1967.
8. Brittingham, T.E., and Chaplin, H.: Febrile transfusion reactions caused by sensitivity to donor leukocytes and platelets. JAMA *165*:819, 1957.
9. McKittrick, J.E.: Banked autologous blood in elective surgery. Am J Surg *128*:137, 1977.
10. Lister, T.A., and Yankee, R.A.: Blood component therapy. Clin Haematol *7*:407, 1978.
11. Slichter, S.J.: Controversies in platelet transfusion therapy. Ann Rev Med *31*:509, 1980.
12. McCullough, J.: Leukapheresis and granulocyte transfusion: CRC Crit Rev Clin Lab Sci *91*:275, 1979.
13. Peskin, G.W., O'Brien, K, and Rabiner, S.F.; Stroma-free hemoglobin solution: The "ideal" blood substitute? Surgery *66*:185, 1969.
14. Tremper, K.K., Friedman, A.E., Levine, E.M., et al.: The preoperative treatment of severely anemic patients with a perfluorochemical oxygen-transport fluid, Fluoscl-DA. N Eng J Med *307*:277, 1982.
15. Oberman, H.A. (ed.): Standards for Blood Banks and Transfusion Services. 10th Ed. Washington, D.C.; American Association of Blood Banks, 1981.
16. Miller, R., Robbins, T.O., Tong, M.J. and Barton, S.L : Coagulation defects associated with massive blood transfusion. Ann Surg *174*:794, 1971.

17. Collins, J.A.: Massive blood transfusion. Clin Haematol *5*:201, 1976.
18. Snyder, E.L., Underwood, P.S., Spivack, M., et al.: An in vivo evaluation of microaggregate blood filtration during total hip replacement. Ann Surg *190*:75, 1979.
19. Wolf, P.L., McCarthy, L.J., and Hafleigh, B.: Extreme hypercalcemia following blood transfusions combined with intravenous calcium. Vox Sang *19*:544, 1970.
20. Lee, Y.C.P., Richman, H.G., and Visscher, M.B.: [Ca^{++}] and [K^{+}] interrelations influencing mechanical and electrical events in cardiac activity. Am J Physiol *210*:499, 1966.
21. Howland, W.S., Bellville, J.W., and Zucker, M.B.: Massive blood transfusion. V. Failure to demonstrate citrate intoxication. Surg Gynecol Obstet *105*:529, 1957.
22. Goldfinger, D.: Acute hemolytic transfusion reactions—a fresh look at pathogenesis and considerations regarding therapy. Transfusion *17*:85, 1977.
23. Wenz, B., Gurtlinger, K.F., O'Toole, A.M., et al.: The preparation of granulocyte-poor red blood cells by microaggregate filtration. Vox Sang *39*:282, 1980.
24. Vyas, G.N., Holmdahl, L., Perkins, H.A., et al.: Serologic specificity of human anti-IgA and its significance in transfusion. Blood *34*:573, 1969.
25. Engelfriet, C.P.: Post-transfusion purpura: A serochemical study. Br J Haematol *49*:521, 1981.
26. Holland, P.: Current status of post-transfusion hepatitis. Pathobiol Ann *10*:135, 1980.
27. Alter, H.J.: Dominant role of non-A, non-B in the pathogenesis of post-transfusion hepatitis. A clinical assessment. Clin Gastroenterol *9*:155, 1980.
28. Zuckerman, A.J.: Priorities for immunization against hepatitis B. Br Med J *285*:686, 1982.
29. Yeager, A.S., Hafleigh, E.B., Bradley, J.S., et al.: Prevention of transfusion-acquired cytomegalovirus infections in newborn infants. J Pediatr *98*:281, 1981.

Chapter 12
THROMBOEMBOLIC DISEASE

Russell K. Laros, Jr.

Thromboembolic disease is the leading nonobstetric cause of postpartum death. As management of sepsis and eclampsia has improved, pulmonary embolism has made a relatively greater impact and in some series is second only to abortion as a cause of maternal mortality.[1] Fortunately, it is also a disease in which early recognition and proper treatment can dramatically improve the outcome. However, the pregnant patient is unique in that she is actually two patients, and therefore, the usual diagnostic and therapeutic maneuvers must be modified so as not to adversely affect the fetus.

In this chapter we will (1) review the techniques used in making the diagnosis of deep venous thrombosis (DVT) and pulmonary embolism; (2) consider anticoagulant and ancillary therapy for these disorders; (3) discuss in detail the use of heparin in both full anticoagulant and prophylactic dosages; (4) discuss in detail the use of coumarin for anticoagulation; and (5) discuss alternative therapy such as fibrinolytic agents and vena caval interruption.

INCIDENCE AND PATHOPHYSIOLOGY

INCIDENCE

Although thrombophlebitis is serious because of its potentially fatal consequences, fortunately it is quite rare in young women. The reported incidence varies between 0.018 and 0.29% during gestation and between 0.1 and 1.0% post partum.[2] Puerperal patients outnumber antepartum patients by approximately three to one. The difficulty of making an accurate diagnosis accounts for the wide variation in the incidence noted by these reports. Although thrombophlebitis can be seen at any stage of gestation, it appears to increase in frequency as pregnancy advances.[3] After delivery, DVT is most frequently seen on the second postpartum day (DVT appears in 55% of patients within the first three days), but it may occur up to four weeks after delivery.[3]

The incidence of pulmonary embolism depends on whether or not DVT is adequately treated. If untreated, as many as 24% of patients with antenatal DVT will have pulmonary embolism, with a mortality rate of approximately 15%.[2] If patients are treated with anticoagulants, embolization will occur in only 4.5%, and the mortality rate is less than 1%.[4] The importance of proper treatment with anticoagulation agents is clear.

PATHOPHYSIOLOGY

Over a century ago, Virchow described a triad of factors that play an essential role in the initiation of intravascular coagulation: injury to the vessel wall, stasis, and changes in local clotting factors. During pregnancy thrombosis may occur without any known abnormality of the endothelium. However, vein distensibility increases during the first trimester,[5] and by the third trimester the velocity of venous flow in the lower extremities is reduced by half, in part because the gravid uterus provides a mechanical impediment to venous return.[6] This tendency toward stasis is augmented if the patient requires periods of prolonged bed rest, as is the case in pre-eclampsia, threatened abortion, or premature labor.

As discussed in Chapter 8, levels of fibrinogen, factor VIII, and other vitamin K–dependent clotting factors are increased during pregnancy.[7] There is also evidence of decreased fibrinolytic activity and reduced levels of available circulating plasminogen activator.[8] It is interesting that although pregnancy would appear to be a "hypercoagulable state," the increased risk of thromboembolism seems to be confined primarily to the postpartum period. The risk is enhanced by cesarean section (a ninefold increase over vaginal delivery), instrument delivery, advanced maternal age, increased parity, and suppression of lactation by estrogens.[9] Other risk factors reported include a history of prior thromboembolism or trauma, infection, obesity, congestive heart failure, dehydration, shock, disseminated cancer, dysproteinemia, polycythemia vera, and anemia (especially sickle cell).[9, 10]

Overall, the risk of thromboembolism during pregnancy and post partum is 5.5 times greater than that for nonpregnant controls.[11] With the availability of effective contraceptives, more women are delaying childbearing, and a concomitant increase in the incidence of pulmonary emboli can be expected because of the increase in maternal age.

DIAGNOSIS

Because thromboembolism can be fatal, early and accurate diagnosis is essential. Unfortunately, specific diagnosis, especially during pregnancy, can be difficult. Anticoagulation, although an invaluable therapeutic tool, is not without hazard. Therefore, the physician should be certain of the diagnosis before committing a patient to a lengthy course of treatment.

DEEP VENOUS THROMBOSIS

The signs and symptoms most commonly used to diagnose deep venous thrombosis (DVT) are listed in Table 12–1. Leg swelling is a measured difference in leg circumference of greater than 2 cm. A positive Homans' sign is pain in the calf when the great toe is passively dorsiflexed. A positive Lowenberg test is pain in the calf or thigh when a blood pressure cuff is rapidly inflated to 180 mm Hg pressure. Unfortunately, many of the complaints listed occur as normal physiologic changes of pregnancy. Haeger found that not only are none of these symptoms or signs specific but also that their presence in limbs with and without thrombosis occurs with approximately equal frequency.[12] Forty-five percent of patients thought to have clinically

Table 12–1. Signs and Symptoms of Deep Venous Thrombosis

Muscle pain
Tenderness
Swelling
Homans' sign
Positive Lowenberg test

certain DVT had an entirely normal venous system according to venography. Conversely, venograms done on patients with pulmonary emboli may demonstrate clots in a totally asymptomatic limb.[13] In only 10% of patients is the diagnosis of DVT made prior to fatal pulmonary embolism.[14] It appears that the more symptomatic the thrombus, the more tightly adherent it is to the vessel wall.

Septic pelvic thrombophlebitis may be even more difficult to diagnose, and the only signs may be chills and a hectic febrile course.[15] Pelvic examination is frequently unrevealing, and the diagnosis is usually made on the basis of failure to respond to a 48- to 72-hour regimen of adequate antibiotic therapy (including coverage of anaerobes).

Venography

Diagnosis of DVT during pregnancy is further hampered because the physician is restricted to those methods that do not harm the fetus. Venography is the reference standard against which all other methods are compared. Although it is the most specific procedure, it has limitations. It is invasive, expensive, and difficult to interpret unless all the deep veins are filled adequately. It cannot be used to demonstrate the pelvic venous plexus. It cannot be repeated frequently, and the contrast material may cause chemical phlebitis. Further, venography has not been used frequently during pregnancy because of possible hazards to the fetus. However, it is often the only definitive study available, and the fetus can be protected by shielding of the maternal abdomen.[11]

Isotope Scanning

^{125}I fibrinogen uptake scanning is useful in evaluating the lower extremities below the midthigh. Unfortunately, it loses sensitivity in the upper thigh and pelvis because of the increased background radioactivity levels in the femoral artery and bladder.[16] This is a significant deficiency, because the majority of serious pulmonary emboli are thought to originate from deep veins in the iliofemoral region. This method should rarely be used during pregnancy, because free isotopic iodine crosses the placenta and concentrates in the fetal thyroid.

Impedance Plethysmography

This technique utilizes temporary occlusion of venous return by inflation of a thigh cuff. The occlusion results in an increase in the venous volume of the calf. Release of the cuff results in a rapid decrease in volume as the blood drains proximally. If venous obstruction is present, the rate of outflow is diminished. These changes in blood volume can be detected by measuring electrical resistance in the calf.[17–19]

Clarke-Pearson and associates have documented the reliability of this technique in the gynecologic patient[18] and suggest that it may also be a sensitive and specific test during pregnancy.[19] However, only a few cases of documented DVT during pregnancy have been studied with this technique, and its ultimate place in the diagnostic armamentarium remains unclear.

Doppler Ultrasound

Doppler flow studies are an alternative, noninvasive test for proximal vein occlusion. A 5-MHz transducer is placed over the vein. Venous flow produces a characteristic low-pitched sound that is abolished by venous occlusion. Again, there are no data available delineating the specificity of this technique during pregnancy.

Blood Tests for Thrombosis

Several tests are available that reflect the formation of intravascular fibrin.[20] They are invariably positive when thrombosis has occurred. Unfortunately, they are also positive in the presence of hematomas or inflammatory exudates containing fibrin. The assays for fibrinopeptide A and fibrin-fibrinogen degradation product fragment E are the most sensitive.

A Noninvasive Approach to Diagnosis of DVT

Hirsh and colleagues have analyzed the cost effectiveness of clinical diagnosis, venography, and noninvasive testing in patients with symptomatic DVT.[21] Their data indicate that clinical diagnosis is not cost-effective and that the ideal approach in the nonpregnant individual is to combine impedance plethysmography and leg scanning as an alternative to venography. In pregnancy, we prefer venography to assure the diagnosis, unless the clinical features are pathognomonic, e.g., phlegmasia cerulea dolens.

PULMONARY EMBOLISM

Clinical Signs and Symptoms

Although small emboli may go unrecognized by the patient, the hallmark of pulmonary embolism is dyspnea. The major sign is tachypnea. Table 12–2 shows the signs and symptoms most frequently encountered.[22] Small emboli become lodged more peripherally and may produce infarction accompanied by pleural signs, including cough, hemoptysis, pleuritic chest pain with splinting, and a friction rub. However, the majority of emboli do not produce infarction, and these symptoms are absent. Leg discomfort and shortness of breath may be the result of uterine enlargement in the third trimester but also may indicate multiple small emboli. Also, multiple small emboli can mimic a major embolus. Massive pulmonary embolism, defined for clinical purposes as occlusion of at least 50% of the pulmonary arterial circulation, may present with symptoms suggesting a myocardial infarction, including hypotension and occasionally syncope or convulsions.

Tachycardia or a few atelectatic rales may be the only finding on physical examination. However, massive emboli may produce right-sided heart failure with jugular venous distention, an enlarged liver, a left parasternal heave, and fixed splitting of the second heart sound. Cardiac auscultation during normal pregnancy may reveal a variety of "functional" murmurs or an increase in P_2; thus these findings are valuable only if they are clearly new.

Table 12–2. Signs and Symptoms of Pulmonary Embolism

Sign or Symptom	%*
Tachypnea	89
Dyspnea	81
Pleuritic pain	72
Apprehension	59
Cough	54
Tachycardia	43
Hemoptysis	34
Temperature (> 37°C)	34

* % of patients with proven pulmonary embolism having these findings.

Electrocardiogram

The ECG is abnormal in 90% of patients; however, tachycardia alone is the most common abnormality. Nonspecific T-wave inversion is found in 40%, and the classic right axis shift with strain pattern ($S_1Q_3T_3$) is found in those patients with extensive embolization.

Arterial pO_2

An arterial partial pressure of O_2 (PaO_2) of higher than 80 mm Hg in the patient breathing room air makes pulmonary embolism unlikely. However, 11.5% of patients with proven pulmonary embolism have a PaO_2 of between 80 and 90 mm Hg, and thus it seems more prudent to use a level of 90 mm Hg as excluding the diagnosis of pulmonary embolism.[22]

Lung Scanning and Pulmonary Arteriography

Because pulmonary embolism is a diagnosis of such consequence, if it cannot be excluded on the basis of a normal PaO_2, a lung scan should be done. The agent of choice is microspheres on macroaggregates labeled with technetium ($^{99}mT_c$), which has a half-life of six hours. Because a one-mCi dose given to the mother yields a fetal dose of only about 2 mrad, a perfusion scan is a safe procedure during pregnancy. The likelihood of visualizing a pulmonary embolus depends on the nature of the abnormality observed on the scan. The specificity of the lung scan is significantly improved if coupled with a ventilation study. This is especially true if the perfusion defects are not typical of embolization or if they are accompanied by chest film abnormalities suggesting consolidation.[23]

Pulmonary angiography is indicated if surgical intervention is contemplated. In attempting to assess anticoagulation failures requiring caval interruption, it is the only method capable of reliably distinguishing between recurrent embolism and fragmentation and distal migration of the original clot.

Other Laboratory Studies

Laboratory examinations are typically unrevealing, although the white count, serum LDH and bilirubin levels, and erythrocyte sedimentation rate may each be elevated. Fibrin split products are always present; however, they can be found in uncomplicated pregnancy and in most postoperative patients. Their absence, however, essentially excludes the possibility of embolism.[20] When a family history of repeated thromboembolism is encountered, the level of antithrombin III should be studied to rule out familial antithrombin III deficiency.[24]

MANAGEMENT

Anticoagulation therapy, which will be discussed later, is the mainstay of therapy for deep thrombophlebitis with or without pulmonary embolism. However, for both entities there are a number of additional modalities useful in achieving symptomatic relief.

DEEP VENOUS THROMBOSIS

Bed rest with elevation of the involved extremity is valuable initially, because it promotes venous return and decreases edema. The Trendelenburg position, obtained by elevating the foot of the bed approximately eight inches, is preferable to using pillows, which may impede femoral flow because they flex the hip. The patient may be supplied with a foot board and instructed in the performance of hourly flexion and extension exercises of both lower extremities. However, as soon as symptoms permit, the patient should be encouraged to ambulate, since bed rest itself may enhance venous stasis. There is no evidence that bed rest will prevent embolus detachment. Sitting with legs dependent is contraindicated.

Application of moist heat to involved areas can be beneficial. Although moist heat is more effective than dry heat, it is useless unless hot packs are replaced as frequently as they cool.

Analgesic drugs may be required, but those that affect platelet function (e.g., aspirin) must be avoided while anticoagulants are being used. Anti-inflammatory drugs, although useful agents, are generally contraindicated during pregnancy. By decreasing prostaglandin levels, indomethacin can cause premature closure of the ductus arteriosus and consequent pulmonary hypertension.[25] In animal studies phenylbutazone exhibits evidence of embryotoxicity and appears in breast milk.[26] In addition, it potentiates the effects of the coumarin anticoagulants.

When correctly designed, elastic stockings increase the velocity of venous flow. The pressure gradient should decrease from ankle to thigh without a constricting garter at the top. Certain brands designed for ambulatory patients may be overly compressive in the recumbent position. Elastic bandages, once in vogue, are best avoided because they are often wrapped incorrectly, with the greatest pressure ending up at the top and thus impeding venous return.

PULMONARY EMBOLISM

If an embolic source can be traced to the lower extremities, the above measures can be employed. In addition, specific treatment of the embolus is required. Oxygen therapy is particularly important during pregnancy, because even if the mother survives, the fetus may die or be damaged secondary to maternal hypoxia. The maternal PaO_2 should be maintained above 70 mm Hg. Positive pressure administration may be required if pulmonary edema is present. Meperidine or morphine may be used for pain and apprehension. Bed rest is indicated for at least five to seven days, allowing time for the initial organization of the clot. Straining bowel movements are best avoided, and stool softeners may prove helpful.

A vasoactive amine such as isoproterenol or dopamine is indicated for treatment of shock. The objective is to increase the mean arterial pressure and the flow through the pulmonary vasculature. Isoproterenol (mix 1 mg in 500 ml of normal saline, yielding 2 μg per ml) is given at 2 to 8 μg per minute and dopamine (200 mg in 500 ml of normal saline yielding 400 μg per ml) is started at 200 μg per minute. Administration of both fluids and vasoactive amines should be monitored via a Swan-Ganz catheter measuring pulmonary artery and wedge pressures. Aminophylline and digoxin may also be useful. Aminophylline decreases reflux bronchospasm and has a diuretic action that is particularly useful if pulmonary edema is present. Digoxin can be administered if heart failure is present but is rarely of benefit. Aminophylline (250 mg in 500 ml of normal saline, yielding 500 μg per ml) is infused rapidly over 20 minutes to give a dose of 4 to 5 mg per kg of body weight. The infusion is then slowed to 12 to 15 μg/kg/min. The dosage is adjusted to achieve a serum concentration of 10 to 20 μg per ml. Antibiotics are not indicated unless a septic embolus is suspected.

ANTICOAGULATION

Currently, three major types of therapeutic agents are available for treating thrombosis. Each is directed at a different portion of the coagulation process. They consist of (1) agents that interfere with platelet adhesion and aggregation, (2) agents that interfere with fibrin formation, and (3) agents that facilitate clot lysis.

Agents that interfere with fibrin formation are by far the most important in treating thromboembolism, and in the United States they are heparin and the coumarin derivatives. Heparin is the preferred agent in the initial treatment of thromboembolism, while for long-term management in the nonpregnant state conversion to a coumarin derivative is usually ideal. For reasons to be discussed later, we feel that heparin is the preferred drug throughout pregnancy.

Heparin

Heparin is a naturally occurring mucopolysaccharide organic base found within mast cells of most mammals. In plasma it combines with an α-globulin known as antithrombin III to become a potent inhibitor of thrombin (thus preventing conversion of fibrinogen to fibrin) and to increase the circulating levels of activated factor X (Xa) inhibitor.[27] Heparin does not have a direct antiplatelet effect, nor will it stimulate fibrinolysis or directly lyse thrombi.[28] Because of its large size and negative charge, it does not cross the placenta or appear in breast milk, both advantages when anticoagulation is required during pregnancy or lactation. If necessary, heparin effects can be reversed rapidly by administering protamine sulfate in a dose of 1 mg per 100 U of administered heparin. (When using constant infusion methods, twice the amount necessary to neutralize the hourly dose should be sufficient.) No more than 50 mg should be given over any 10-minute period, since protamine itself can cause bleeding.

Heparin is used primarily to prevent either initiation or propagation of venous thromboembolism. Three different dosage ranges are commonly used, as outlined in Table 12–3.

Medium-Dose Therapy. There is now clear evidence that monitoring the dosage of heparin affects the recurrence rate of thrombotic events.[29] Although presumed, it is less clear that monitoring affects hemorrhagic complications. A variety of clotting studies are available for monitoring circulating heparin levels. After reviewing the literature on control of heparin therapy, Estes[30] and Godal[31] both agree that partial thromboplastin times (PTT, aPTT, whole blood thromboplastin time [WBPTT]) are

Table 12–3. Heparin Regimens

Dosage (USP U/24 h)	Route	Clinical Indications
Medium: 20,000–60,000	Continuous intravenous or intermittent subcutaneous	Active thromboembolism; disseminated intravascular coagulation
High: 60,000–100,000	Continuous intravenous	Massive pulmonary embolism
Low: 10,000–15,000	Intermittent subcutaneous or continuous intravenous	Elective pelvic surgery; disseminated intravascular coagulation

more sensitive and accurate tests than is the Lee-White clotting time (LWCT). Although a number of investigators have favored the aPTT, there is evidence that aPTTs greater than 70 sec are poorly reproducible and hence unreliable when assessing higher degrees of anticoagulation.[32] The thrombin clotting time (TCT) also seems to satisfy the requirements for accuracy and ease of performance and is the method preferred by some.[32]

Optimal anticoagulation is usually obtained with a circulating heparin level of 0.3 U per ml (TCT, 2.5 × control; aPTT, 2.5 to 3.0 × control). Spontaneous hemorrhage frequently occurs if the concentration exceeds 0.6 U per ml for periods of time exceeding 12 hours.[33] The circulating level is a balance between input of new drug, rapid metabolism, and excretion either directly by the kidneys or indirectly by diffusion into extravascular spaces to be metabolized slowly. The half-life of heparin is 1.5 hours,[30] and a stable circulating level is most easily achieved by giving a loading dose followed by a continuous intravenous infusion. Because normal individuals vary widely in their responses to a given dose, the rate of infusion should be varied to achieve an aPTT within the therapeutic range regardless of the amount of heparin this requires. Table 12–4 gives a schema for continuous intravenous infusion for DVT.

The clinical impression that there is an increased requirement for heparin during pregnancy has been confirmed in the laboratory.[34] This relative resistance during pregnancy is in part caused by an increased volume of distribution, a decrease in plasma albumin concentration, and a significant increase in factors VII, VIII, IX, X, and fibrinogen. Although ineffective when taken orally, heparin is well absorbed after subcutaneous administration. The intramuscular route should not be used because of the high incidence of hematoma formation at the injection site. While a steady circulating level can most easily be obtained by continuous intravenous administration, either the intermittent intravenous or the subcutaneous route can be used. However, intermittent administration produces peaks and valleys in the circulating heparin activity that lead to seven times as many major bleeding complications as continuous infusion.[35] When an intermittent regimen is chosen, the total daily dose is 400 to 500 U/kg/day in divided doses. The intravenous dose should be given every six hours and the subcutaneous every eight or 12 hours. In most cases this will provide an average anticoagulant activity of 0.3 U per ml. Initially, monitoring should be performed frequently (aPTT three to four times daily). Blood samples should be obtained two hours prior to the next dose and levels should not exceed 0.3 U (TCT, 2 × control; aPTT, 2.5 × control) following an intravenous bolus or 0.2 U (TCT, 1.5 × control; aPTT, 2 × control) following a subcutaneous injection. Once a stable dose is obtained, monitoring can be decreased to daily or every other day.

Table 12–4. Anticoagulation with Medium-Dose Heparin

Loading dose:	5000 U intravenously by rapid administration.
Continuous infusion:	Hourly rate of 15 to 20 U/kg/hr. Adjust rate to achieve TCT of 2.5 × control (aPTT 2.5 to 3 × control).
Long-term anticoagulation:	150 to 250 U/kg/12 hr. Adjust dose to achieve TCT of 1.5 to 2 × control 2 hr prior to next dose (aPTT 2 to 2.5 × control).

Before initiating therapy, a baseline hematocrit value, platelet count, PT, and aPTT or TCT should be obtained. Heparin should be avoided if the platelet count is less than 50,000 × $10^9/l$ or if platelet function is inadequate.

Heparin may be mixed in 250 ml of physiologic saline or glucose and saline and then administered using an infusion pump. Ideally, to avoid accidental overdose, no more than a six-hour infusion volume should be connected to the patient's intravenous line.

Continuous intravenous heparin should be maintained for seven to 14 days for active thromboembolic disease or until symptoms have resolved and there is no evidence of recurrence. At this point the patient may be switched to subcutaneous heparin or oral coumarin if long-term management is indicated. Long-term heparinization is accomplished using a schedule of 150 to 250 U/kg every 12 hours for pulmonary embolism and DVT. The patient is instructed in self-administration using the 40,000 U per ml preparation of heparin, a tuberculin syringe, and a 25-gauge 5/8-inch needle to inject deep into the subcutaneous fat of the anterior abdominal wall. Local hematoma formation can be reduced by applying ice to the site for several minutes prior to injection, and the site should be changed daily. Intramuscular injections are forbidden, and the patient must be cautioned against the concomitant use of aspirin. While some have advocated an intermittent intravenous dose schedule for long-term maintenance,[35] we see no advantage and in fact several disadvantages to this technique as compared with a subcutaneous regimen. There is ample data supporting the practicality, safety, and efficacy of chronic heparin therapy in ambulatory pregnant[36, 37] and nonpregnant patients.[38]

Indications for anticoagulant therapy beyond the acute episode include recurrence and pulmonary embolization. We usually treat an acute first episode of thrombophlebitis during pregnancy for three to six weeks and institute prophylaxis during labor, delivery, and the immediate postpartum state. If pulmonary embolization has occurred, therapy would be extended to six months. Similarly, therapy should be extended for patients with iliofemoral venous thrombosis and recurrent venous thrombosis and should include either therapeutic or prophylactic doses during labor, delivery, and the early puerperium.

High-Dose Therapy. In patients with massive pulmonary embolism, a high dose of heparin should be used during the first 24 hours of treatment. The initial loading dose should be 10,000 to 15,000 U, followed by an hourly dose sufficient to yield a total dose of 60,000 U during the first 24 hours.[22, 39] While there are no guidelines from clinical trials, it has been suggested that high doses are beneficial by relieving vasospasm. Additionally there is evidence that a patient's heparin requirement is related to the extent of thrombosis.[40] The high dose should be reduced to the medium dose range after 12 to 24 hours of treatment.

Low-Dose Therapy. In recent years the prophylactic use of heparin in "minidoses" to prevent thromboembolism has received a considerable amount of attention. The rationale for using low doses centers on the concept that a critical concentration of factor Xa (activated factor X) is required for thrombus formation. Factor Xa is the major component of the complex that activates prothrombin and lies at the point at which both intrinsic and extrinsic pathways converge to form the final common pathway of the clotting cascade. Heparin markedly enhances the action of the major plasma inhibitor of factor Xa, antithrombin III. It takes much less heparin to inhibit factor Xa than to prevent clotting once thrombin has been formed.

Standard regimens employ only 5000 U subcutaneously every eight or 12 hours. This dose is insufficient to do more than minimally prolong the aPTT; consequently, there is no need to monitor dosage and no increase in hemorrhagic complications or intraoperative transfusion requirements. The only adverse effect reported is a slight increase in the number of wound hematomas. Multiple studies confirm that low-dose heparin prophylaxis in patients undergoing abdominothoracic surgery markedly decreases the incidence of DVT.[41–45] More important, there is proof from a multicenter trial that the incidence of fatal pulmonary emboli is reduced as well.[44] Unfortunately, prophylaxis is not as efficacious in major hip surgery.

Following baseline hematologic studies, the prophylactic regimen we prefer is 5000 U given subcutaneously two hours prior to surgery and then repeated every 12 hours until the patient is fully ambulatory. Available evidence in general abdominal surgery shows no greater efficacy and a higher incidence of bleeding complications when an every eight hour regimen is used.[41] If possible, the patient should not receive anti-platelet-aggregating agents (dipyridamole, clofibrate, ASA) for five days prior to surgery, because low-dose heparin potentiates the aspirin-induced prolongation of the bleeding time observed in certain individuals.[46] When these agents are avoided, there is no apparent increase in operative blood loss or postoperative hematoma formation.[46–48]

An alternative low-dose method is the adjusted dose technique.[49] In this regimen heparin is given every 12 hours in a dose adjusted to prolong the midinterval aPTT to 1½ times control. After initial adjustment, the subcutaneous dose of heparin is fixed, and no additional coagulation monitors are performed. This method has been shown to be as effective as therapeutic doses of warfarin in prevention of recurrent thromboembolism.[49] It has also been shown to be effective in reducing the frequency of DVT in patients undergoing hip replacement surgery.[50]

The newest technique for preventing postoperative DVT is a dihydroergotamine-heparin combination.[51] Dihydroergotamine mesylate, 0.5 mg, plus 5000 U of heparin, was found to be more effective than either minidose heparin or dihydroergotamine alone.

If a woman has had one pregnancy that was complicated by a pulmonary embolus, a strong argument can be made for the necessity of prophylaxis during subsequent pregnancies. In one study, two of every 20 patients with pregnancy-related pulmonary emboli had a history of this complication.[51]

We believe that prophylactic doses of heparin should be used at the time of labor and delivery under the following circumstances: (1) in patients with previous pulmonary emboli, (2) in patients with previous thrombophlebitis, and (3) in patients at high risk for phlebitis, i.e., individuals with severe varicosities who are undergoing cesarean section.

The safety of minidose heparin during pregnancy has been amply documented.[52] While it seems reasonable to extend the efficacy data from nonpregnant to pregnant subjects, as yet there really are no data documenting its efficacy during pregnancy.

When conduction anesthesia is anticipated for delivery, the regimen is changed so that the first heparin dose is given in early labor. The epidural catheter is placed when appropriate, after obtaining a TCT in the normal range. The second dose of heparin is not given until after the catheter is removed.

Side-Effects. The major risk of heparin therapy is hemorrhage. Recent reports show an incidence of approximately 4% in properly monitored nonsurgical patients receiving heparin via the intravenous route.[29] Heparin causes osteoporosis when administered in doses higher than 15,000 U per day for more than six months.[53] This usually is not a problem during pregnancy, since patients rarely require antepartum therapy for periods this long. However, this complication has been reported and warrants concern.[54] It can be prevented by concomitant administration of calcium gluconate (1.5 g daily). Other rare effects of heparin include hypotension, alopecia, allergic reactions, pain at the injection site, and thrombocytopenia. The last, apparently an immune phenomenon, is characterized by a decline in platelets between the third and eighth days following initiation of therapy, reaching its nadir in two or three days, with recovery usually following within five days of discontinuing the drug.[55, 56] In most patients the platelet count returns to normal even if heparin is continued.[57]

A prospective study of 120 nonpregnant patients treated with porcine heparin revealed only a 3% incidence of thrombocytopenia.[58] In two of the four patients who did develop thrombocytopenia, a cause other than heparin for the fall in platelet count was found.

Heparin is contraindicated in threatened abortion, or if suspicion of significant risk of intracranial hemorrhage exists (e.g., in the eclamptic patient or the patient with severe hypertension). Hemoptysis from pulmonary infarction is not a contraindication.

Coumarin Agents

Of the various coumarin derivatives available, sodium warfarin is the most widely used in managing thromboembolic disease. Its therapeutic efficacy lies in its ability to inhibit the actions of vitamin K. Vitamin K functions in the liver as a cofactor in the synthesis of four essential clotting factors: factors VII, IX, X, and prothrombin.

A small molecule loosely bound to albumin, warfarin easily crosses the placenta and is excreted in breast milk.[59] For these reasons its use during pregnancy can be extremely hazardous. If it is administered during the first trimester (especially the fourth through eighth weeks), a fetal syndrome that phenotypically resembles the Conradi-Hünermann type of chondrodysplasia congenita punctata may result.[60] These children are born with multiple congenital anomalies, including nasal cartilage hypoplasia, stippling of bones, slight intrauterine growth retardation, and brachydactyly.

Recent reports indicate that warfarin may cause birth defects even if first administered in the second and third trimesters. Three children with microcephaly, bifrontal narrowing, mental retardation, and ophthalmologic abnormalities have been reported.[61–64] It is postulated that the first trimester anomalies may be secondary to either a direct teratogenic effect, or warfarin, or a vitamin K deficiency effect, while the second and third trimester defects could result from fetal hemorrhage.

The primary problem of warfarin administration during the last two trimesters has been fetal and placental hemorrhage resulting in fetal death. In a collected series of 214 patients, there were 25 fetal deaths or a fetal mortality rate of 11.7%.[65] However, the great majority of such events appears to be secondary to the trauma of delivery itself.[66] In a prospective study of 23 women with heart valve prostheses who conceived 40 times, the fetal wastage exceeded 80%.[67]

Although we and most authors believe that coumarin therapy is contraindicated during pregnancy, Hall and associates state that two thirds of pregnant women to whom coumarin derivatives were administered yielded normal infants, and that heparin was not a clearly superior alternative.[68] We disagree with their conclusions and feel that coumarin derivatives should be used during pregnancy only in patients who are either unable to master self-administration of heparin or who exhibit allergic reactions. In such cases heparin should be used for the acute episode and until 14 weeks of gestation, at which point warfarin can be substituted. Warfarin should be stopped and heparin substituted well in advance of labor. The patient should be fully informed of the potential risks of using coumarin (and all other vitamin K antagonists) during pregnancy.

Evidence suggests that the antithrombotic effect of warfarin is largely related to reduction in circulating levels of factors IX and X, while untoward bleeding seems more closely related to the levels of factor VII. High loading doses tend to greatly depress factor VII (which has a half-life of only six hours) and produce bleeding. Thus, a good therapeutic dosage schedule aims at a smooth reduction in circulating levels of all of these factors. The usual anticoagulating dose of warfarin is 10 to 15 mg daily until a therapeutic prolongation of the prothrombin time is achieved (1.5 to 2.5 $\times$ control). Thereafter, a maintenance dose of 3 to 20 mg daily is utilized, with re-evaluation of the prothrombin time once or twice weekly. During the first five to seven days of warfarin therapy heparin is continued. Since heparin can prolong the prothrombin time by 2 to 4 secs, the prothrombin time should be at least 2.5 times the control value by the time it is discontinued. Alternatively, heparin can be withdrawn in gradual decrements.

It is important to remember that a number of drugs affect the activity of the coumarin derivatives.[69] Agents increasing the activity of warfarin include salicylates, phenothiazines, phenylbutazone, and antibiotics, while ethyl alcohol and barbiturates decrease its activity. Fever, diarrhea, and change in intake of leafy green vegetables also decrease the effect of a given dose.

As mentioned previously, warfarin should be discontinued and heparin therapy resumed well in advance of labor. The average half-life for disappearance of the drug is 44 hours.[59] It is not known exactly how long it takes for the effects of oral anticoagulation on the fetus to wear off, but it is thought to be somewhere between three and 14 days.[70] If spontaneous labor occurs while the patient is still taking warfarin, its effects can be reversed by administering vitamin K and fresh frozen plasma. A single dose of 5 mg vitamin K_3 given orally or subcutaneously begins to normalize the prothrombin time within six hours. Higher doses (e.g., 25 to 50 mg) normalize the prothrombin time slightly more rapidly but also render the patient refractory to reanticoagulation for a period of 10 days to two weeks.

Because there is some experimental and clinical evidence that vitamin K crosses the placenta, its administration may enhance the rate of return of fetal clotting factors as well.[71] Immediately after delivery the infant is given 1 mg of vitamin K intramuscularly. If the newborn shows signs of bleeding or is less than 35 weeks of gestation or if it was a difficult instrument delivery, fresh frozen plasma, 5 mg per kg, may be required as well.

Patients already taking coumarin agents and desiring to conceive (e.g., patients with prosthetic heart valves) should be switched to heparin prior to conception. Patients who inadvertently receive oral agents during the first trimester must be advised of the risks involved and given the option of terminating the pregnancy.

Intrapartum, Intraoperative, and Postpartum Anticoagulation

Selected patients—those with recent pulmonary embolization, recent iliofemoral thrombosis, and heart valve prostheses—should be continued on high-dose heparin during delivery or surgery. These patients should be hospitalized in anticipation of delivery and converted to a regimen of continuous intravenous heparin. The dose should be adjusted to achieve a circulating heparin level of 0.1 to 0.2 U/ml (aPTT 1.5 × control; TCT 2 × control) during labor and delivery. Continuing this regimen does not increase the incidence of postpartum hemorrhage in a normal delivery. However, there is a slight increase in the incidence of episiotomy hematoma, and it may contribute to blood loss in patients with uterine atonia or retained placenta.[70] Conduction anesthesia is contraindicated in these patients.

Full doses of heparin should be reinstituted six hours after delivery or surgery to reattain a circulating level of 0.2 to 0.4 U/ml. Warfarin may be started (if the patient is not nursing) as soon as the patient resumes oral intake. Heparin is then discontinued five to seven days later, as described above. Oral agents should be continued for three to six months post partum, depending on the seriousness of the condition. Clotting factors tend to return to normal approximately eight weeks after delivery.[72] Warfarin may be monitored successfully on an outpatient basis, as described by Davis and associates. In 263 patients followed over a five-year period using serial hematocrit readings, prothrombin times, and urinalyses, major bleeding episodes developed in only 4% and minor bleeding in another 4%.[73]

A study of 68 patients with deep venous thrombosis indicated that the administration of therapeutic doses of warfarin was superior to long-term administration of low-dose heparin in preventing new episodes of thromboembolism.[74] Whether this therapeutic advantage is also true if coumarin is compared with long-term, medium-dose heparin administration has not yet been studied. As discussed, adjusted dose heparin has been shown to be superior to warfarin.[49]

There is controversy as to the safety of allowing women who are taking warfarin to breast-feed. While some authors state that warfarin passes into breast milk,[76] a recent study by Orme and associates disputes this finding.[75] Their study of 13 mothers showed only minute levels of warfarin in breast milk and none in the plasma of the seven infants who were being breast-fed. Despite these findings, at present we discourage breast-feeding in women taking warfarin. As more data become available, this recommendation may change.

Estrogen suppression of lactation is contraindicated because of a tenfold increase in venous thrombosis in mothers over the age of 25.[77] Although the issue of whether or not oral contraceptives predispose to thromboembolism is still heatedly debated,[77–80] we recommend that patients use an alternative method of birth control. Patients who smoke are encouraged to stop. Wearing of elastic stockings and elevation of the foot of the bed are continued at home as long as any edema of the lower extremities persists.

ALTERNATIVE THERAPY

Fibrinolytic Agents

Two fibrinolytic agents, streptokinase (SK) and urokinase (UK), have undergone extensive clinical trials and are now available for use. Both agents act to increase plasmin formation and thus the rate of clot lysis.[81] In acute DVT, SK produces total clot lysis in 30 to 50% of patients. Both SK and UK produce rapid resolution of pulmonary emboli, evident on angiography, as noted by improvement in pulmonary hemodynamics.[82, 83] Both agents are contraindicated during pregnancy and for the first ten days post partum. Urokinase should not be used in patients who are anticoagulated, and SK must be used with great caution, as the combination of SK and heparin greatly enhances the risk of overanticoagulation and bleeding.

Antiplatelet Agents

These drugs may play a role in arterial thromboembolism, but there is as yet no definitive evidence that they are effective in the treatment or prophylaxis of venous thromboembolism.[84] Dextran, the most widely used of these agents, must be administered intravenously, but it is less effective than low-dose subcutaneous heparin for prophylaxis.[85]

Surgical Intervention

Surgery is reserved for those patients for whom anticoagulants are contraindicated or have failed after an adequate course of therapy. Lower extremity thrombectomy is justified only if the patient is threatened by impending gangrene due to phlegmasia cerulea dolens.[72] It does not reduce subsequent chronic venous insufficiency, because the majority of vessels so treated do not remain patent on long-term follow-up. Inferior vena caval ligation, plication, clipping, or insertion of an umbrella is not indicated unless recurrent, life-threatening embolization persists despite adequate anticoagulation. A minor recurrence is observed in approximately 10% of patients during the first few days of heparin therapy and should not be considered a failure of therapy.[86] Bilateral ligation of the femoral veins is not fully protective because of the frequent involvement during pregnancy of the pelvic and gluteal veins, which drain into the iliacs above the inguinal ligament. If a pelvic source of embolism is suspected, the left ovarian vein may also require ligation.

Pulmonary embolectomy may be life-saving but should be considered only in those patients with angiographically demonstrated massive embolization to the main pulmonary artery with persistent inadequate cardiac output refractory to appropriate measures. In such situations the maternal outcome is of primary concern. Evans and coworkers describe a patient who underwent interruption of the inferior vena cava, pulmonary angiography, peripheral venography, laparotomy, and thoracotomy on cardiopulmonary bypass with subsequent delivery of a normal baby.[87]

SPECIAL GYNECOLOGIC PROBLEMS

OVARIAN HEMORRHAGE DURING ANTICOAGULANT THERAPY

Intraperitoneal hemorrhage secondary to rupture of an ovarian cyst has been reported as a rare complication of anticoagulant therapy. Twenty-nine laparotomies were performed on 25 patients because of hemoperitoneum secondary to ruptured ovarian cysts.[88,89] The patients were receiving a coumarin derivative in 21 instances. This distribution of cases undoubtedly reflects the greater usage of coumarin agents for long-term therapy rather than a therapeutic advantage of heparin. Seventeen of the 21 patients for whom a pathologic diagnosis was given had a ruptured corpus luteum.

The clinical presentation of acute onset of lower abdominal pain followed by distention should suggest the diagnosis of a ruptured cyst in any menstruating woman who is receiving anticoagulant therapy. Culdocentesis is useful in confirming the impression of intraperitoneal hemorrhage. While ovarian conservation is warranted, bilateral oophorectomy should be considered in situations in which the patient has a lifelong indication for anticoagulation.

SEPTIC PELVIC THROMBOPHLEBITIS

Septic thrombophlebitis is a serious complication of pyogenic pelvic infections. Findings on pelvic examination are often not diagnostic, and recognition depends on a high index of suspicion in postpartum, postabortion, and postoperative patients who develop a spiking fever that persists despite adequate antibiotic therapy.[15, 90–92]

When the presumptive diagnosis of septic thrombophlebitis is made, the patient is started on a medium-dose heparin regimen. If the diagnosis is correct, the fever should defervesce within 12 to 36 hours. Thus heparin is both a diagnostic and a therapeutic tool. In the absence of a significant temperature response, a reassessment of the cause of the fever is indicated.

While there is general agreement as to initiation of therapy, there are no data dealing with how long to continue therapy. Our practice has been to treat these patients in a manner identical to treatment for cases of acute, uncomplicated deep venous thrombosis. Thus, a medium-dose heparin regimen is started, and the patient is then converted to a coumarin agent, which is continued for a total course of anticoagulation of three to six weeks.

WHICH PATIENTS SHOULD RECEIVE PROPHYLACTIC ANTICOAGULATION?

The data presented above make it clear that minidose heparin is effective in preventing postoperative DVT. This benefit is achieved at minimal cost and with little risk of increased bleeding. However, there are low risk groups of patients who should not receive antithrombotic prophylaxis. Conversely, there are patients at very high risk who should almost always receive minidose heparin or its equivalent.

Table 12–5 displays a system of risk scoring that identifies a low, medium, and high risk population of patients for thromboembolic diseases.[93] Table 12–6 validates the importance of the risk scoring system by demonstrating the observed incidence of DVT and PE in each risk group. Certainly all high and many medium risk patients should receive prophylactic anticoagulation.

There continues to be interest in physical methods of prophylaxis. These methods are aimed at preventing stasis and pooling in the venous system of the legs and pelvis. Early studies of patients wearing elastic stockings showed no benefit.[93] More recent studies of graded static compression of the legs show a significant reduction of DVTs.[94]

Intermittent pneumatic compression used only during surgery has generally not been effective.[95] However, if compression is continued in the postoperative period for 24 hours, it effectively reduces DVTs.[96–98] In a recent study of patients undergoing major gynecologic surgery, intermittent pneumatic compression was superior to heparin in preventing pulmonary embolism.[99] Additional studies are necessary to deter-

Table 12–5. Risk Classification for Thromboembolic Disease

Risk	Clinical State
Low	Uncomplicated surgery; age <40; no other factors
Intermediate*	Surgery longer than 30 min; age ≥ 40; myocardial infarction; heart failure
High	Age $\geq$ 40 plus; previous DVT or PE, cancer, stroke, or major orthopedic surgery

* Risk increased by obesity, malignancy, varicosities, prolonged bed rest, and previous PE or DVT.

Table 12–6. Incidence of Thromboembolic Disease in Various Risk Groups

	Risk		
Event	**Low**	**Moderate**	**High**
Calf DVT	2	10–40	40–80
Proximal DVT	0.4	2–8	10–20
Clinical DVT	0.2	1–8	5–10
Fatal DVT	0.002	0.1–0.4	1–5

mine the place of this modality as compared with various heparin regimens. Cost, convenience of use, and effectiveness all need to be considered.

REFERENCES

1. Arthurs, H.: Maternal deaths from pulmonary embolism. J Obstet Gynecol Br Cwlth *75*:1309, 1968.
2. Wessler, S.: Medical management of venous thrombosis. Ann Rev Med *27*:313, 1976.
3. Aaro, L.A., and Juergens, J.L.: Thrombophlebitis associated with pregnancy. Am J Obstet Gynecol *109*:1128, 1971.
4. Villasanta, U.: Thromboembolic disease in pregnancy. Am J Obstet Gynecol *93*:142, 1965.
5. McCausland, A.M., Hyman, C., Winsor, T., et al.: Venous distensibility during pregnancy. Am J Obset Gynecol *81*:472, 1961.
6. Wright, H.P., Osborn, S.B., and Edmonds, D.G.: Changes in the rate of flow of venous blood in the leg during pregnancy, measured with radioactive sodium. Surg Gynecol Obstet *90*:481, 1950.
7. Todd, M.E., Thompson, J.H., Bowie, E.J.W., et al.: Changes in blood coagulation during pregnancy. Mayo Clin Proc *40*:370, 1965.
8. Nilsson, I. and Kullander, S.: Coagulation and fibrinolytic studies during pregnancy. Acta Obstet Gynecol Scand *46*:273, 1967.
9. Editorial: Venous thromboembolism and anticoagulants in pregnancy. Br Med J *4*:421, 1975.
10. Rickles, F.R., and Edwards, R.L.: Activation of blood coagulation in cancer. Blood *62*:14, 1983.
11. Bonnar, J.: Venous thromboembolism. *In* Recent Advances in Obstetrics and Gynecology. London, Churchill Livingstone, 1979.
12. Haeger, K.: Problems of acute deep venous thrombosis. Angiology *20*:219, 1969.
13. Cranley, J.J., Canos, A.J., and Sull, W.J.: The diagnosis of deep venous thrombosis—fallibility of clinical symptoms and signs. Arch Surg *111*:34, 1976.
14. Coon, W.W.: The spectrum of pulmonary embolism: Twenty years later. Arch Surg *111*:398, 1976.
15. Duff, P., and Gibbs, R.S.: Pelvic vein thrombophlebitis: Diagnostic dilemma and therapeutic challenge. Obstet Gynecol Surv *38*:365, 1983.
16. Gallus, A.S.: ^{125}I-fibrinogen leg scanning. *In* Prophylactic Therapy of Deep Vein Thrombosis and Pulmonary Embolism. Edited by J. Fratantoni and S Wessler. Bethesda, Md, NIH, 1975, p. 83.
17. Toy, P.T.C.Y., and Schrier, S.L.: Occlusive impedance plethysmography. West J Med *129*:89, 1978.
18. Clarke-Pearson, D.L., and Creasman, W.T.: Diagnosis of deep venous thrombosis in obstetrics and gynecology by impedance phlebography. Obstet Gynecol *58*:52, 1981.
19. Clarke-Pearson, D.L., and Jelovsek, F.R.: Alterations of occlusive cuff impedance plethysmography results in the obstetric patient. Surgery *89*:594, 1981.
20. Hirsh, J.: Blood tests for the diagnosis of venous and arterial thrombosis. Blood *57*:1, 1981.
21. Hull, R., Hirsh, J., Sackett, D.L., et al.: Cost effectiveness of clinical diagnosis, venography, and noninvasive testing in patients with symptomatic deep-vein thrombosis. N Engl J Med *304*:1561, 1981.
22. Sasahara, A.A., Sharma, G.V.R.K., Barsamian, E.M., et al.: Pulmonary thromboembolism. JAMA *249*:2945, 1983.
23. Hull, R.D., Hirsh, J., Carter, C.J., et al.: Pulmonary angiography, ventilation lung scanning, and venography for clinically suspected pulmonary embolism with abnormal perfusion lung scan. Ann Intern Med *98*:891, 1983.
24. Mackie, M., Bennett, B., Ogston, D., et al.: Familial thrombosis: Inherited deficiency of antithrombin III. Br Med J *1*:136, 1978.
25. Heymann, M.A., Rudolph, A.M., and Silverman, N.H.: Closure of the ductus arteriosus in premature infants by inhibition of prostaglandin synthesis. N Engl J Med *295*:530, 1976.
26. Physician's Desk Reference, 39th Ed. Oradell, NJ, Medical Economics Company, 1985, p. 956.
27. Rosenberg, R.D.: Actions and interactions of antithrombin and heparin . N Engl J Med *292*:146, 1975.
28. Wessler, S., and Gitel, S.N.: Heparin: New concepts relevant to clinical use. Blood *53*:525, 1979.
29. Basu, D., Gallus, A., Hirsh, J., et al.: A prospective study of the value of monitoring heparin treatment with the activated partial thromboplastin time. N Engl J Med *287*:324, 1972.
30. Estes, J.W.: Kinetics of the anticoagulant effect of heparin. JAMA *212*:1492, 1970.

31. Godal, H.C.: Heparin assay methods for the control of in vivo heparin effects. Thromb Diath Haemor *33*:77, 1974.
32. Penner, J.A.: Experience with a thrombin clotting time assay for measuring heparin activity. Am J Clin Pathol *61*:645, 1974.
33. Salzman, E., Deykin, D., Shapiro, R., et al.: Management of heparin therapy: Controlled prospective trial. N Engl J Med *292*:1046, 1975.
34. Whitfield, L.R., Lele, A.S., and Levy, G.: Effect of pregnancy on the relationship between concentration and anticoagulant action of heparin. Clin Pharmacol Ther *34*:23, 1983.
35. Hill, W.C., and Pearson, J.W.: Outpatient intravenous heparin therapy for antepartum iliofemoral thrombophlebitis. Obstet Gynecol *37*:785, 1971.
36. Spearing, G., Fraser, J., Turner, G., et al.: Long-term self-administered subcutaneous heparin in pregnancy. Br Med J *1*:1457, 1978.
37. Howell, R., Fidler, J., Litsky, E., et al.: The risk of antenatal subcutaneous heparin prophylaxis: A controlled trial. Br J Obstet Gynaecol *90*:1124, 1983.
38. Stillman, R.M., Chapa, L., Stark, M.L., et al.: A ten year study of heparin therapy for thrombophlebitis in ambulatory patients. Surg Gynecol Obstet *145*:193, 1977.
39. Sutton, G.C.: The management of pulmonary embolism. *In* Thromboembolism: Aetiology, Advances in Prevention and Management. Edited by AN Nicolaides Lancaster, Medical and Technical Publishing, 1975.
40. White, T.M., Bernene, J.L., and Marino, A.M.: Continuous heparin infusion requirements. JAMA *241*:2717, 1979.
41. Gallus, A.S., Hirsch, J., Tuttle, R.J., et al.: Small subcutaneous doses of heparin in prevention of venous thrombosis. N Engl J Med *288*:545, 1973.
42. Nicolaides, A.N., Desai, S., Douglas, J.N., et al.: Small doses of subcutaneous sodium heparin in preventing deep venous thrombosis after major surgery. Lancet *2*:890, 1972.
43. Kakkar, V.V., Nicolaides, A.N., Field, E.S., et al.: Low doses of heparin in prevention of deep-vein thrombosis. Lancet *2*:669, 1971.
44. Kakkar, V.V., Corrigan, T.P., and Fossard, D.P.: Prevention of fatal postoperative pulmonary embolism by low doses of heparin: An international multicentre trial. Lancet: *2*:45, 1975.
45. Wessler, S.: Heparin as an antithrombotic agent—Low dose prophylaxis. JAMA *236*:389, 1976.
46. Gurewich, V., Nunn, T., Kuriakos, T.T.X., et al.: Hemostatic effects of uniform, low-dose subcutaneous heparin in surgical patients. Arch Intern Med *138*:41, 1978.
47. Ballard, R.M., Bradley-Watson, P.J., Johnstone, F.D., et al.: Low doses of subcutaneous heparin in the prevention of deep vein thrombosis after gynaecologic surgery J Obstet Gynaecol Br Cwlth *80*:469, 1973.
48. Gjonnaess, H., and Abildgaard, V.: Bleeding in gynecologic surgery: Influence of low dose heparin. Int J Gynaecol Obstet *14*:9, 1976.
49. Hull, R., Delmore, T., Carter, C., et al.: Adjusted subcutaneous heparin versus warfarin sodium in the long-term treatment of venous thrombosis. N Engl J Med *306*:189, 1982.
50. Leyvraz, P.F., Richard, J., Bachmann, F., et al.: Adjusted versus fixed-dose subcutaneous heparin in the prevention of deep-vein thrombosis after total hip replacement. N Engl J Med *309*:954, 1983.
51. Sasahara, A.A.: Dihydroergotamine-heparin prophylaxis of postoperative deep vein thrombosis: A multicenter trial. JAMA *251*:2960, 1984.
52. Baskin, H.F., Murray, J.M., and Harris, R.E.: Low-dose heparin for prevention of thromboembolic disease in pregnancy. Am J Obstet Gynecol *129*:590, 1972.
53. Griffith, G.C., Nichols, G., Asher, J.D., et al.: Heparin osteoporosis. JAMA *193*:185, 1965.
54. DeSwiet, M., Ward, P.D., Fidler, J., et al.: Prolonged heparin therapy in pregnancy causes bone demineralization. Br J Obstet Gynaecol *90*:1129, 1983.
55. Babcock, R.B., Dumper, C.M., and Scharkman, W.B.: Heparin-induced immune thrombocytopenia. N Engl J Med *295*:237, 1976.
56. Wahl, T.O., Lipschitz, D.A., and Stechschulte, D.J.: Thrombocytopenia associated with antiheparin antibody. JAMA *240*:2560, 1978.
57. Johnson, R.A., Lazarus, K.H., and Henry, D.H.: Heparin-induced thrombocytopenia. Am J Hematol *17*:349, 1984.
58. Power, P.J., Cuthbert, D., and Hirsh, J.: Thrombocytopenia found uncommonly during heparin therapy. JAMA *241*:2396, 1979.
59. Wessler, S., and Gitel, S.N.: Warfarin. N Engl J Med *311*:645, 1984.
60. Shaul, W.L., and Hall, J.G.: Multiple congenital anomalies associated with oral anticoagulants. Am J Obstet Gynecol *127*:191, 1977.
61. Quenneville, G., Barton, B., McDevitt, E., et al.: The use of anticoagulants for thrombophlebitis during pregnancy. Am J Obstet Gynecol *77*:1135, 1959.
62. Sherman, S., and Hall, B.D.: Warfarin and fetal abnormality. Lancet *1*:692, 1976.
63. Larson, M., and Reid, M.: Warfarin and fetal abonormality. Lancet *1*:1356, 1976.
64. Stevenson, R.E., Burton, O.M., Ferlauto, G.J., et al.: Hazards of oral anticoagulants during pregnancy. JAMA *243*:1549, 1980.

65. Laros, R.K., Jr.: Anticoagulants: Indications and use. Contemp Obstet Gynecol *5*:67, 1975.
66. Bloomfield, D.K.: Fetal deaths and malformations associated with the use of coumarin derivatives in pregnancy. Am J Obstet Gynecol *107*:883, 1970.
67. Lutz, D.J., Noller, K.L., Spittell, J.A., et al.: Pregnancy and its complications following cardiac valve prostheses. Am J Obstet Gynecol *131*:460, 1978.
68. Hall, J.G., Pauli, R.M., and Wilson, K.M.: Maternal and fetal sequelae of anticoagulation during pregnancy. Am J Med *68*:122, 1980.
69. Koch-Weser, J., and Sellers, E.M.: Drug interactions with coumarin anticoagulants. N Engl J Med *285*:547, 1971.
70. Pridmore, B.R., Murray, K.H., and McAllen, P.M.: The management of anticoagulant therapy during and after pregnancy. Br J Obstet Gynaecol *82*:740, 1975.
71. Hirsh, J., Cade, J.F., and Gallus, A.S.: Anticoagulants in pregnancy: A review of indications and complications. Am Heart J *83*:301, 1972.
72. Gurll, N., Hefand, Z., Salzman, E.F., et al.: Peripheral venous thrombophlebitis during pregnancy. Am J Surg *121*:449, 1971.
73. Davis, F.B., Estruch, M.T., Samson-Corvera, E.B., et al.: Management of anticoagulation in outpatients. Arch Intern Med *137*:197, 1977.
74. Hull, R., Delmore, T., Genton, E., et al.: Warfarin sodium versus low-dose heparin in the long-term treatment of venous thrombosis. N Engl J Med *301*:855, 1979.
75. Orme, M.L.E., de Swiet, M., Serlin, M.J., et al.: May mothers given warfarin breast-feed their infants? Br Med J *1*:1564, 1977.
76. Oseid, B.J.: Breast feeding and infant health. Clin Obstet Gynecol *18*:149, 1975.
77. Daniel, D.G., Campbell, H., and Turnbull, A.C.: Puerperal thromboembolism and suppression of lactation. Lancet *2*:287, 1967.
78. Goldzieher, J.W., and Dozier, T.S.: Oral contraceptives and thromboembolism: A reassessment. Am J Obstet Gynecol *123*:878, 1975.
79. Correspondence: Oral contraceptives and thromboembolism. Am J Obstet Gynecol *125*:1057, 1976.
80. Correspondence: Oral contraceptives and thromboembolism. Am J Obstet Gynecol *126*:607, 1976.
81. Porter, J.M., and Goodnight, S.H.: The clinical use of fibrinolytic agents, Am J Surg *134*:217, 1977.
82. Urokinase Pulmonary Embolism Trial Study Group, Urokinase pulmonary embolism trial: Phase 1, JAMA *229*:2163, 1970.
83. Urokinase Pulmonary Embolism Trial Study Group, Urokinase pulmonary embolism trial: Phase 2. JAMA *229*:1606, 1974.
84. Genton, E., Gent, M., Hersh, J., et al.: Platelet-inhibiting drugs in the prevention of clinical thrombotic disease. N Engl J Med *293*:1296, 1975.
85. Macintyre, I.M.C., Vasilescu, C., Jones, D.R.B., et al.: Heparin versus dextran in the prevention of deep-vein thrombosis: A multi-unit controlled trial. Lancet *2*:118, 1974.
86. Sherry, S.: Thromboembolic diseases. *In* Textbook of Medicine. Edited by P.B. Beeson and W. McDermott. 14th Ed. Philadelphia, W.B. Saunders Company, 1975.
87. Evans, G.L., Dalen, J.E., and Dexter, L.: Pulmonary embolism during pregnancy. JAMA *206*:320, 1968.
88. Waxman, M., and Baird, G.J.: Corpus luteum hemorrhage: Cause of abdominal pain in patients receiving anticoagulant therapy. JAMA *239*:2270, 1978.
89. Peters, W.A., Thiagarajah, S., and Thornton, W.N.: Ovarian hemorrhage in patients receiving anticoagulant therapy. J Reprod Med *22*:82, 1979.
90. Ledger, W.J., and Peterson, E.P.: The use of heparin in the management of pelvic thrombophlebitis. Surg Gynecol Obstet *131*:1115, 1970.
91. Josey, W.E., and Staggers, S.R.: Heparin therapy in septic pelvic thrombophlebitis. Am J Obstet Gynecol *120*:228, 1974.
92. Cohen, M.B., Pernoll, M.L., Gevirtz, C.M., et al.: Septic pelvic thrombophlebitis: An update. Obstet Gynecol *62*:83, 1983.
93. Farquharson, D.I.M., and Orr, J.W.: Prophylaxis against thromboembolism in gynecologic patients. J Reprod Med *29*:845, 1984.
94. Holford, C.P.: Graded compression for preventing deep venous thrombosis. Br Med J *2*:969, 1976.
95. Smith, R.C., Elton, R.A., Orr, J.D., et al.: Dextran and intermittent pneumatic compression in prevention of postoperative deep vein thrombosis: Multiunit trial. Br Med J *1*:952, 1978.
96. Skillman, J.J., Collins, R.E., Coe, N.P, et al.: Prevention of deep vein thrombosis in neurosurgical patients. Surgery *83*:354, 1978.
97. Coe, N.P., Collins, R.E., Klein, L.A., et al.: Prevention of deep vein thrombosis in urologic patients. Surgery *83*:230, 1978.
98. Salzmen, E.W., Ploetz, J., Bettman, M., et al.: Intraoperative external pneumatic calf compressions to afford long-term prophylaxis against deep vein thrombosis in urologic patients. Surgery *87*:239, 1980.
99. Jobson, V.W., Homesley, H.D., and Welander, C.E.: Comparison of heparin and intermittent calf compression for prevention of pulmonary embolism. Gynecol Oncol *15*:143, 1983.

INDEX